1988

UROLOGY ANNUAL

Volume 2

1988

UROLOGY ANNUAL

Volume 2

Series Editor

Stephen N. Rous, A.B., M.D., M.S. (Urology), F.A.C.S., F.A.A.P.

Professor and Chairman, Department of Urology
Medical University of South Carolina
Charleston, South Carolina

APPLETON & LANGE
Norwalk, Connecticut/San Mateo, California

0-8385-9319-4

Notice: Our knowledge in clinical sciences is constantly changing. As new information becomes available, changes in treatment and in the use of drugs become necessary. The author(s) and the publisher of this volume have taken care to make certain that the doses of drugs and schedules of treatment are correct and compatible with the standards generally accepted at the time of publication. The reader is advised to consult carefully the instruction and information material included in the package insert of each drug or therapeutic agent before administration. This advice is especially important when using new or infrequently used drugs.

88 89 90 91 92 / 10 9 8 7 6 5 4 3 2 1

Prentice-Hall of Australia, Pty. Ltd., Sydney
Prentice-Hall Canada, Inc.
Prentice-Hall Hispanoamericana, S.A., Mexico
Prentice-Hall of India Private Limited, New Delhi
Prentice-Hall International (UK) Limited, London
Prentice-Hall of Japan, Inc., Tokyo
Prentice-Hall of Southeast Asia (Pte.) Ltd., Singapore
Whitehall Books Ltd., Wellington, New Zealand
Editora Prentice-Hall do Brasil Ltda., Rio de Janeiro

ISBN: 0-8385-9319-4
ISSN: 0889-6283

Production Editor: Elizabeth C. Ryan

PRINTED IN THE UNITED STATES OF AMERICA

Contributors

Joseph Addonizio, M.D.
Director of Urology, Westchester County Medical Center; Professor and Chairman, Department of Urology, New York Medical College, Valhalla, New York

David M. Barrett, M.D.
Consultant, Department of Urology, Mayo Clinic and Mayo Foundation; Professor of Urology, Mayo Medical School, Rochester, Minnesota

G. William Bates, M.D.
Dean, College of Medicine; Professor of Obstetrics and Gynecology, Medical University of South Carolina, Charleston, South Carolina

J.M. Brisset, M.D.
Department of Urology, CMC de la Porte de Choisy, Paris, France

Anton J. Bueschen, M.D.
Professor and Director, Division of Urology, University of Alabama at Birmingham, Birmingham, Alabama

Muhammad Choudhury, M.D.
Chief, Section of Urologic Oncology, Westchester County Medical Center; Assistant Professor of Urology, New York Medical College, Valhalla, New York

J. Dory
Engineer, EDAP Company, Marne la Vallée, France

Charles T. Fitts, M.D.
Professor of Surgery, Medical University of South Carolina, Charleston, South Carolina

William L. Furlow, M.D.
Center for Urological Treatment and Research, Nashville, Tennessee

Benad Goldwasser, M.D.
Department of Urology, Chaim Sheba Medical Center, Tel-Hashomer, Israel

Michael M. Lieber, M.D.
Consultant, Department of Urology, Mayo Clinic and Mayo Foundation; Professor of Urology, Mayo Medical School, Rochester, Minnesota

Abe M. Macher, M.D.
Commander, United States Public Health Service; Director, Collaborative Center for the Investigation of AIDS Pathology, Washington, D.C.

John J. Mulcahy, M.D., M.S., Ph.D., F.A.C.S.
Associate Professor of Urology, Indiana University Medical Center, Indianapolis, Indiana

Kaoru Nakamura, M.D.
Sony Research Fellow, Department of Urology, New York Medical College, Valhalla, New York

Leroy M. Nyberg, Jr., Ph.D., M.D.
Associate Professor of Surgery (Urology), Department of Surgery, Division of Urology, University of Connecticut Health Center, Farmington, Connecticut

Norman E. Peterson, M.D.
Associate Director of Surgery, Division Chief, Urology, Denver General Hospital, Denver, Colorado

Leslie M. Rainwater, M.D.
Resident, Department of Urology, Mayo Clinic, Rochester, Minnesota

Martin I. Resnick, M.D.
Professor and Chairman, Division of Urology, Case Western Reserve University, School of Medicine, Cleveland, Ohio

G. Alan Rose, M.A., D.M., F.R.C.P., F.R.C. Path., F.R.S.C.
Consultant Chemical Pathologist to St. Peters' Hospitals, London; Consultant Chemical Pathologist to the Royal National Orthopedic Hospital, Stanmore, Middlesex, United Kingdom

P.H. Thibault, M.D.
Department of Urology, Hospital Tenon, Paris, France

W.R. Turner, Jr., M.D.
Professor of Urology of Pediatrics, Medical University of South Carolina, Charleston, South Carolina

G. Vallancien, M.D.
Department of Urology, CMC de la Porte de Choisy, Paris, France

Winfred L. Wiser, M.D.
Professor and Chairman, Department of Obstetrics and Gynecology, University of Mississippi School of Medicine, Jackson, Mississippi

Contents

Preface

This volume, the second in a projected annual series, attempts to offer comprehensive presentations of various topics that, in the Editor's opinion, are—or should be—of considerable interest to practicing urologists. For each topic, the Editor has made every effort to recruit well-recognized experts to either author or co-author the manuscript.

Perhaps the "hottest" current topic in urology, and even in all of medicine, is the acquired immune deficiency syndrome (AIDS). The first chapter in this volume is therefore devoted to AIDS and it has been written with specific relevance to those aspects of AIDS that are germane to urologists. The next two chapters concern flow cytometry, arguably the wave of the future for diagnosis and prognosis of urothelial cancers. These are followed by two chapters in the always interesting area of prostatic cancer, one concerning the use of luteinizing hormone-releasing hormone (LH-RH) analogues for treatment, the other covering the role of ultrasound in diagnosis. Extracorporeal shock-wave lithotripsy (ESWL) continues to be of interest to urologists and the next paper describes a new and different type of lithotripter with great promise for the future. Two chapters on the current management of erectile dysfunction and the role of artificial urinary sphincters follow, and then a chapter on urethral trauma. Newer insights into the etiology and management of calcium oxalate stones is offered next and this is followed by an informative discussion on diagnosing and caring for intersex problems. The burgeoning role of nuclear imaging in urology is then presented and is followed by an extraordinarily lucid and easy to follow paper on the etiologies and management of shock. The final chapter is an up-to-date and comprehensive review of neonatal circumcision.

As the reader goes through this book, the Editor hopes that any suggestions, thoughts, or ideas for future inclusion will be noted and sent to him; these might include entirely new subjects or those that the reader would like to see covered again, perhaps from a different perspective.

This book may serve as a yearly compendium of what is important and timely to the practicing urologist; it may also serve as a reference book for urology residents and for those seeking detailed information, presented by experts, on the subjects covered.

It is hoped that the reader will enjoy this book as much as the Editor has enjoyed working with the chapter authors in its development.

Stephen N. Rous, M.D.

The Acquired Immune Deficiency Syndrome (AIDS)
A Guide for Urologists

Commander Abe M. Macher

DEFINITION OF AIDS

The acquired immune deficiency syndrome (AIDS) is a devastating new disease that has afflicted more than 33,000 Americans. Patients with illnesses that, in retrospect, were manifestations of AIDS were first described in the summer of 1981.[1,2] A case definition of AIDS for national reporting was first published by the Centers for Disease Control (CDC) in September 1982.[3,4] The definition included a list of diseases used as indicators of underlying cellular immunodeficiency.

Since the 1982 definition was published, a retrovirus, the human immunodeficiency virus (HIV), also referred to as human T-lymphotropic virus type III (HTLV-III)/lymphadenopathy-associated virus (LAV), has been recognized as the cause of AIDS.[5–7] All patients with antibodies to HIV must be considered capable of transmitting the AIDS virus. The clinical manifestations of infection by HIV may be directly attributable to infection with this virus or the result of secondary conditions occurring as a consequence of immune dysfunction caused by the underlying infection with HIV. The range of manifestations may include none, nonspecific signs and symptoms of illness, autoimmune and neurologic disorders, a variety of opportunistic infections, and several types of malignancy. AIDS was defined for national reporting before its etiology was known and encompassed only certain secondary conditions that reliably reflected the presence of a severe immune dysfunction. Laboratory tests to detect antibody to HIV made it possible to include additional serious conditions in the syndrome, as well as to further improve the specificity of the definition used for reporting cases. In June 1985, the CDC[8] issued a revision of the case definition of AIDS for national reporting. CDC defines a case of AIDS as an illness characterized by:

I. One or more of the opportunistic diseases listed below that are at least moderately indicative of underlying cellular immunodeficiency
II. Absence of all known underlying causes of cellular immunodeficiency (other than infection by HIV) and absence of all other causes of reduced resistance reported to be associated with at least one of those opportunistic diseases

Despite having the above, patients are *excluded* as AIDS cases if they have negative results on testing for serum antibody to HIV, do not have a positive culture for HIV, and have both a normal or high number of T-helper lymphocytes and a normal or high ratio of T-helper to T-suppressor lymphocytes. A single negative test for HIV may be applied here if it is an antibody test by enzyme-linked immunoabsorbent assay (ELISA), immunofluorescent, or Western blot methods, because such tests are very sensitive. Viral cultures are less sensitive but more specific, and so may be relied on if positive but not if negative. If multiple antibody tests have inconsistent results, the result applied to the case definition should be that of the majority. A positive culture, however, would over-rule negative antibody tests. In the *absence* of any test results, patients satisfying all other criteria in this definition are included as cases.

This general case definition may be made more explicit by specifying:

I. The particular diseases considered at least moderately indicative of cellular immunodeficiency, which are used as indicators of AIDS
II. The known causes of cellular immunodeficiency, or other causes of reduced resistance reported to be associated with particular diseases, which would disqualify a patient as an AIDS case

This specification is as follows:

I. *Diseases at least moderately indicative of underlying cellular immunodeficiency (indicators of AIDS):*
   In the following list of diseases, the required diagnostic methods with positive results are shown in parentheses. "Microscopy" may include cytology.
   A. *Protozoal and helminthic infections*
      1. Cryptosporidiosis, intestinal, causing diarrhea for over 1 month (on histology or stool microscopy)
      2. *Pneumocystis carinii* pneumonia (on histology or microscopy of a touch imprint, bronchial washings, or sputum)
      3. Strongyloidiasis, causing pneumonia, central nervous system in-

fection, or infection disseminated beyond the gastrointestinal tract (on histology)

4. Toxoplasmosis, causing infection in internal organs other than liver, spleen, or lymph nodes (on histology or microscopy of a touch imprint)

B. *Fungal infections*
   1. Candidiasis, causing esophagitis (on histology or microscopy of a "wet" preparation from the esophagus, or endoscopic or autopsy findings of white plaques on an erythematous mucosal base, but not by culture alone)
   2. Cryptococcosis, causing central nervous system or other infection disseminated beyond lungs and lymph nodes (on culture, antigen detection, histology, or India ink preparation of cerebrospinal fluid)

C. *Bacterial infections*
   1. *Mycobacterium avium* or *intracellulare* (*M. avium* complex), or *M. kansasii,* causing infection disseminated beyond lungs and lymph nodes (on culture)

D. *Viral infections*
   1. Cytomegalovirus, causing infection in internal organs other than liver, spleen, or lymph nodes (on histology or cytology, but not by culture or serum antibody titer)
   2. Herpes simplex virus, causing chronic mucocutaneous infection with ulcers persisting more than 1 month, or pulmonary, gastrointestinal tract (beyond mouth, throat, or rectum), or disseminated infection (but not encephalitis alone) (on culture, histology, or cytology)
   3. Progressive multifocal leukoencephalopathy (presumed to be caused by papovavirus) (on histology)

E. *Cancer*
   1. Kaposi's sarcoma (on histology)
   2. Lymphomas limited to the brain (on histology)

F. *Other opportunistic infections with positive test for HIV:*
   In the absence of the above opportunistic diseases, any of the following diseases is considered indicative of AIDS if the patient had a positive test for HIV:
   1. Disseminated histoplasmosis (on culture, histology, or cytology)
   2. Bronchial or pulmonary candidiasis (on microscopy or visualization grossly of characteristic white plaques on the bronchial mucosa, but not by culture alone)
   3. Isosporiasis, causing chronic diarrhea (over 1 month) (on histology or stool microscopy)

G. *Chronic lymphoid interstitial pneumonitis:*
   In the absence of the above opportunistic diseases, a histologically confirmed diagnosis of chronic (persisting over 2 months) lymphoid

interstitial pneumonitis in a child (under 13 years of age) is indicative of AIDS unless tests for HIV are negative. A positive test for HIV may consist of a reactive test for antibody to HIV or a positive culture (isolation of HIV from a culture of the patient's peripheral blood lymphocytes). If multiple antibody tests have inconsistent results, the result applied to the case definition should be that of the majority done by the ELISA, immunofluorescent, or Western blot methods. A positive culture, however, would over-rule negative antibody titers. The histologic examination of lung tissue must show diffuse interstitial and peribronchiolar infiltration by lymphocytes, plasma cells with Russell bodies, plasmacytoid lymphocytes, and immunoblasts. Histologic and culture evaluation must not identify a pathogenic organism as the cause of this pneumonia

H. *Non-Hodgkin's lymphoma with positive test for HIV:*
If the patient had a positive test for HIV, then the following histologic types of lymphoma are indicative of AIDS, regardless of anatomic site:
1. Small noncleaved lymphoma (Burkitt's tumor or Burkitt-like lymphoma), but not small cleaved lymphoma
2. Immunoblastic sarcoma (or immunoblastic lymphoma) or B-cell or unknown immunologic phenotype (not of T-cell type). Other terms which may be equivalent include diffuse undifferentiated non-Hodgkin's lymphoma, large cell lymphoma (cleaved or noncleaved), diffuse histiocytic lymphoma, reticulum cell sarcoma, and high-grade lymphoma

Lymphomas should not be accepted as indicative of AIDS if they are described in any of the following ways: low grade, of T-cell type (immunologic phenotype), small cleaved lymphoma, lymphocytic lymphoma (regardless of whether well or poorly differentiated), lymphoblastic lymphoma, plasmacytoid lymphocytic lymphoma, lymphocytic leukemia (acute or chronic), or Hodgkin's disease (or Hodgkin's lymphoma).

II. *Known causes of cellular immunodeficiency or other causes of reduced resistance (which would disqualify a patient as an AIDS case):*
Known causes of reduced resistance to diseases indicative of immunodeficiency are listed in the left column, while the diseases that may be attributable to these causes (rather than to the immunodeficiency caused by HIV infection) are listed in the right column.

Known Causes of Reduced Resistance	Diseases Possibly Attributable to the Known Causes of Reduced Resistance
Systemic corticosteroid therapy	Any infection diagnosed during or within 1 month after discontinuation of the corticosteroid therapy, unless symptoms specific for an infected anatomic

Known Causes of Reduced Resistance	Diseases Possibly Attributable to the Known Causes of Reduced Resistance
Systemic corticosteroid therapy (cont.)	site (e.g., dyspnea for pneumonia, headache for encephalitis, diarrhea for colitis) began before the corticosteroid therapy
	Any cancer diagnosed during or within 1 month after discontinuation of more than 4 months of long-term corticosteroid therapy, unless symptoms specific for the anatomic sites of the cancer (as described above) began before the long-term corticosteroid therapy
Other immunosuppressive or cytotoxic therapy	Any infection diagnosed during or within 1 year after discontinuation of the immunosuppressive therapy, unless symptoms specific for an infected anatomic site (as described above) began before the therapy
	Any cancer diagnosed during or within 1 year after discontinuation of more than 4 months of long-term immunosuppressive therapy, unless symptoms specific for the anatomic site of the cancer (as described above) began before the long-term therapy
Cancer of lymphoreticular or histiocytic tissue such as lymphoma (except for lymphoma localized to the brain), Hodgkin's disease, lymphocytic leukemia, or multiple myeloma	Any infection or cancer, if diagnosed after or within 3 months before the diagnosis of the cancer of lymphoreticular or histiocytic tissue
Age 60 years or older at diagnosis	Kaposi's sarcoma, but not if the patient has a positive test for HIV
Age under 28 days (neonatal) at diagnosis	Toxoplasmosis or herpes simplex virus infection, as described above
Age under 6 months at diagnosis	Cytomegalovirus infection, as described above
An immunodeficiency atypical of AIDS, such as one involving hypogammaglobulinemia or angio-	Any infection or cancer diagnosed during such immunodeficiency

(*continued*)

Known Causes of Reduced Resistance	Diseases Possibly Attributable to the Known Causes of Reduced Resistance
immunoblastic lymphadenopathy; or an immunodeficiency of which the cause appears to be a genetic or developmental defect, rather than HIV infection	
Exogenous malnutrition (starvation due to food deprivation, not malnutrition due to malabsorption or illness)	Any infection or cancer diagnosed during or within 1 month after discontinuation of starvation

GENITOURINARY MANIFESTATIONS

The genitourinary lesions in patients with AIDS reflect involvement by the aforementioned opportunistic infections and malignancies. Cytomegalovirus, *M. avium-intracellulare, M. tuberculosis, M. kansasii, Cryptococcus neoformans, Histoplasma capsulatum, Coccidioides immitis, Nocardia* species, and *Salmonella typhimurium* have been cultured from the urine of patients with AIDS. Cultures of semen may be positive for cytomegalovirus and may contain hepatitis B virus antigen. Histopathologic examination of tissue sections have revealed infection by cytomegalovirus in adrenal, kidney, urinary bladder, testis, epididymis, and seminal vesicle. Disseminated fungal, mycobacterial, and nocardial infections have involved kidney and adrenal. The penis is a frequent site of condyloma acuminatum and of infection by herpes simplex. Kaposi's sarcoma, the most common neoplasm in patients with AIDS, may be in adrenal, kidney, epididymis, seminal vesicle, penis, and scrotum. B-cell lymphomas may involve kidney. Atrophy, fibrosis and arrest of spermatic maturation are common changes in testis.

Condyloma acuminatum is a frequent anogenital lesion in homosexual patients with AIDS. Herpes simplex is also a frequent cause of anogenital infection in patients with AIDS. Kaposi's sarcoma may cause lesions involving the penis and scrotum. Kaposi's sarcoma most frequently involves mucocutaneous sites in patients with AIDS. Being a vascular tumor, Kaposi's sarcoma presents as an erythematous or violaceous macular, papular, or nodular process. The earliest flat, macular lesions (patch stage) may be mistaken for pityriasis rosea, purpura, pigmented nevi, early melanomas, flat hemangiomas, progressive pigmented purpuric eruptions, or secondary syphilis. The mucocutaneous lesions of Kaposi's sarcoma are usually asymptomatic, may be single or multiple, and sometimes appear simultaneously or sequentially. As these tumors evolve, the flat lesions become elevated, developing into plaques or papules (plaque stage). These raised lesions may resemble the eruptions of secondary syphilis, lichen planus, sarcoidosis, eruptive xanthomas, hemangiomas, urticaria pigmentosa, junctional or dysplastic nevi, chronic inflammatory reactions to insect bites, papular urticaria, dermatofibromas, pyogenic granulomas, glomus tumors, cutaneous lymphomas, basal cell carcinomas, cutaneous metastases of internal tumors, and angiosarcomas. Eventually, lesions of the plaque stage may enlarge, coalesce, and become elevated nodules (nodular stage). Visceral lesions of Kaposi's sarcoma may also appear in conjunction with mucocutaneous disease. As a multifocal tumor, lesions of Kaposi's sarcoma may also appear in the adrenal gland, kidney, epididymis, and seminal vesicle.[9–11]

In addition to Kaposi's sarcoma, AIDS patients have an increased incidence of extranodal non-Hodgkin's lymphomas. These tumors may present in the kidneys of patients with AIDS.[12,13]

Gonorrhea and syphilis are common in homosexual patients with AIDS and we have seen one patient with syphilitic orchitis. Autopsy specimens of testis may reveal a moderate to striking degree of atrophy and maturation arrest of sperm. The basement membranes of the seminiferous tubules are thickened and fibrous scars may be present.[14] Kidneys may have focal and segmental glomerulosclerosis.[15]

Many patients with AIDS have clinically significant infections with cytomegalovirus. Although cytomegalovirus infects a wide range of tissues and organs, the most common sites of infection are lung, adrenal, eye (chorioretinitis), central nervous system, gastrointestinal tract, and blood. In the patient with AIDS, cytomegalovirus is disseminated in the bloodstream, from which it can be isolated. In the lung, cytomegalovirus causes focal or diffuse interstitial pneumonitis. Infection of adrenal may cause bilateral hemorrhagic necrosis with preferential involvement of the medullas. The extent to which massive adrenal necrosis plays a role in the terminal hypotensive episodes in some patients with AIDS is still under investigation. Cytomegalovirus is also in semen and urine. Cytomegaloviral inclusions are especially common in the tissue sections of seminal vesicle. Infection by cytomegalovirus of epididymis may cause symptomatic epididymitis.

Disseminated infection by *M. avium-intracellulare* is uniquely common in patients with AIDS. Before AIDS, this ubiquitous environmental saprophytic bacillus was an uncommon pathogen of man. *M. avium-intracellulare* may be cultured from urine, blood, and bone marrow of patients with AIDS. Disseminated foci of infection by *M. avium-intracellulare* are found in adrenal and kidney.

Cryptococcal, histoplasmal, and coccidioidal infections disseminate in patients with AIDS and *C. neoformans, H. capsulatum,* and *C. immitis* may be cultured from urine and blood. Histopathologic tissue sections may reveal involvement of adrenal and kidney.

Patients with AIDS have a predilection for developing salmonellosis with bacteremia by *S. typhimurium. S. typhimurium* has been cultured from urine of these patients.[16]

Homosexual male patients have an increased incidence of genital scabies and such patients with AIDS may present with the "Norwegian" type of scabies.

Thus, the genitourinary system of a patient with AIDS may reflect any of a number of infectious and malignant processes that afflict this unique population of immunoincompetent individuals.

RECOMMENDATIONS FOR PREVENTING TRANSMISSION OF INFECTION BY HIV TO HEALTH CARE WORKERS

Persons at increased risk of acquiring infection with HIV include homosexual and bisexual men, intravenous drug abusers, persons transfused with contaminated blood or blood products, heterosexual contacts of persons with HIV infection, and children born to infected mothers. HIV is transmitted through sexual contact, parenteral exposure to infected blood or blood components, and perinatal transmission from infected mother to neonate. HIV has been isolated from blood, semen, saliva, tears, breast milk, and urine and is likely to be isolated from some other body fluids, secretions, and excretions, but epidemiologic evidence has implicated only blood and semen in transmission.

The epidemiology of infection by HIV is similar to that of hepatitis B virus (HBV) infection. Both viruses are transmitted through sexual contact, parenteral exposure to contaminated blood or blood products, and perinatal transmission from infected mothers to their offspring. Thus, some of the same major groups at high risk for HBV infection (e.g., homosexual men, intravenous drug abusers, persons with hemophilia, infants born to infected mothers) are also the groups at highest risk for infection by HIV. Neither HBV or HIV has been shown to be transmitted by casual contact in the workplace, contaminated food or water or airborne or fecal–oral routes.

HBV infection is an occupational risk for health care workers, but this risk is related to degree of contact with blood or contaminated needles. Health care workers who do not have contact with blood or needles contaminated with blood are not at risk for acquiring HBV infection in the workplace. Current evidence indicates that, despite epidemiologic similarities of HBV and HIV infection, the risk for HBV transmission in health care settings far exceeds that for HIV transmission. The risk of acquiring HBV infection following a needlestick from an HBV carrier ranges from 6 to 30 percent, far in excess of the risk of HIV infection following a needlestick involving a source patient infected with HIV, which is less than 1 percent. Therefore, recommendations for the control of HBV infection should, if followed, also effectively prevent spread of HIV.

Using the HBV model, the highest risk for transmission of HIV in the workplace would involve parenteral exposure to a needle or other sharp instrument contaminated with blood of an infected patient. The risk to health care workers of acquiring HIV infection in the workplace has been evaluated in several studies. In five separate studies, a total of 1498 health care workers had been tested for antibody to HIV. In these studies, 666 (44.5 percent) of the health care workers had direct parenteral (needlestick or cut) or mucous membrane exposure to patients with AIDS or HIV infection. Most of these exposures were to blood rather than to other body fluids. None of the health care workers whose initial serologic tests were negative developed subsequent evidence of HIV infection following their exposures. Twenty-six health care workers in these five studies were seropositive when first tested; all but three of these persons belonged to groups recognized to be at increased risk for AIDS. Since one was tested anonymously, epidemiologic information was available on only two of these three seropositive health care workers. Although these two health care workers were reported as probable occupationally related HIV infection, neither had a preexposure nor an early postexposure serum sample available to help determine the onset of infection. One case reported from England describes a nurse who seroconverted following an accidental parenteral exposure to a needle contaminated with blood from a patient with AIDS.

In spite of the extremely low risk of transmission of HIV infection, even when needlestick injuries occur, more emphasis must be given to precautions targeted to prevent needlestick injuries in health care workers caring for any patient, since such injuries continue to occur even during the care of patients who are known to be infected with HIV. The following precautions, issued by the CDC[17] in November 1985, apply to preventing transmission of HIV and other bloodborne infections and should be used routinely:

1. Sharp items (needles, scalpel blades, and other sharp instruments) should be considered as potentially infective and be handled with extraordinary care to prevent accidental injuries.
2. Disposable syringes and needles, scalpel blades, and other sharp items should be placed into puncture-resistant containers located as close as practical to the area in which they are used. To prevent needlestick injuries, needles should not be recapped, purposefully bent, broken, removed from disposable syringes, or otherwise manipulated by hand.
3. When the possibility of exposure to blood or other body fluids exists, routinely recommended precautions should be followed. The anticipated exposure may require gloves alone, as in handling items soiled with blood or equipment contaminated with blood or other body fluids, or may also require gowns, masks, and eye-coverings when performing procedures involving more extensive contact with blood or potentially infective body fluids, as in some dental or endo-

scopic procedures or postmortem examinations. Hands should be washed thoroughly and immediately if they accidentally become contaminated with blood.

4. To minimize the need for emergency mouth-to-mouth resuscitation, mouth pieces, resuscitation bags, or other ventilation devices should be strategically located and available for use in areas where the need for resuscitation is predictable. No transmission of HBV infection during mouth-to-mouth resuscitation has been documented. Because of the theoretical risk of salivary transmission of HIV during mouth-to-mouth resuscitation, however, special attention should be given to the use of disposable airway equipment or resuscitation bags and the wearing of gloves when in contact with blood or other body fluids. Resuscitation equipment and devices known or suspected to be contaminated with blood or other body fluids should be used once and disposed of or be thoroughly cleaned and disinfected after each use.
5. Pregnant health care workers are not known to be at greater risk of contracting HIV infections than health care workers who are not pregnant; however, if a health care worker develops HIV infection during pregnancy, the infant is at increased risk of infection resulting from perinatal transmission. Because of this risk, pregnant health care workers should be especially familiar with precautions for preventing transmission of HIV.

There have been no reports of HIV transmission from a health care worker to a patient or from a patient to a health care worker during an operative procedure. Nevertheless, special emphasis should be placed on the following precautions, issued by the CDC[18] in April 1986, to prevent transmission of bloodborne agents between all patients and all health care workers who perform or assist in invasive procedures.

1. All health care workers who perform or assist in operative procedures must be educated regarding the epidemiology, modes of transmission, and prevention of HIV infection and the need for routine use of appropriate barrier precautions during procedures and when handling instruments contaminated with blood after procedures.
2. All health care workers who perform or assist in invasive procedures must wear gloves when touching mucous membranes or nonintact skin of all patients and use other appropriate barrier precautions when indicated, e.g., masks, eye-coverings, and gowns, if aerosolization or splashes are likely to occur.
3. All health care workers who perform or assist in invasive procedures must use extraordinary care to prevent injuries to hands caused by needles, scalpels, and other sharp instruments or devices during procedures; when cleaning used instruments; during disposal of used needles; and when handling sharp instruments following pro-

cedures. After use, disposable syringes and needles, scalpel blades, and other sharp items must be placed in puncture-resistant containers for disposal. To prevent needlestick injuries, needles should not be recapped, purposefully bent or broken, removed from disposable syringes, or otherwise manipulated by hand.

4. No health care worker who has exudative lesions or weeping dermatitis should perform or assist in invasive procedures or other direct patient care activities or handle equipment used for patient care.

MANAGEMENT OF PARENTERAL AND MUCOUS MEMBRANE EXPOSURES TO HIV BY HEALTH CARE WORKERS

If a health care worker has a parenteral, e.g., needlestick or cut, or mucous membrane, e.g., splash to the eye or mouth, exposure to blood or other body fluids, the source patient should be assessed clinically and epidemiologically to determine the likelihood of HIV infection. If the assessment suggests that infection may exist, the patient should be informed of the incident and requested to consent to serologic testing for evidence of HIV infection. If the source patient has AIDS or other evidence of infection, declines testing, or has a positive test, the health care worker should be evaluated clinically and serologically for evidence of HIV infection as soon as possible after the exposure, and, if seronegative, retested after 6 weeks and on a periodic basis thereafter, e.g., 3, 6, and 12 months following exposure, to determine if transmission has occurred. During this follow-up period, especially the first 6 to 12 weeks, when most infected persons are expected to seroconvert, exposed health care workers should receive counseling about the risk of infection and follow U.S. Public Health Service recommendations for preventing transmission of AIDS. If the source patient is seronegative and has no other evidence of HIV infection, no further follow-up of the health care worker is necessary.

STERILIZATION, DISINFECTION, HOUSEKEEPING, AND WASTE DISPOSAL TO PREVENT TRANSMISSION OF HIV

Sterilization and disinfection procedures currently recommended for use in health care facilities are adequate to sterilize or disinfect instruments, devices, or other items contaminated with blood or other body fluids from individuals infected with HIV. Instruments or other nondisposable items that enter normally sterile tissue or the vascular system or through which blood flows should be sterilized before reuse. Surgical instruments used on all patients should be decontaminated after use rather than just rinsed with water. Decontamination can be accomplished by machine or by hand cleaning by trained personnel wearing appropriate protective attire and using appropriate chemical germicides. Instruments or other nondisposable items that touch intact mucous membranes should receive high level disinfection.

Several liquid chemical germicides commonly used in laboratories and health care facilities have been shown to kill HIV at concentrations much lower than are used in practice. When decontaminating instruments or medical devices, chemical germicides that are registered with and approved by the U.S. Environmental Protection Agency (EPA) as "sterilants" can be used either for sterilization or for high level disinfection depending on contact time; germicides that are approved for use as "hospital disinfectants" and are mycobactericidal when used at appropriate dilutions can also be used for high level disinfection of devices and instruments. Germicides that are mycobactericidal are preferred because mycobacteria represent one of the most resistant groups of microorganisms; therefore, germicides that are effective against mycobacteria are also effective against other bacterial and viral pathogens. When chemical germicides are used, instruments or devices to be sterilized or disinfected should be thoroughly cleansed before exposure to the germicide, and the manufacturer's instructions for use of the germicide should be followed.

Laundry and dishwashing cycles commonly used in hospitals are adequate to decontaminate linens, dishes, glassware, and utensils. When cleaning environmental surfaces, housekeeping procedures commonly used in hospitals are adequate; surfaces exposed to blood and body fluids should be cleaned with a detergent followed by decontamination using an EPA-approved hospital disinfectant that is mycobactericidal. Individuals cleaning up such spills should wear disposable gloves.

In addition to hospital disinfectants, a freshly prepared solution of sodium hypochlorite (household bleach) is an inexpensive and very effective germicide. Concentrations ranging from 5000 ppm (a 1:10 dilution of household bleach) to 500 ppm (a 1:100 dilution) sodium hypochlorite are effective, depending on the amount of organic material, e.g., blood or mucus, present on the surface to be cleaned and disinfected.

Sharp items should be considered as potentially infective and should be handled and disposed of with extraordinary care to prevent accidental injuries. Other potentially infective waste should be contained and transported in clearly identified impervious plastic bags. If the outside of the bag is contaminated with blood or other body fluids, a second outer bag should be used. Recommended practices for disposal of infective waste are adequate for disposal of waste contaminated by HIV. Blood and other body fluids may be carefully poured down a drain connected to a sanitary sewer.

CONCLUSION

As the AIDS pandemic continues, urologists will be examining and operating on more of these patients in the future. Patients with AIDS may be afflicted by any of a number of infectious and malignant complications. Guidelines have been developed to minimize the possibility of spread of the AIDS virus (HIV) to health care workers. All personnel in offices, clinics, and hospitals should be made aware of these guidelines.

REFERENCES

1. Centers for Disease Control: *Pneumocystis* pneumonia—Los Angeles. Morbid Mortal Weekly Rep 30:250, 1981
2. Centers for Disease Control: Kaposi's sarcoma and *Pneumocystis* pneumonia among homosexual men—New York City and California. Morbid Mortal Weekly Rep 30:305, 1981
3. Centers for Disease Control: Hepatitis B virus vaccine safety: Report of an interagency group. Morbid Mortal Weekly Rep 31:465, 1982
4. Centers for Disease Control: Update on acquired immune deficiency syndrome (AIDS)—United States. Morbid Mortal Weekly Rep 31:507, 1982
5. Barre-Sinoussi F, Chermann J, Rey F, et al: Isolation of a T-lymphotropic retrovirus from a patient at risk for acquired immune deficiency syndrome (AIDS). Science 220:859, 1983
6. Popovic M, Sarngadharan M, Reed E, et al: Detection, isolation, and continuous production of cytopathic human T-lymphotropic retrovirus (HTLV-III) from patients with AIDS and pre-AIDS. Science 224:497, 1984
7. Gallo R, Salahuddin S, Popovic M, et al: Frequent detection and isolation of cytopathic retroviruses (HTLV-III) from patients with AIDS and at risk for AIDS. Science 224:500, 1984
8. Centers for Disease Control: Revision of the case definition of acquired immunodeficiency syndrome for national reporting—United States. Morbid Mortal Weekly Rep 34:373, 1985
9. Krigel R, Friedman-Kien A: Kaposi's sarcoma in AIDS. In Devita V, Hellman S, Rosenberg S (eds): AIDS—Etiology, Diagnosis, Treatment and Prevention. Philadelphia, Lippincott, 1985, pp 185–211
10. Gottlieb G, Ackerman A: Kaposi's sarcoma: An extensively disseminated form in young homosexual men. Hum Pathol 13:10, 1982
11. Safai B, Parris A, Urmacher C: Histopathology of Kaposi's sarcoma and other neoplasms. In Ebbesen P, Biggar R, Melbye M (eds): AIDS—A Basic Guide for Clinicians. Munksgaard, Copenhagen, 1984, p 113
12. Ziegler J, Beckstead J, Volberding P, et al: Non-Hodgkin's lymphoma in 90 homosexual men. Lancet 2:631, 1982
13. Macher A, De Vinatea M, Daly M, et al: AIDS case for diagnosis. Milit Med 151:M73, 1986
14. Reichert C, Kelly V, Macher A: Pathologic features of AIDS. In Devita V, Hellman S, Rosenberg S (eds): AIDS—Etiology, Diagnosis, Treatment and Prevention. Philadelphia, Lippincott, 1985, pp 111–160
15. Rao T, Filippone E, Nicastri A, et al: Associated focal and segmental glomerulosclerosis in the acquired immunodeficiency syndrome. N Engl J Med 310:669, 1984
16. Smith P, Macher A, Bookman M, et al: *Salmonella typhimurium* enteritis and bac-

teremia in the acquired immune deficiency syndrome. Ann Intern Med 102:207, 1985
17. Centers for Disease Control: Summary: Recommendations for preventing transmission of infection with human T-lymphotropic virus type III/lymphadenopathy-associated virus in the workplace. Morbid Mortal Weekly Rep 34:681, 1985
18. Centers for Disease Control: Recommendations for preventing transmission of infection with human T-lymphotropic virus type III/lymphadenopathy-associated virus during invasive procedures. Morbid Mortal Weekly Rep 35:221, 1986

Flow Cytometry in Bladder Cancer

Muhammad Choudhury, Kaoru Nakamura, and Joseph Addonizio

Flow cytometry is a rapidly developing type of microscopy which evaluates the biologic characteristics of individual cells by analyzing their constituents, particularly DNA, which is present in abnormally large amounts in cancer cells. Instead of being examined on a glass slide after staining with dyes specific for a cellular component, the cells are suspended in liquid; and the amount of dye in individual cells is measured as they flow in single file through a narrowly focused beam of light to which the dye responds by emitting light.[1,2] Thus, flow cytometry provides an objective measure of the amount of the cell component in the sample.

Bladder tumors are composed of cells with large, hyperchromatic nuclei because of an abnormally high DNA content as a result of chromosomal alterations. Flow cytometry measures the amount of DNA and attempts to correlate it with the presence or absence of tumor in the bladder and with the degree of tumor aggressiveness. Even with the measurement of DNA alone, flow cytometry of bladder cancer has achieved a degree of diagnostic accuracy similar to that of conventional cytology.[2] Measurement of other cellular components and features, such as RNA, nuclear size, and proliferation rate, are also being developed or evaluated.

This chapter reviews the need for new methods of predicting the behavior of bladder tumors, the theoretical foundation of flow cytometry as now practiced, the techniques needed, and the results of the test.

IS THERE A NEED FOR A NEW DIAGNOSTIC TEST FOR BLADDER TUMORS?

Most clinicians would agree that the answer to this question is unequivocally "yes." Both the present diagnostic studies and the available predictive tests have drawbacks.

Cystoscopy has long been a standard method of diagnosis and follow-up of bladder cancer. However, it has two significant limitations. First, it is unable to detect microscopic disease. Second, tumors may be overlooked even by the experienced endoscopist, especially if they are in areas of the bladder that are difficult to examine. The availability of the flexible cystoscope has reduced this problem but not eliminated it. A less significant drawback of cystoscopy is its invasiveness.

Urine cytology has proved a powerful diagnostic and prognostic tool in many cases. However, it, too, has several important limitations. First, even for high grade urothelial cancers, the diagnostic accuracy may be as low as 62 percent.[3] Second, the exfoliated cells of a low grade bladder tumor differ so subtly from normal urothelium that their identification poses a challenge for even the most experienced cytopathologist. As a result, the diagnostic accuracy for these low grade tumors may be as low as 32 percent.[3] Of course, an experienced cytopathologist is not always available. Finally, prior instrumentation of the genitourinary tract, urinary calculi, and trabeculation may cause alterations in the bladder epithelium that make cytologic diagnosis even more difficult.[4]

At present, the most widely used method for diagnosing bladder cancer and predicting its behavior is histologic examination of biopsy specimens obtained from the tumor, from epithelium near the tumor and suspicious-looking mucosa, and from randomly selected areas of the mucosa. All of the drawbacks of cystoscopy are again involved. Moreover, the biopsied area may not be representative of the entire tumor. Even if it is, histologically identical tumors may differ significantly in their clinical courses.[5] Other problems are introduced because histopathologic classification is subjective, and even experienced pathologists do not always rate tumors identically.[6] An attempt to improve the accuracy of prediction by measuring the presence of ABH blood group antigens on the surface of tumor cells has had some good results, but the test is not entirely objective, nor is it easy to perform reproducibly.[7,8]

The ideal test for the presence and aggressiveness of bladder tumors would have several features. First, it would be objective. Second, it would give quantitative results. Third, it would reflect the nature of all the tumor cells analyzed. Finally, it would be relatively simple to perform and would be reproducible. Flow cytometric measurement of the DNA content of tumor cells appears to satisfy these criteria.[9]

THE CELL CYCLE AND ITS IMPORTANCE IN FLOW CYTOMETRY

The biologic basis of DNA flow cytometry is the fact that most tumor cells have abnormal amounts of DNA because of chromosomal duplications, translocations, and other alterations. To understand the data produced by DNA cytometry, it is helpful to understand the cell's reproductive (mitotic) cycle (Fig. 1).

After completing mitosis (M), cells spend several hours in the Gap 1 (G_1) phase. External conditions determine whether the cell remains in this phase and thus in a proliferative cycle or switches into the resting (Gap 0, or G_0) stage. About 90 percent of somatic cells are normally in the G_1/G_0 phase.

The G_1 cells that continue in proliferative cycle eventually enter the phase of DNA synthesis (S). It is during this time that the chromosome complement is duplicated. There is then a second Gap (G_2) phase, followed by the overt chromosome rearrangements of mitosis and cell division. A normal cell thus enters the S phase with a diploid amount of DNA (that is, 46 chromosomes), referred to as 2C, and enters mitosis with twice this amount (tetraploid amount; 4C). Because fewer than 10 percent of normal human cells are in mitosis at any given time, 90 percent of a normal population will have a diploid amount of DNA and less than 10 percent a tetraploid

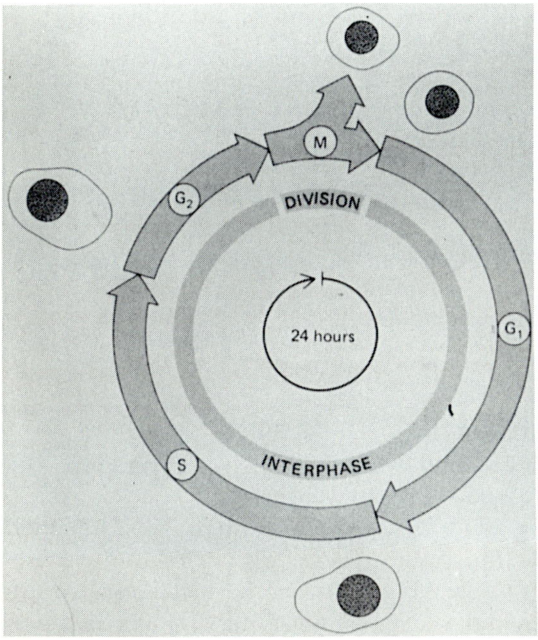

Figure 1. A cell cycle diagram. After cell division (at the top of the circle) cells spend several hours in the G_1 phase. After G_1, during S phase, they synthesize DNA. Then there is the second "gap," G_2 phase, followed by chromosomal rearrangement in mitosis, and another division.

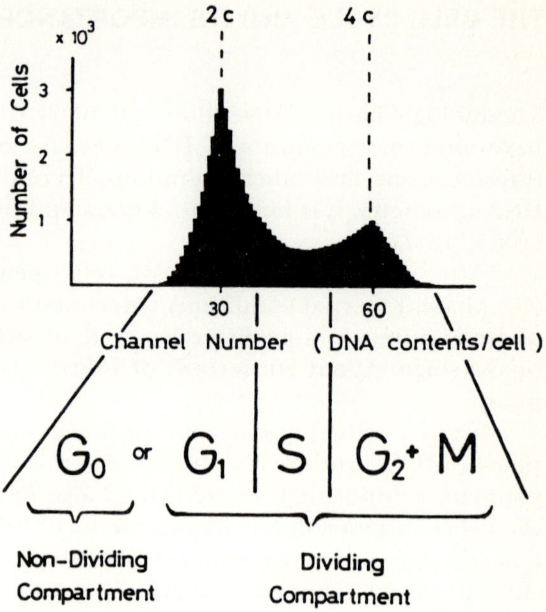

Figure 2. Relationship of the DNA histogram to various stages of the cell cycle. The ordinate represents the number of cells in each channel. The abscissa shows the relative DNA content of cells in an arbitrary unit. The peak to the left represents G_1/G_0 cells with a normal diploid (2C) DNA content. The peak to the right represents normal G_2+M cells with a tetraploid (4C) DNA content. In between these peaks are the cells in the S (synthesis) phase of the cell cycle.

amount. Other distributions of diploidy and tetraploidy, and other amounts of DNA, such as three or five times ploidy (3C or 5C; aneuploidy) indicate an abnormal population of cells (Fig. 2). In flow cytometry, the value of 2C is determined by measurement of the DNA content of blood lymphocytes or granulocytes.[10]

TECHNIQUE OF FLOW CYTOMETRY

There are three basic steps to flow cytometry:

1. Specimen collection and preparation
2. Cell staining
3. Measurement in the flow cytometer

Each step will be described briefly.

Specimen Collection and Preparation

Cells for flow cytometry can be obtained by either biopsy or irrigation. The two types of specimen are prepared somewhat differently.

Biopsy specimens weighing 200 to 500 mg are immediately immersed in cold RPMI-1640 culture medium containing 10 percent fetal bovine serum (GIBCO; Grand Island, NY). The sample is minced mechanically and suspended in the same medium, and a suspension of individual cells is prepared nonenzymatically by filtering the minced tissue through 125-μm nylon mesh. The filtrate is washed with the aid of a tuberculin syringe fitted with a 26-gauge needle and centrifuged at 900 rpm for 5 minutes. The resulting pellet contains 3×10^5 to 5×10^5 cells.

Irrigation specimens are obtained by rinsing the bladder with 50 ml of saline through a urethral catheter or cystoscope for 5 to 10 minutes. The specimen should be refrigerated until it can be processed, which should be within 12 to 24 hours. The specimen is sieved through a 64-μm nylon mesh to remove tissue fragments and cell clusters and then concentrated by centrifugation. The pellet is resuspended in Hank's balanced salt solution at a concentration of approximately 10^6 cells/ml.

Before staining, cells are resuspended by brief vortexing.

Staining

The cells are stained with dyes known as fluorochromes, which bind quantitatively to a specific cell component such as DNA and which emit light at a characteristic wavelength after exposure to high intensity light.

No single flow cytometry staining procedure is universally accepted, and the choice among the alternatives is determined in part by the goal of the study as well as by what equipment is available. If measurement of cellular DNA is the primary objective and an ultraviolet light source is available, a one-step stain with DAPI (4,6-diamidino-2-phenylindole), a specific DNA fluorochrome, is satisfactory.[11] Collste et al and Devonec et al prefer the metachromatic dye acridine orange for bladder irrigation specimens, as it stains DNA and RNA differentially, permitting measurement of both.[11,12]

Measurement

Flow cytometers are available from several companies. We use the Orthosystem 50-H Multiparameter Flow Cytometer equipped with an Ortho 2150 computer (Ortho Diagnostics, Inc.; Westwood, MA) (Fig. 3). The chief components are:

1. A source of high intensity, narrowly focused light, usually a laser or a mercury arc lamp, of carefully controlled wavelength
2. A flow chamber designed to cause the cells to make their transit past the sensor in single file
3. A photoelectronic sensor
4. A computer that controls data collection and performs operator-directed analysis and statistical manipulations of the data

Cells stained with the fluorochrome are induced to pass across the flow chamber by means of a pressure gradient. At a specific point along the way, the cells cross the high intensity light beam, which excites the stain to emit fluorescent light. This emission is sensed, quantified, and stored by the photoelectric equipment.[13] Photosensors convert the light emission signals into

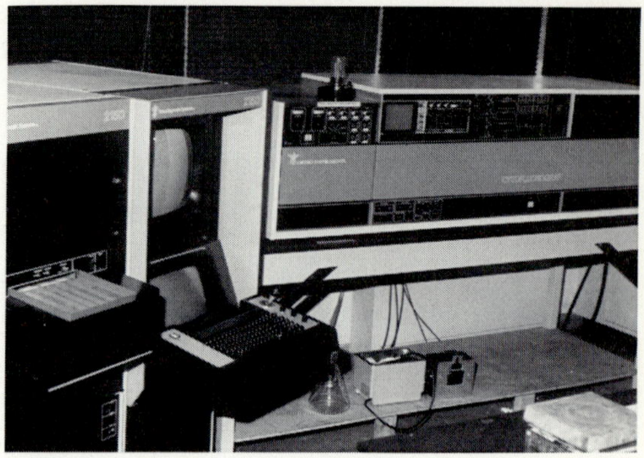

Figure 3. Flow cytometer.

distribution histograms of the amount of the stained cell component in the entire population (Fig. 4). If DNA is being measured, typical characteristics that can be measured objectively include the degree of aneuploidy and percentage of cells in S phase, an indicator of proliferative activity. For each specimen, data are analyzed for a large number of cells (10^4 to 10^6).

Interpretation of the Results

The data from flow cytometry are displayed graphically in various ways. If a single feature such as DNA content is being studied, the distribution of ploidy is shown as a histogram. Figure 5 shows the histograms for various stages in the cell cycle. When tumor cells are studied, the picture is more complex because of the presence of aneuploid cells (Fig. 6). In this example, there is a tetraploid cell line with more than 15 percent hyperdiploid ($>2C$) cells.

Another way to analyze the data is to determine what percentage of cells is dividing; for most cancers, this figure is above that for normal cells. The proliferation index is the ratio of cells in the S and G_2/M phases to the total number of cells in the specimen. For most normal cell populations, this ratio is less than 1:10.

Yet another measure is the DNA index (DI), which is the degree of aneuploidy. The DI represents the ratio of the fluorescence intensity of the aneuploid cells to that of the diploid cells. A diploid population has a DI of 1.0; aneuploid populations have higher DIs, with greater degrees of aneuploidy producing higher numbers.[14]

Tachibana et al recently introduced a method of measuring the relative mean DNA content of cell populations by calculating what they called the heterogeneity index (HI) and heterogeneity index score (HIS).[15] The former is calculated by dividing the total DNA content by the number of cells. The formula for HIS is:

$$(\mathrm{HI} \times 100) - 200$$

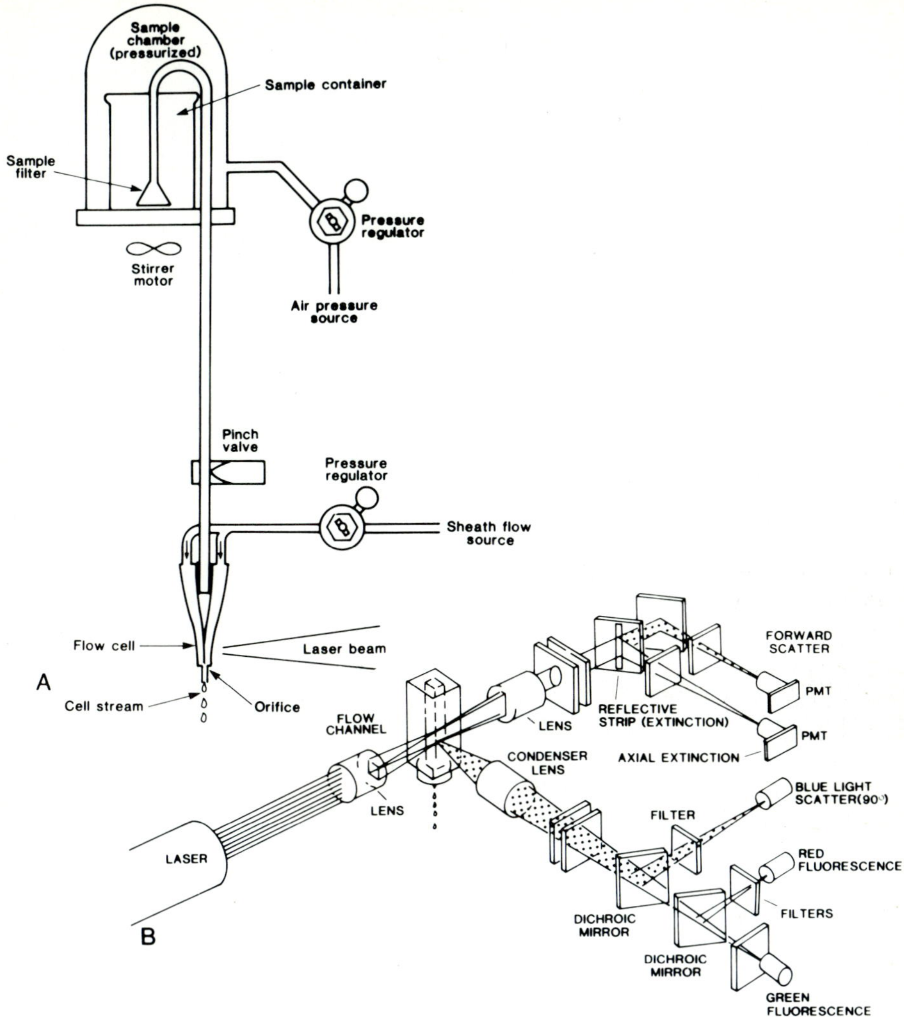

Figure 4. Diagrammatic representation of the flow cytometer. **A.** A suspension of bladder epithelial cells, stained with the flourescent dye acridine orange, is placed in the sample container, then forced under pressure into a narrow stream of cells through the flow cell. Within the flow cell (or flow channel), the cell stream is narrowed further, into a single file of cells, and centered at the focus of the argon ion laser beam by a laminar sheath of saline or water. The water sheath keeps the cells from touching the channel wall, and prevents it from being blocked. On emerging from the channel, the cell stream breaks into droplets that can be charged and deflected electrostatically to sort a particular subpopulation of cells. **B.** The flow channel is rectangular, with optically flat surfaces. As each cell flows through the narrowly focused laser light, it emits a fluorescence flash that is collected at 90 degrees; the red and green components are separated by dichroic mirrors and optical filters, measured by separate photomultipliers, and recorded by computer. The blue laser light absorbed by the cell (extinction) or scattered in a forward direction, or at 90 degrees, gives information about cell size and granularity and can be measured simultaneously by other photomultipliers. *(From Melamed MR, 1984, p 599, with permission.[2])*

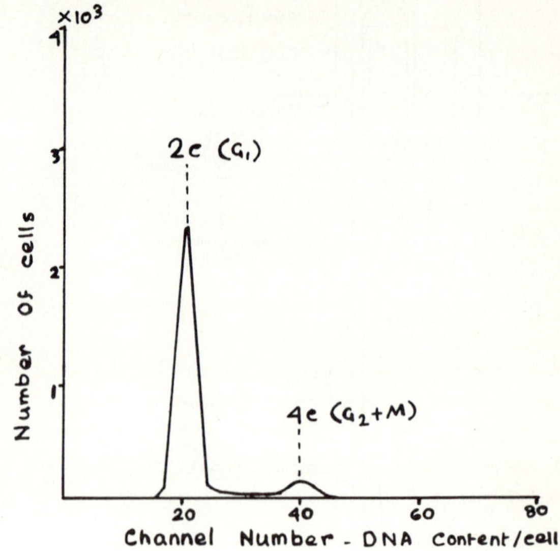

Figure 5. DNA histogram of normal bladder epithelium. The ordinate represents the number of cells. The abscissa shows the relative DNA content of cells. The peak to the left represents G_1 cells with the same DNA content as normal lymphocytes (2C). To the right at twice the channel number G_2+M cells are seen, containing twice the amount of DNA (4C). Between these two peaks are the cells in S phase.

The mean HIS of normal bladder mucosa is 9.805, that of grades I and II tumors is 23.576, and that of grade III tumors 160.965.

In a sense, then, flow cytometry is an automated version of a traditional measure of malignancy, the mitotic index. Flow cytometry is more accurate, however, because it does not depend on human eyesight and patience to locate and identify mitotic figures and because it identifies dividing cells before there are visible changes. Flow cytometry is also much faster.

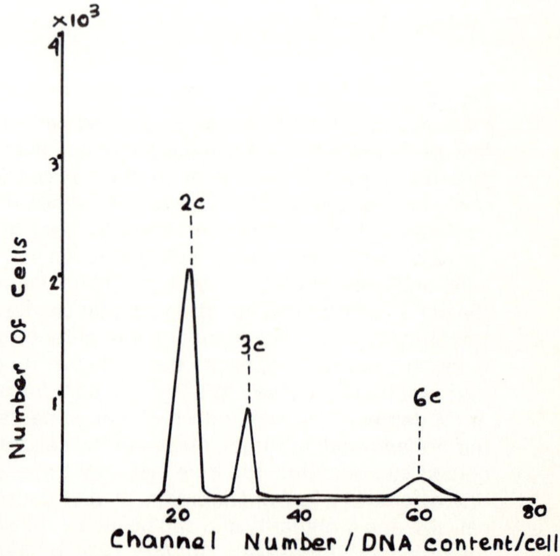

Figure 6. DNA histogram of a bladder tumor. Peak to the left represents the normal G_1 cells. The second peak at about channel 30 with a triploid (3C) DNA content, represents G_1 phase of tumor cells. Tumor cells in the G_2+M phase have hexaploid (6C) DNA content, which is seen at channel number 60 on the graph.

CRITERIA FOR DIAGNOSIS OF BLADDER CANCER BY FLOW CYTOMETRY

In 1982, Klein et al proposed that a bladder specimen should be said to contain cancer if (1) it contained an aneuploid cell population, or (2) it contained a tetraploid line and more than 15 percent hyperdiploid cells.[16] They considered a specimen suspicious for cancer if it contained more than 10 percent hyperdiploid cells with no aneuploidy or 10 to 15 percent hyperdiploid cells with a tetraploid component. A specimen with less than 10 percent hyperdiploid cells and no aneuploidy was considered normal.[16] Using these criteria, investigators at Memorial Sloan-Kettering Cancer Center identified 93 percent of 158 histologically proved bladder carcinomas, including 86 percent of the noninvasive papillary carcinomas. The false-negative rate was 7 percent.[17] The same investigators demonstrated a 2 percent false-positive rate in benign bladder disease and showed that chronic cystitis influenced the result by increasing the number of suspicious looking specimens to 34 percent.[16]

ADVANTAGES AND DISADVANTAGES OF FLOW CYTOMETRY

Few hospitals have the luxury of employing a highly skilled cytopathologist; flow cytometry offers the equivalent of highly accurate conventional cytology.[2] Moreover, the results are objective, quantitative, and easy to retain and compare with later findings.

At the same time, flow cytometry has some significant disadvantages. The first is the cost of the instruments and the need for engineering assistance to maintain and modify both the computer and the flow cytometer. A lesser disadvantage is the need for specialized methods of specimen preparation. Finally, voided urine specimens are not suitable for analysis; one must obtain irrigation or biopsy specimens. Because cystoscopy is often necessary in patients suspected of having or known to have bladder cancer, and because of the simplicity of irrigating the bladder through a urethral catheter, however, obtaining the specimen is not usually a significant problem.

CLINICAL USES OF FLOW CYTOMETRY IN BLADDER CANCER

Diagnosis

Flow cytometric DNA measurements are approximately as good as urine cytology in diagnosing bladder cancer, with the detection rate in both tests being approximately 90 percent if papillomas (grade I transitional cell carcinomas) are excluded.[2,13] The best results are obtained with flat carcinoma in situ; in the reports by Klein et al, 69 of 71 (97 percent) of such tumors were correctly identified. Invasive carcinomas were identified by flow cytometry in 48 of 52 patients (92 percent) and noninvasive papillary carcinomas in 30 of 35 (86 percent). These results are as good as those that can be expected with conventional cytology.[2,18,19] Devonec and colleagues compared flow cytometry and conventional cytology in 84 outpatients who had had prior conservative treatment for low stage bladder tumors and found the former to be a more sensitive measure of cytologic abnormalities.[20]

Cytologically benign papillomas are more difficult to detect by flow cytometry. When DNA measurement alone was used, these lesions were detected in only one third of the cases in which they were known to be present, with another one third of the cases producing suspicious findings (10 to 15 percent hyperdiploid cells). When both DNA and RNA are measured, however, an acceptable detection rate (83 percent) can be achieved.[21]

Follow-up of Patients with Bladder Tumors

One of the most important applications of flow cytometry may be in the follow-up of patients after treatment. Because the measure is objective, reproducible, and graphic, it is easy to compare a sequence of studies over time and so document changes in the aneuploid or hyperdiploid populations or in the distribution of DNA and RNA content. For example, Klein et al[19] followed 98 outpatients treated conservatively for low stage bladder tumors with cystoscopy, conventional cytology, and flow cytometry for 2 years. The cytometry results agreed with the results of the other studies in 80 percent of the examinations, and on occasion abnormalities in flow cytometry antedated development of visible tumors by as much as 12 months. The false-positive rate for flow cytometry was 5.8 percent and the false-negative rate 8.3 percent as judged by the results of the other studies.[19] Devonec et al found flow cytometry to be a more sensitive indicator of cytologic abnormalities than conventional cytology after conservative treatment of low stage tumors.[20]

Monitoring Response to Treatment

If a treatment for bladder cancer is effective, one would expect the number of abnormal cells in a specimen obtained by irrigation to disappear. Staiamo-Coico et al studied 22 patients treated with intravesical bacillus Calmette-Guérin (BCG) for low stage bladder cancer, monitoring their response by cystoscopy, conventional cytology, and flow cytometry. Twelve patients remained clinically free of disease for at least 15 months, and in all but one of these, flow cytometry data had reverted to normal, with a decrease in hyperdiploid cells and disappearance of aneuploid stem lines. Ten patients had recurrences, which were anticipated by flow cytometry in six cases and suspected in another.[22] Klein et al evaluated 28 patients with grades II and III stage T3 bladder cancer before and after delivery of 2000 rad of radiation precystectomy. Four of the five patients downstaged by radiation had normalization of flow cytometry. In the remaining patients, in whom there was no change in stage, eight had normalization of their flow cytometry results. Had cystectomy been delayed, downstaging might have taken place.[23]

Prognostic Indicator

Tumor progression or recurrence can often be predicted from flow cytometry results. Gustafson et al[24] discussed 20 patients with carcinoma in situ and aneuploidy in bladder washing specimens. In seven cases, more than one aneuploid cell line was present, and in all of these patients the disease progressed. There was no progression in the remaining 13 patients, who had single aneuploid stem lines.[24] The same authors studied 222 patients with superficial bladder tumors treated by surgery alone. In the 175 patients with a normal diploid pattern in flow cytometry, the recurrence rate was 0.52 ± 0.58 per year, whereas in the 47 patients with aneuploidy the rate was 1.54 ± 0.78.[25] The DNA pattern might, therefore, be an early indicator of future tumor behavior and thus be useful in the selection of treatment.

Gustafson and colleagues studied 229 patients with grade I (n = 51) or grade II (n = 178) stage Ta and T1 tumors treated by surgery alone. None of the 175 patients with diploid tumors had disease progression, but progression occurred in 19 of the 54 with aneuploidy, 11 of whom died. Thus, all tumors that progressed were aneuploid, but not all aneuploid tumors progressed.[26]

CONCLUSION

Flow cytometry is based on the known propensity of malignant cells for developing chromosomal abnormalities. The method is quantitative and reproducible and allows comparison of changes in a tumor over time. The principal inhibitor of its wider use is the cost of the equipment needed.

REFERENCES

1. Melamed MR, Klein FA: Flow cytometry of urinary bladder irrigation specimens. Hum Pathol 15:302, 1984
2. Melamed MR: Flow cytometry of the urinary bladder. Urol Clin North Am 11:599, 1984
3. Friedell GH, Hawkins IR, Ahmed SW, et al: The role of urinary tract cytology in the detection and clinical management of bladder cancer. In Bonney WW (ed): Bladder Cancer. Baltimore, Williams & Wilkins, 1982, pp 49–62
4. Dean PJ, Murphy WM: Importance of urinary cytology and future role of flow cytometry. Urology 26(suppl):11, 1985
5. Cummings KB: Carcinoma of the bladder: Predictors. Cancer 45:1849, 1980
6. Ooms EC, Anderson WA, Alons CL, et al: Analysis of the performance of pathologists in the grading of bladder tumors. Hum Pathol 14:140, 1983

7. Catalona WJ: Practical utility of specific red cell adherence test in bladder cancer. Urology 18:113, 1981
8. Limas C, Lange PH: A, B, H antigen detectability in normal and neoplastic urothelium: Influence of methodological factors. Cancer Res 42:2476, 1982
9. Frankfurt OS, Huben RP: Clinical application of DNA flow cytometry for bladder tumors. Urology 23(suppl):29, 1984
10. Bohm N, Sandritter W: DNA in human tumors: A cytophotometric study. Curr Top Pathol 60:151, 1975
11. Devonec M, Darzynkiewicz Z, Kostyrka-claps ML, et al: Flow cytometry of low stage bladder tumors. Cancer 49:109, 1982
12. Collste LA, Darzynkiewicz Z, Traganos F, et al: Flow cytometry in bladder cancer detection and evaluation using acridine orange metachromatic nucleic acid staining of irrigation cytology specimens. J Urol 123:478, 1980
13. Stephenson RA, Herr HW: Flow cytometry in urologic oncology. Urol Clin North Am 13:525, 1986
14. Barlogie B, Raber MN, Schumann J, et al: Flow cytometry in clinical cancer research. Cancer Res 43:3982, 1983
15. Tachibana M, Addonizio JC, Chiao JW, et al: Heterogeneity index score (HIS): New computerized method for classification of human bladder carcinomas using flow cytometry. Urology 26:356, 1985
16. Klein FA, Herr HW, Sogani PC, et al: Flow cytometry of normal and non-neoplastic disease of the bladder: An estimate of the false positive rate. J Urol 127:946, 1982
17. Klein FA, Herr HW, Sogani PC, et al: Detection and follow-up of carcinoma of the urinary bladder by flow cytometry. Cancer 50:389, 1982
18. Klein FA, Herr HW, Whitmore WF, et al: An evaluation of automated flow cytometry in detection of carcinoma in situ of the bladder. Cancer 50:1003, 1982
19. Klein FA, Whitmore WF, Herr HW, et al: Flow cytometry follow-up of patients with low stage bladder tumors. J Urol 128:88, 1982
20. Devonec M, Darzynkiewicz Z, Kostyrka-claps ML, et al: Flow cytometry of low stage bladder tumors. Cancer 49:109, 1982
21. Klein FA, Melamed MR, Whitmore WF, et al: Characterization of bladder papilloma by two parameter DNA-RNA flow cytometry. Cancer Res 42:190, 1982
22. Staiamo-Coico L, Huffman J, Wolf R, et al: Monitoring intravesical Bacillus Calmette-Guérin treatment of bladder carcinoma with flow cytometry. J Urol 133:786, 1985
23. Klein FA, Whitmore WF, Wolf RM: Presumptive down staging from preoperative irradiation for bladder cancer as determined by flow cytometry: Preliminary report. Int J Radiat Oncol Biol Phys 9:487, 1983
24. Gustafson H, Tribukair B, Esposti PL: The prognostic value of DNA analysis in primary carcinoma-in-situ of the urinary bladder. Scand J Urol Nephrol 16:141, 1982
25. Gustafson H, Tribukair B, Esposti PL: DNA pattern, histological grade and multiplicity related to recurrence rate in superficial bladder tumor. Scand J Urol Nephrol 16:135, 1982
26. Gustafson H, Tribukair B, Esposti PL: DNA profile and tumor progression in patients with superficial bladder tumors. Urol Res 10:13, 1982

New Uses for Old Nuclei
DNA Ploidy Pattern and Prognosis for Patients with Genitourinary Neoplasms

Leslie M. Rainwater and Michael M. Lieber

For approximately the past 50 years, the prognosis for patients with genitourinary malignancies has been determined by ascertaining tumor clinical and pathologic stage, histologic grade, and cell type. A search for additional biologic markers of tumor behavior and patient prognosis has gone on steadily for the past several decades. Except for a few laboratory tests such as the measurement of serum acid phosphatase by enzymatic or radioimmunoassay, of serum prostate-specific antigen by radioimmunoassay and determination of the tumor markers alpha-fetoprotein and beta-human chorionic gonadotopin (HCG) by serum radioimmunoassay for germ cell testicular tumors, however, tumor stage, grade, and cell type have remained the essential core variables for managing patients with urologic malignancies.

It now seems likely that determination of *the nuclear DNA histogram or ploidy pattern* soon will come to have an essential role as well in the routine evaluation of many urologic and nonurologic human cancers. The major practical advance which has made routine determination of DNA ploidy patterns possible was the description in 1983 by David Hedley and colleagues from Sydney, Australia, of a method of extracting nuclei from archival paraffin-embedded tumor blocks and of using such formalin-fixed and paraffin embedded tissue for measuring DNA ploidy patterns successfully.[1–4] Since formalin fixation and paraffin embedding is routinely used in the preparation of histologic sections for pathologic diagnosis after tumor resection, the same specimen substrates used to make histologic sections can be routinely used for the determination of nuclear DNA ploidy patterns. In the past 2 years, the Urology Research Laboratory at the Mayo Clinic has extensively applied Hedley's method to the study of nuclear DNA ploidy patterns of urologic cancers resected at the Mayo Clinic over the past half century. The methods used, the results found, and, particularly, the correlations between nuclear DNA ploidy patterns and prognosis constitute the subjects of this review.

TECHNOLOGIC INTRODUCTION

Nuclear DNA ploidy pattern refers to the aggregate histogram pattern of total DNA content of the nuclei of a given tissue sample, measured in this instance by flow cytometry (FCM). In a flow cytometric ploidy analysis, approximately 2×10^4 cells or nuclei individually have the relative quantity of DNA in their nuclei measured by rapid fluorometric methods. With modern FCM instruments using lasers and sophisticated computers, such measurements of $\sim 2 \times 10^4$ nuclei can be performed in a matter of minutes.

Much simpler technologic efforts to quantitate the DNA content of normal and tumor cells began about 40 years ago. In the late 1940s, Caspersson described the use of ultraviolet illumination and string electrometers in the study of nucleic acid and protein metabolism during both normal and abnormal cell growth.[5] Friedman's observations that nuclei of malignant cells stained more intensely than nuclei of normal cells[6] were applied in the Mellors and Silver Microfluorometric Scanner in 1951.[7] This device was capable of automatic searching and detecting of cancer cells on microscopic slides. Also, in the early 1950s, sheath flow systems[8] were developed for the accurate instrumental counting and sizing of blood cells.[9] With the introduction and elaboration of computerized storage and statistical analysis of such data, automated differential cytology became a common clinical tool. Finally, use of the single mercury arc lamp[10] or argon ion laser[11] for excitation of fluorescence of cancer cells in a flow system was completed by development of multiple laser source multiparameter flow cytometer systems approximately 10 years ago.[12] In 1988, commercially available flow cytometers can be easily used to determine a number of physical and biologic parameters of fresh normal and malignant cells, including cell size, nuclear size, DNA, RNA, and protein content, and the distribution of cells in the various parts of the reproductive cell cycle such that as G_0, G_1, S, and G_2/M stages. An excellent current book by Shapiro[13] describes much of the technologic and instrumental background FCM methodology.

In flow cytometer systems, biologic particles, such as individual cells or individual nuclei, linearly travel through a laminar flow sheath system to have various optical properties such as light scatter or dye fluorescence measured quickly by an elaborate electronic system. Such methodology works particularly well for blood cells, marrow cells, or already monodispersed tumor cell sources such as cells from bladder washings which come ready to be stained and put in the flow cytometer. Solid tissues or solid tumors require some sort of mechanical and/or enzymatic digestion in order to generate a single cell suspension which can then be studied on the flow cytometer. While FCM studies commonly have been done over the past decade, these investigations have required processing of fresh tumor tissues immediately as they became available. This time factor associated with the use of fresh tissues somewhat limited the practical uses of FCM in clinical oncology including uro-oncology. What was needed was a simple and reliable methodology which enabled some parameters, particularly DNA content of tumor cells, to be measured in fixed tumor tissues using FCM. The elegant methodologic advances by Hedley and his group beginning in 1983 provided straightforward techniques for extracting nuclei from formalin-fixed paraffin-embedded archival tissue specimens in a way that allowed for subsequent successful staining of nuclear DNA and flow cytometric analysis.[1–4] By this relatively easy technique, it at once became possible to correlate the integrated nuclear DNA content of a large tumor cell sample, i.e., its ploidy pattern, with tumor behavior and patient prognosis, using specimens which had been removed surgically even decades before. For common tumor types such as renal cell carcinoma or adenocarcinoma of the prostate, large numbers of tumors with long clinical follow-up could be readily assembled, to determine if the nuclear DNA ploidy patterns measured correlated with tumor behavior and patient prognosis. For rare tumor types such as Wilms' tumor, squamous cell carcinoma of the male urethra, and adrenal pheochromocytoma, the ability to apply FCM ploidy analysis to archival tumor specimens has allowed investigation of this variable in tumor systems where analysis of fresh material and correlation with prognosis would take decades of prospective study.

SPECIMEN PREPARATION AND TECHNIQUES

The modified Hedley methodology for analyzing the nuclear DNA ploidy pattern of formalin-fixed paraffin-embedded archival tumor specimens used in our laboratory has been as follows[14]: Two or three 40- to 50-μm thick sections are cut using a standard microtome from the paraffin-embedded tissue block. These thick sections are placed in a 10-ml glass culture tube and then are dewaxed using two changes of Histoclear (National Diagnostics, Somerville, NJ) 3 ml for 10 minutes at room temperature, and then are rehydrated in a sequence of ethanol/water solutions of 3 ml of 100, 90, 70 percent ethanol for 5 minutes at room temperature. The dewaxed tissue pellet is then washed twice in distilled water and resuspended in 1 ml of 0.5 percent pepsin and normal saline adjusted to pH 1.5. These specimens are incubated at 37°C for 90 minutes in a tissue culture incubator with intermittent vortex mixing. This is followed by low speed centrifugation to pellet the nuclei and the pepsin-containing supernatant is removed. With the nuclei freed from their paraffin blocks by these simple maneuvers, they are ready to be stained for analysis in the flow cytometer system. Our laboratory has used the fluorescent dye propidium iodide, which binds to DNA and gives a quantitative fluorescent measurement of nuclear DNA content. Our laboratory has used this specific methodology described by Vindelv[15,16] which works for nuclei digested from archival pathologic material or from fresh cells obtained by bladder washings or from enzymatically digested solid tumors. This method is as follows: Briefly, 0.9 ml of a solution (solution A) containing 0.015 g trypsin dissolved in 500 ml of stock solution [2 g trisodium citrate, 2 ml Nonidet P-40, 1.044 g spermine tetrahydrochloride, and 0.121 g Tris (hydroxymethyl)-aminomethane] adjusted to pH 7.6 were added to 0.1 ml of cell suspension in citrate buffer and mixed gently for 10 minutes. Then, 0.75 ml of a solution (solution B) containing 0.25 g trypsin inhibitor and 0.05 g ribonuclease A dissolved in 500 ml of stock solution adjusted to pH 7.6 were mixed gently for 10 minutes. Finally, 0.75 ml of a solution (solution C) containing 0.208 g propidium iodide and 0.580 g spermine tetrahydrochloride dissolved in 500 ml of stock solution adjusted to pH 7.6 were added. The solution of propidium iodide was protected against light with tinfoil during preparation, storage, and the staining procedure. The solutions were mixed and the sample was filtered through a 30-μm pore diameter nylon mesh filter to eliminate nuclear clumps.

INSTRUMENTATION AND DATA ANALYSIS

Our laboratory has used a Becton Dickinson FACS IV Flow Cytometer and Cell Sorter equipped with a 5-watt argon ion laser run at a wavelength of 514 nm to excite propidium iodide fluorescence. This instrument is interfaced with a Consort 40 Minicomputer which was programmed to perform Dean and Jett mathematical analysis of the cell cycle.[17] In the FCM instrument, monodispersed nuclei or cells are arranged into a single file through the use of a narrow capillary tube dispensing the particles into a larger capillary tube. A sheath of fluid passes around the particles maintaining them in a laminar flow and confining the particles to the central region of the tube. The cells or nuclei, moving in single file, pass through the beam of the argon ion laser which excites fluorescence from the propidium iodide-stained DNA. The resultant dye fluorescence, directly proportional to particle DNA content, is detected by a photomultiplier tube, and is nearly instantaneously electronically quantitated as the cells pass through the flow cytometer instrument.[13]

Typically, about 2×10^4 individual tumor cell nuclei have been analyzed for each given sample of tissue studied in this laboratory. For normal tissues studied, almost all the nuclei sampled are in the G_0/G_1 phase of the cell cycle and contain a normal or diploid or 2C amount of DNA. These nuclei produce a large sharp peak on the typical DNA histogram which is the final output from the flow cytometer (Fig. 1). A small second peak re-

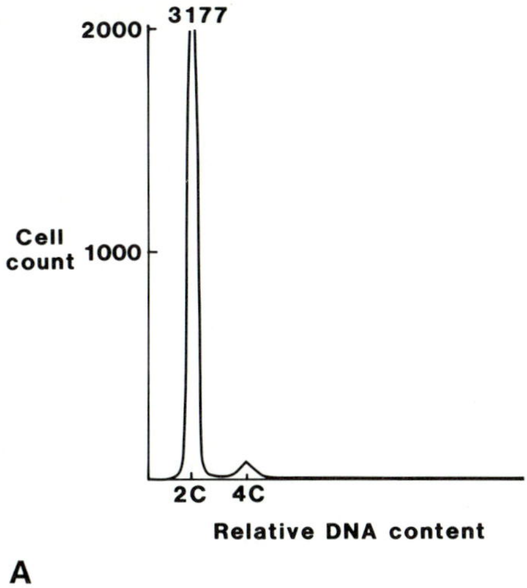

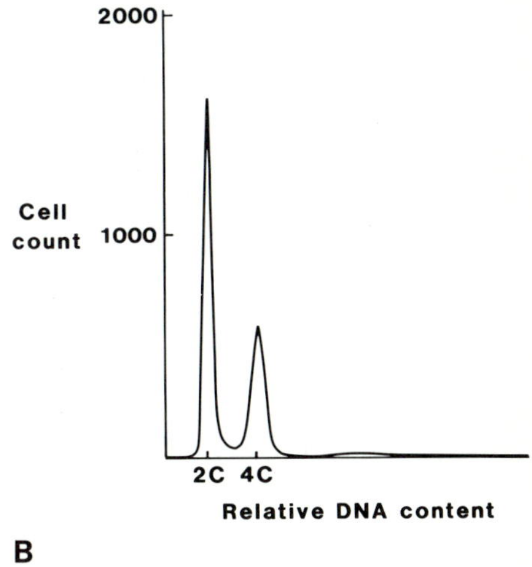

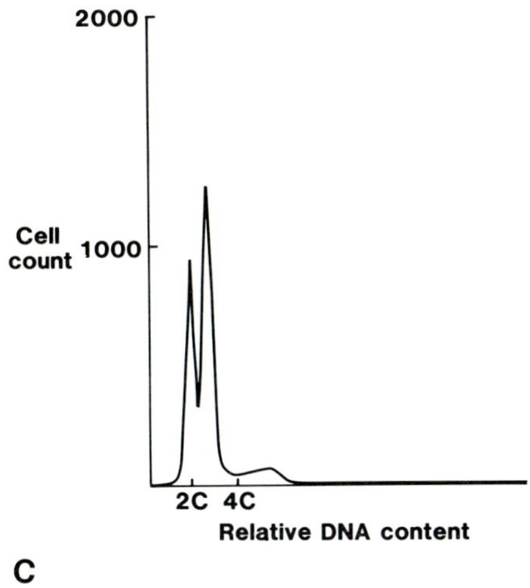

Figure 1. Representative nuclear DNA histogram patterns. Y axis shows cell nuclei count per channel on flow cytometer used. **A.** Pattern of normal or DNA diploid. **B.** DNA tetraploid pattern. **C.** DNA aneuploid pattern.

flecting twice as much DNA in nuclei also is found on the normal DNA histogram. This 4C peak represents cells which contain twice as much DNA in their nucleus, already having gone through the process of DNA synthesis (S phase) and are now G_2 cells ready to proceed through cell division or mitosis. The small number of cells in cycle and going through the DNA synthesis or S phase cells occupy the trough between the 2C and 4C peaks on the DNA histogram. Such normal tissue DNA peak patterns or ploidy patterns illustrated and described also are commonly found in all of the urologic cancer samples which we have studied in the laboratory so far.

In tumor cells, however, two other common DNA histogram patterns have been observed. In one variation, the relative number of nuclei in the 4C peak is markedly increased compared to that found in normal tissues.

When the number of nuclei in the 4C peak is more than three standard deviations above that seen in normal control tissue, our research group commonly has classified such tumors as "DNA tetraploid" and abnormal. In addition, many tumor cell populations contain cell nuclei with a DNA content which are neither 2C or 4C but lie somewhere in between. DNA ploidy patterns or histograms with such abnormal DNA stem lines are classified as "DNA aneuploid."[18] For DNA aneuploid pattern histograms, a so-called "DNA index" is calculated as a ratio of the channel number for the peak channel of the abnormal DNA cells to the peak channel of the DNA normal 2C cells.

It is important to note once again that the pattern generated by the flow cytometer represents an integrated histogram showing the amount of stained DNA fluorescence for a very large number of nuclei or cells studied for a given tissue sample. The individual data points in the histograms are the amount of stained DNA fluorescence from single nuclei. At present, we truly have little understanding of the genetic changes which determine the "gross" nuclear DNA content abnormalities measured by this instrument. Virtually none of the urologic tumor types described below have been adequately studied by cytogenetics to determine characteristic chromosomal changes which make a transformed tumor cell different from a normal cell of the same tissue. At a more microscopic level, the actual mutational changes in the genes responsible, the so-called "oncogenes," for perturbing the characteristics of cell proliferation and invasiveness in malignant tumors are just beginning to be defined. As demonstrated below, however, whatever these cytogenetic and oncocytogenetic changes may be, they commonly result in major disturbances of tumor cell nuclear DNA content which are measured as obvious DNA aneuploidy or DNA tetraploidy by the FCM instrumentation used. It turns out that this abnormal ploidy pattern phenotype correlates well with urologic tumor biologic behavior and patient prognosis.

FINAL TECHNICAL POINT

We have observed, as have others, that the propidium iodide DNA fluorescence intensity measured from formalin-fixed nuclei is decreased compared to that seen in fresh tissue samples from the same source and is dependent on the duration of formalin fixation.[19] Formalin treatment cross-links nuclear proteins which inhibit use of both intercalating and nonintercalating DNA dyes.[13,19] It is thought that these cross-linkages are broken down by pepsin, allowing stoichiometric binding of the fluorochrome to the DNA, and, thus, giving a good correlation between the DNA ploidy pattern of paraffin-embedded versus fresh unfixed cells from the same tissue. With extended formalin fixation, however, these cross-linkages become so dense that they are inadequately broken by the pepsin treatment used, resulting in low fluorescence intensity of the nuclei studied and in a large coefficient of variation of the histogram peaks. With Bouin's fixative and mercury-based fixatives, even less satisfactory results are found because of fluorescence quenching.[20] In our experience, tissues which have been incubated in acid-formalin for more than several days to several weeks will not give interpretable DNA ploidy patterns when processed using Henley's method as described above with standard staining. Since most routine pathology specimens were fixed only briefly or not at all before paraffin embedding, however, this problem generally has not been a factor in the analysis of routine archival tissue specimens embedded in paraffin; we have found more than 95 percent of specimens to give high quality DNA histograms by the methods described. Unfortunately, however, it has not been possible to go back to the original formalin-fixed and preserved tissues to obtain additional specimens for correlation studies or for extensive sampling throughout a given volume of a large tumor such as a renal cell carcinoma. However, it is quite possible that the DNA strands of such formalin-fixed materials remain intact; technical extensions of Hedley's methodology may enable such heavily formalin-fixed materials to be studied by similar techniques in the future.

RENAL CELL CARCINOMA

Several research groups have studied DNA ploidy patterns of freshly excised renal cell carcinomas and have found a correlation between ploidy pattern, tumor grade, and tumor stage.[21-26] Otto et al[24] reported 68 patients followed for 1 to 4 years. Thirty-three tumors were DNA diploid and 35 tumors were DNA aneuploid; 21 percent of the DNA diploid tumors and 89 percent of the DNA aneuploid tumors metastasized during the study period. Also investigating fresh renal cell carcinoma tissue studied by FCM, Ljungberg and colleagues[26] prospectively studied 23 patients with metastatic renal cell carcinoma. Although follow-up was limited, 9 of 10 patients with DNA diploid primary tumors were alive compared to only 1 of 13 patients with a DNA aneuploid tumor cell stem line.

Use of Hedley's method to study archival paraffin-embedded tissue blocks has enabled our research group to make fairly extensive studies of renal cell carcinoma. In one investigation, 206 well-differentiated pure clear cell renal carcinoma specimens were analyzed for a group of patients with a minimum clinical follow-up of 7 years postnephrectomy.[14] As expected, tumor nuclear DNA ploidy patterns correlated significantly with tumor histologic grade and tumor pathologic stage. Most important, tumors with abnormal DNA histograms, either DNA tetraploid or DNA aneuploid, had a significantly higher rate of tumor progression and a decreased rate of patient survival, independent of stage and grade. Even though well-differentiated clear cell renal carcinomas as a group have a relatively good prognosis,

10-year survival for patients with tumors with a diploid/normal DNA pattern was 62 percent; for patients with tumors with an abnormal DNA pattern, 10-year survival was only 37 percent, a difference which was highly statistically significant. Moreover, even those patients with well-differentiated clear cell carcinoma who developed metastatic disease and who had a normal DNA pattern in the primary tumor did better than those patients with metastatic disease with an abnormal ploidy pattern in the primary renal tumor. In the group of patients evaluated, 3-year survival after development of metastatic disease was 41 percent for patients with a normal DNA pattern in the primary tumor but only 16 percent for patients with an abnormal DNA histogram pattern.

Other investigators have demonstrated that the measured DNA ploidy pattern occasionally can vary throughout the bulk of a large tumor such as a renal cell carcinoma.[27] They have stressed that multiple samples need to be studied in order to obtain the highest probability of detecting an abnormal ploidy pattern. Since multiple sampling methodology could not be applied in a retrospective study in which we were limited to tissue samples retained in the pathology archives as paraffin-embedded blocks, it seems quite likely that the prognostic use of DNA ploidy analysis for clear cell renal cancer will be further enchanced when multiple areas of tumors are studied in the future in order to yield a higher probability of picking up abnormal ploidy patterns.

Well-differentiated oncocytic renal tumors or renal oncocytomas also have been studied by Hedley's flow cytometric methodology. Eble and Sledge[28,29] found that in a relatively small tumor sample, all of their renal oncocytomas showed typical DNA normal diploid patterns. Our Mayo group restudied the tissue blocks from a large cohort of patients with well-differentiated oncocytic renal tumors which had previously been reported from this institution.[30] Fifty-one typical (grade I) renal oncocytomas and 21 grade II oncocytic renal cancers were analyzed.[31] In the Mayo group, only 50 percent of typical renal oncocytomas had a normal DNA ploidy pattern; 39 percent were classified as DNA tetraploid, and 11 percent as DNA aneuploid. Among the grade II oncocytic renal tumors, 33 percent had a DNA normal pattern, 43 percent were classified as DNA tetraploid, and 24 percent as DNA aneuploid. Despite the common occurrence of abnormal ploidy patterns, however, almost all of the patients with well-differentiated oncocytic renal tumors did well, never developed metastatic cancer, and never died from their tumor.

These results found for two relatively common types of renal neoplasm highlight two features which we have found in a number of other urologic and nonurologic tumor types we have studied to date in our laboratory. First, tumor classes such as renal oncocytoma or gastric or uterine leiomyoma, which are routinely considered to be benign tumors, can have detected a low percentage of abnormal DNA ploidy patterns, usually DNA tetraploid but occasionally DNA aneuploid. Such "abnormal ploidy pattern" histologically benign tumors continue to show benign biologic/clinical behavior. Thus, FCM DNA aneuploid and DNA tetraploid patterns *are not* invariable markers of neoplastic malignancy and cannot easily be used to diagnose malignancy "by machine." Conversely, many individual tumors which show typical standard malignant behavior with local invasion, metastases, and subsequent patient tumor death have DNA diploid or normal patterns. Tumors with DNA diploid patterns individually can be just as aggressive as tumors with abnormal ploidy patterns. *In the aggregate, however, generalizing across a variety of histologic tumor types, malignant tumors with a DNA diploid or normal pattern are much less aggressive than tumors with either a DNA tetraploid or DNA aneuploid pattern.*

Finally, most important, each individual histologic tumor type must be analyzed separately and generalizations about tumor behavior and ploidy pattern cannot be routinely lifted from one human tumor system to another. For example, in a study of carcinoid tumors of the small intestine analyzed in this laboratory by Tsushima et al (unpublished data), although the vast majority of the tumors had metastasized to the regional lymph nodes or liver, almost all of the tumors had a DNA ploidy pattern which was DNA diploid/normal. Such a finding deviates sharply from that found with renal oncocytoma and grade II renal oncocytic tumors,[31] wherein a high incidence of DNA tetraploid and DNA aneuploid patterns were measured but where patients almost invariably had a good prognosis with no evidence of malignant tumor behavior.

WILMS' TUMOR

Since Wilms' tumor is relatively rare in any single medical institution, ploidy analysis of Wilms' tumor has been little studied previously. Tanaka et al[32] presented results of a static cytofluorometric analysis of eight Wilms' tumor specimens. One tumor was DNA diploid while seven tumors were DNA nondiploid. No correlation between the ploidy pattern and patient survival was seen.

Schmidt et al described 59 cases of Wilms' tumor and related pediatric renal neoplasms studied by Hedley's method recently.[33] This group found that the presence of abnormal ploidy patterns correlated with previous prognosis-related groupings. In the Mayo Urology Research Laboratory using paraffin-embedded archival specimens, Hedley technique flow cytometric ploidy analysis was carried out on 56 Wilms' tumor specimens.[34] In the pre-1960 prechemotherapy era, nine patients studied had a 33 percent 5-year survival rate. No correlation between DNA ploidy pattern and survival was found. In the modern adjuvant chemotherapy era, however, nuclear DNA ploidy patterns correlated significantly with patient prognosis. Twenty-eight percent of Mayo Wilms' tumors had a normal DNA pattern, 23 percent had DNA aneuploid peaks, and 49 percent had DNA tetraploid patterns. Patients with DNA diploid and DNA aneuploid tumors for all pathologic stages had 5-year survival rates of 100 percent. Only patients with tumors with DNA tetraploid patterns died of Wilms' tumor in this series. Furthermore, patients with high stage, i.e., stage III or IV, Wilms' tumors with a DNA tetraploid pattern had a 2-year survival rate of just 25 percent. Thus, nuclear DNA ploidy analysis identifies a Wilms' tumor patient group who are at high risk for treatment failure in the current chemotherapy era. Moreover, no correlation was seen between ploidy pattern and Wilms' tumor histology in the group studied at Mayo. Confirmatory studies of these single institution findings in a larger multi-institutional series of Wilms' tumors must be performed. If DNA ploidy analysis can identify a group of Wilms' tumor patients at risk of treatment failure, however, treatment modification would be strongly indicated for these currently poor prognosis patients.

TRANSITIONAL CELL CARCINOMA OF THE RENAL PELVIS

Fresh samples of transitional cell carcinoma of the renal pelvis had not been extensively studied by FCM before the availability of Hedley's methodology. We have recently completed study of 111 samples of transitional cell carcinoma of the renal pelvis which were surgically removed between 1960 and 1975.[35] As has been found for transitional cell carcinoma arising in other sites, particularly the urinary bladder, a good correlation was found between DNA ploidy patterns, histologic grade, tumor stage, and clinical outcome. For grade I tumors (n = 28), there were no DNA aneuploid patterns measured and no patients died of metastatic transitional cell carcinoma. By contrast, 30 of 31 patients with grades III and IV tumors had an abnormal DNA pattern (DNA tetraploid or DNA aneuploid) and 26 (84 percent) died of metastatic transitional cell carcinoma. Most important, for grade II transitional cell carcinomas of the renal pelvis, all patients with tumors with a DNA aneuploid pattern (n = 6) died; this was significantly worse than the survival found for patients with DNA diploid or DNA tetraploid patterns. DNA ploidy analysis identified a special prognostically aggressive group of grade II tumors which were not detectable by light microscopy.

SQUAMOUS CELL CARCINOMA OF THE MALE URETHRA

As noted previously, the ability to analyze tumor ploidy patterns from archival material enables one to study relatively rare tumors in an efficient and useful manner. Tumors such as squamous cell carcinoma of the male urethra are extremely rare even in a large cancer center. It would be difficult to study such a tumor in a systematic way prospectively over many years. With Hedley's methodology, however, we were able to study a group of 30 primary male squamous cell urethral carcinomas resected at the Mayo Clinic between 1950 and 1980.[36] Among many tumor types studied, the association of DNA ploidy patterns with tumor behavior and prognosis is as striking for this group as for any tumor type studied so far. Bulbomembranous urethral tumors had a much higher incidence of abnormal DNA ploidy patterns than penile urethral tumors, 69 and 29 percent respectively. Eighteen percent of tumors exhibiting a DNA diploid pattern and 93 percent of tumors with an abnormal DNA histogram showed subsequent tumor progression ($p < 0.001$). Indeed, none of the grade I or II tumors with a DNA diploid pattern developed local recurrences or distant metastases during the period of clinical observation, whereas 90 percent of the low grade tumors with an abnormal DNA pattern eventually progressed. Patients with tumors with DNA diploid ploidy had a 5- and 10-year disease-free survival rate of 85 percent. In contrast, patients with tumors with abnormal DNA ploidy patterns had 5- and 10-year disease-free survival rates of 20 and 0 percent respectively. Beyond doubt, determination of DNA ploidy patterns by FCM does provide important prognostic information for patients with very rare primary squamous cell carcinoma of the male urethra.

TRANSITIONAL CELL CARCINOMA OF THE BLADDER

Because fresh and monodispersed samples of bladder cancer cells have been easy to obtain clinically, nuclear DNA ploidy analysis by FCM of bladder neoplasms has been extensively investigated during the past decade.[37–39] Indeed, even comparisons of flow cytometric ploidy analysis and cytogenetics for certain bladder cancers already have been reported. Abnormal DNA ploidy patterns correlated well with abnormal chromosome counts and the degree of malignancy.[40,41] Comparison of standard cytologic and flow cytometric analysis of bladder washings found the flow cytometric method to be a more sensitive measure of important malignant abnormalities than conventional visual cytology.[42–44] In combination, both were quite valuable in the conventional cytologic and FCM follow-up of patients with transitional cell carcinoma of the bladder.[45] Certain patients with cytoscopically normal appearing bladder mucosa were found to have abnormal DNA stem lines by FCM analysis; this finding correlated with subsequent histologic examination of random biopsy tissues.[42,43]

In a more global perspective, results of nuclear DNA flow cytometric ploidy analysis of transitional cell carcinoma of the bladder have been shown to correlate well with both tumor grade and tumor stage.[46–48] Grade I tumors tend to be DNA diploid. DNA tetraploid and DNA aneuploid tumors are associated with higher tumor grade and stage. For tumors with abnormal DNA stem lines, DNA tetraploid tumors tend to exhibit less malignant characteristics compared to DNA aneuploid tumors. Muscle invasive tumors often show more than one abnormal DNA aneuploid peak. Similar findings were noted in high grade primary transitional cell carcinoma in situ of the bladder urothelium.[49] Moreover, abnormal nuclear DNA patterns correlated significantly with tumor progression. In patients with superficial bladder cancer determined to have DNA diploid patterns, no patients showed tumor progression with a mean follow-up of 2.6 years. In contrast, 35 percent (19 of 54 patients) with an abnormal DNA ploidy pattern demonstrated tumor progression; 58 percent of patients with tumor progression died. Approximately 50 percent of the tumors showing tumor progression were DNA aneuploid whereas only 10 percent were DNA tetraploid. For 20 patients with primary carcinoma in situ of the bladder, all patients exhibited at least one abnormal DNA stem line when studied by FCM.[49] Seven patients (35 percent) showed disease progression within 2 years. All of these patients had had specimens with more than one abnormal DNA ploidy pattern.

The above highly significant FCM results with transitional cell carcinoma of the urinary bladder were obtained with fresh tumor samples. Since this urologic tumor has been so extensively studied previously using fresh tissue, we have put our laboratory emphasis on other tumor types rather than bladder carcinoma. Using the Hedley technique, however, one study of transitional cell carcinoma of the urinary bladder has been carried out at Mayo. This was a project to see if ploidy patterns of superficial papillary tumors could accurately forecast subsequent development of muscle invasive bladder cancer. Sixty-four superficial papillary (pTA and pT1) bladder carcinomas were analyzed by the Hedley methodology.[50] DNA histograms of these 64 tumors were classified as follows: 45 had a normal DNA pattern, 13 showed a DNA tetraploid pattern, and 6 of the tumors exhibited a DNA aneuploid pattern. Eighty percent of 50 grade I or II tumors but only 36 percent of 14 grade III tumors had a normal DNA pattern. After more than 2 years follow-up, *none of the 45 patients* with a DNA diploid or normal tumor pattern developed a muscle invasive tumor. By contrast, 58 percent (19 patients) with abnormal DNA ploidy patterns subsequently developed a $\geq$ pT2 tumor. Postresection recurrence occurred in 36 percent of patients with DNA normal tumors and 68 percent of patients with DNA ploidy abnormal tumors. Thus, in our experiences, flow cytometric DNA ploidy measurement of nuclei isolated from formalin-fixed paraffin-embedded superficial papillary bladder tumors seems to provide a convenient and important parameter to characterize the subsequent behavior of transitional cell carcinomas of the urinary bladder.

ADENOCARCINOMA OF THE PROSTATE

Although adenocarcinoma of the prostate is the most prevalent urologic malignancy in the United States, only a small number of such prostate carcinoma tumor samples have been studied by flow cytometric methods. Almost all reported methods have used fresh tumor samples. Indeed more than a decade has passed since Bichel et al, in 1977, described the use of FCM analysis of transrectal fine needle prostate aspirates to characterize prostate carcinoma.[51] Their investigations, since confirmed by others,[52,53] demonstrated that the presence of abnormal DNA ploidy patterns, both DNA tetraploid and DNA aneuploid, correlated with increasing histologic anaplasia of the prostate tumors studied. Poorly differentiated prostate carcinomas had almost exclusively abnormal DNA patterns. Moderately differentiated tumors had a mixture of patterns with some tumors being DNA diploid while other tumor specimens were DNA aneuploid or DNA tetraploid. Pontes and colleagues performed FCM analysis on 33 radical prostatectomy specimens.[54] Nuclear DNA ploidy analysis combined with Gleason's score was found to improve predictive value of the histologic grading in high stage lesions. Benson et al studied prostatic tumor cell heterogeneity using multiparameter flow cytometric analysis.[55,56] Both perpendicular and forward light scattering measuring relative internal cell structure and cell size were incorporated into these measurements.

Using paraffin-embedded archival material to perform FCM analysis, Fordham et al recently reported data on 70 patients with prostate adenocarcinoma with up to a 12-year follow-up.[57] These authors found that the prognosis for patients with DNA aneuploid tumors was significantly worse than for patients with DNA diploid tumors. When the results of DNA ploidy analysis were combined with the Gleason scores from histologic grading, it was thought possible to detect which patients would die from their prostate cancers.

Studies of prostate carcinoma from our Mayo laboratory have been somewhat limited to date. Significant results are now available on a group of 121 patients with stage D1 carcinoma of the prostate treated by radical prostatectomy and bilateral pelvic lymphadenectomy with a follow-up of a minimum of 5 years.[58] For this group of patients with metastatic deposits in the pelvic lymph nodes, measured ploidy pattern had a very significant association with the subsequent course of malignant disease. Overall, patients with DNA diploid pattern tumors had a very low chance of showing progressive disease, 7 percent at 5 years. By contrast, patients with either DNA tetraploid or DNA aneuploid pattern prostate tumor showed a 73 percent disease progression rate at 5 years. These differences were highly statistically significant at the $p < 0.0001$ level. Even more dramatic, for those patients with stage D1 prostate cancer with a DNA diploid pattern who underwent early hormonal treatment, *none (0 percent)* showed evidence of disease progression at 5 years. In contrast, the group of patients with D1 prostate cancer *and* an abnormal ploidy pattern who did not undergo early endocrine therapy showed disease progression by 5 years in 93 percent of cases.

These preliminary data from other laboratories and our own suggest that flow cytometric DNA ploidy analysis will come to have an important management role for patients with carcinoma of the prostate. Indeed, adenocarcinoma of the prostate, just like adenocarcinoma of the rectum, in which the vast majority of patients have intermediate grade tumors, is the class of clinical tumor problems for which flow cytometric ploidy analysis is most likely to make an important contribution to patient management. For tumor types in which a wide variety of histologic grades are seen, e.g., transitional cell carcinomas of the urinary tract, such a good correlation is seen between DNA ploidy pattern and tumor grading that the independent contribution of DNA ploidy analysis to patient prognosis is usually not strongly significant. When almost all tumor samples of a given histologic type are of intermediate histologic grade, FCM ploidy analysis has the potential to become a much more important independent variable of prognosis.

ADRENAL TUMORS

Tumors of the adrenal gland, both adrenocortical tumors and pheochromocytomas arising from the adrenal medulla, are also quite rare tumors. Flow cytometric ploidy studies of these tumors have been rarely reported. Neoplasms of endocrine tissue origin, however, are notoriously difficult to categorize by light microscopy and this has seemed a very promising area in which to apply flow cytometric ploidy analysis. Klein et al[59,60] reported five adrenal cortical carcinomas, all of which were found to have a DNA aneuploid stem line. One pheochromocytoma was found to have a DNA tetraploid cell population. In a study using paraffin-embedded archival material, Bowlby et al[61] described results of six adrenal cortical carcinomas investigated. For these tumors, 83 percent were DNA aneuploid and 50 percent subsequently died of disease with a follow-up of 1 to 96 months. All of 16 adrenal cortical adenomas studied were DNA diploid.

In the Urology Research Laboratory at the Mayo Clinic, the Hedley methodology has been used to study a series of adrenal pheochromocytomas, aldosteronomas arising from the adrenal cortex, and adrenal cortical carcinomas. Seventy-five adrenal pheochromocytomas were studied by Hedley's technique.[62] Twenty-three tumors showed a normal DNA histogram, 31 showed a significant increase in the DNA tetraploid peak, and 21 showed a DNA aneuploid pattern. There were 62 pheochromocytoma patients who had a minimum of 10 years of clinical follow-up. *All* of the 18 patients in this group with a diploid/normal DNA histogram followed a benign clinical course. However, 31 percent of 26 patients with tumors classified as DNA tetraploid and 39 percent of the 18 patients having a DNA aneuploid tumor had evidence of malignancy. These two groups had significantly more malignant tumors ($p < 0.05$, $p < 0.02$, respectively) than the normal DNA group. Thus, FCM DNA ploidy measurements provide very useful prognostic information for patients with pheochromocytomas.

We investigated a group of adrenal aldosteronomas made up of 20 benign and 6 malignant primary aldosteronomas.[63] Eighty-five percent of benign aldosteronomas had a normal DNA histogram, 10 percent had a DNA tetraploid pattern, and 5 percent had a DNA aneuploid pattern. The three benign aldosteronomas with abnormal DNA histograms with a follow-up of from 12 to 20 years, were significantly larger than the tumors with normal DNA histograms. All six primary malignant aldosteronomas were found to have abnormal DNA histograms with 50 percent DNA tetraploid and 50 percent DNA aneuploid. No patients with tumors with DNA tetraploid patterns died of disease with a follow-up of from 1 to 28 years. Two patients with tumors with DNA aneuploid stem lines died of metastatic adrenal cortical carcinoma while one is alive without evidence of disease 21 years postoperatively.

A group of 52 adrenal cortical carcinomas was also intensively studied in our laboratory using the Hedley technique.[64] For these rare, highly malignant adrenal tumors, 17 percent had a normal DNA pattern, 25 percent showed a DNA tetraploid pattern, and 58 percent of tumors showed DNA aneuploid patterns. Among the DNA aneuploid patterns, 18 percent of tumors had typical one abnormal stem line histograms and 12 tumors showed at least two stem lines of abnormal DNA pattern cells. For low stage adrenal cortical carcinomas resected completely, the 5-year disease-free survivals of patients with DNA normal and DNA tetraploid tumors were 67 and 25 percent, respectively. For patients with one stem line and two stem line DNA aneuploid tumors, the 5-year survival rates were 60 and 0 percent. For high stage tumors that were unable to be completely removed surgically, survival experience was not significantly associated with DNA ploidy pattern. Although adrenal cortical carcinoma is generally a markedly aggressive neoplasm with poor prognosis, nuclear DNA ploidy patterns do identify certain groups of patients with this malignancy with relatively favorable prognoses.

CONCLUSION AND FUTURE DIRECTIONS

Because analysis of archival tumor samples enables investigators to look back to a group of tumors and their hosts treated many years ago, the association of DNA ploidy pattern measured by the Hedley technique with tumor behavior and patient prognosis has become established in a very short time. The results found are conceptually different from those determined in standard prospective clinical trials of malignancy. In the studies carried out in our laboratory, patients selected for study have had a minimum of 5 years of postresection follow-up to allow for tumor behavior to become manifest. Many patients have had 10 to 20 years of clinical follow-up. Because of this uniquely powerful chronologic feature of such archival studies, one can state with confidence that flow cytometric ploidy analysis of tumor tissues will without doubt and very quickly come to be an important tool in the day-to-day clinical management of patients with a variety of genitourinary cancers including the variety of renal parenchymal tumors, adrenal tumors, urothelial tumors, and prostate carcinomas; this conclusion is based only on the early studies which have been performed so far.

The use of FCM to study archival tumor specimens is truly in its infancy. At present, only nuclear DNA content has been extensively measured in genitourinary tumors. It is already apparent that numerous other tumor parameters can be measured on the nuclei extracted from archival samples by the Hedley technique. Using monoclonal antibody techniques, the content of oncogene products such as the c-myc oncogene[65] and other internuclear antigens can be quantitated by FCM at the same time that nuclear DNA content is being measured. Many additional uses for old (nonfresh) tumor nuclei will be found in the future as quantitative pathologists and other investigators begin to explore what must be a very rich motherlode of prognostic variables for genitourinary and other human malignancies. One can already state with considerable confidence that the study of formalin-fixed paraffin-embedded tumor tissues is already important and will go on to increasing levels of sophistication, just as the scientific investigation of Egyptian mummies has advanced considerably over the past several centuries.

With the demonstrated success of flow cytometric ploidy analysis on old tumor samples, and the strong association found between ploidy pattern and tumor behavior, increasing attention can be turned again to the use of this methodology to study fresh tumor cells. For fresh cells with their cell membranes and proteins intact, many types of cell surface and cytoplasmic antigens identified by monoclonal antibody technique can be quantitated by FCM.[66] In addition, detailed parameters of the cell cycle can be investigated in fresh living cells through techniques such as BrDU labeling and monoclonal staining for BrDU-labeled DNA.[67,68] Flow cytometric studies of *both fixed and fresh* tumor specimens are certain to be significant investigative tools in the future.

Because the Hedley ploidy analysis technique can be performed on tumor tissues formalin fixed and paraffin-embedded for routine light microscopy, a rapid transfer of this particular technique from the medical center research laboratory into routine clinical urologic practice must be expected in 1988.

REFERENCES

1. Hedley DW, Friedlander ML, Taylor IW, et al: Method for analysis of cellular DNA content of paraffin-embedded pathological material using flow cytometry. J Histochem Cytochem 31:1333, 1983
2. Hedley DW, Rugg CA, Ng ABP, Taylor IW: Influence of cellular DNA content

on disease-free survival of stage II breast cancer patients. Cancer Res 44:5395, 1984

3. Friedlander ML, Hedley DW, Taylor IW, et al: Influence of cellular DNA content on survival in advanced ovarian cancer. Cancer Res 44:397, 1984
4. Hedley DW, Friedlander ML, Taylor, IA: Application of DNA flow cytometry to paraffin-embedded archival material for the study of aneuploidy and its clinical significance. Cytometry 6:327, 1985
5. Caspersson TO: Cell Growth and Cell Function. New York, Norton, 1950
6. Friedman HP Jr: The use of ultraviolet light and fluorescent dyes in the detection of uterine cancer by vaginal smear. Am J Obstet Gynecol 59:852, 1950
7. Mellors RC, Silver R: A microfluorometric scanner for the differential detection of cells: Application to exfoliative cytology. Science 114:356, 1951
8. Crosland-Taylor PJ: A device for counting small particles suspended in fluid through a tube. Nature 171:37, 1953
9. Coulter WH: High speed automatic blood cell counter and cell size analyzer. Proc Natl Electronics Conf 12:1034, 1956
10. Culett HR, Bonner WA, Barrett J, et al: Automated separation of mammalian cells as a function of intracellular fluorescence. Science 166:747, 1969
11. Van Dilla MA, Trujillo TT, Mullaney DF, et al: Cell microfluorometry: A method for rapid fluorescence measurement. Science 163:1213, 1969
12. Shapiro HM, Schildkraut ER, Curbelo R, et al: Cytomat-R: A computer-controlled multiple laser source multiparameter flow cytophotometer system. J Histochem Cytochem 25:836, 1977
13. Shapiro HM: Practical Flow Cytometry. New York, Alan R. Liss, 1985
14. Rainwater LM, Hosaka Y, Farrow GM, Lieber, MM: Well-differentiated clear cell renal carcinoma: Significance of nuclear deoxyribonucleic acid patterns studied by flow cytometry. J Urol 137:15, 1987
15. Vindelv LL: Flow microfluorometric analysis of nuclear DNA in cells from solid tumors and cell suspension: A new method for rapid isolation and staining of nuclei. Virch Arch B Cell Pathol 24:227, 1977
16. Vindelv LL, Christensen IJ, Nissen NI: A detergent-trypsin method for the preparation of nuclei for flow cytometric DNA analysis. Cytometry 3:323, 1983
17. Dean PN, Jett JH: Mathematical analysis of DNA distributions derived from flow microfluorometry. J Cell Biol 60:523, 1974
18. Hiddemann W, Schumann J, Andreef M, et al: Convention on nomenclature for DNA cytometry. Cancer Genet Cytogenet 13:181, 1984
19. Schutte B, Reynders MMJ, Bosman FT, Blijham GH: Flow cytometric determination of DNA ploidy level in nuclei isolated from paraffin-embedded tissue. Cytometry 6:26, 1985
20. Hedley DW, Friedlander ML, Taylor IW, et al: DNA flow cytometry of paraffin-embedded tissue (letter to the editor). Cytometry 5:660, 1984
21. Linden WA, Kollerman M, Konig K: Flow cytometric and autoradiographic studies of human kidney carcinomas surgically removed after preirradiation. Br J Cancer 41 (suppl IV):177, 1980
22. Baisch H, Otto U, Konig K, et al: DNA content of human kidney carcinoma cells in relation to histological grading. Br J Cancer 45:878, 1982
23. Bennington JL, Mayall BH: DNA Cytometry on four-micrometer sections of paraffin-embedded human adrenocarcinomas and adenomas. Cytometry 4:31, 1983

24. Otto U, Baisch H, Huland H, Kloppel G: Tumor cell deoxyribonucleic acid content and prognosis in renal cell carcinoma. J Urol 132:237, 1984
25. Chin JL, Pontes JE, Frankfurt OS: Flow cytometric deoxyribonucleic acid analysis of primary metastatic human renal cell carcinomas. J Urol 133:582, 1985
26. Ljungberg B, Stenling R, Roos G: Prognostic value of deoxyribonucleic acid content in metastatic renal cell carcinoma. J Urol 136:801, 1986
27. Ljungberg B, Stenling R, Roos G: DNA content in renal cell carcinoma with reference to tumor heterogeneity. Cancer 56:503, 1985
28. Eble JN, Sledge G: Euploidy of renal oncocytomas: Analysis of cellular DNA content using flow cytometry. Lab Invest 51:20A, 1985
29. Eble JN, Sledge G: Cellular deoxyribonucleic acid content of renal oncocytomas: Flow cytometric analysis of paraffin-embedded tissues from eight tumors. J Urol 136:522, 1986
30. Lieber MM, Tomera KM, Farrow GM: Renal oncocytoma. J Urol 125:481, 1981
31. Rainwater LM, Farrow GM, Lieber MM: Flow cytometry of renal oncocytoma: Common occurrence of deoxyribonucleic acid polyploidy and aneuploidy. J Urol 135:1167, 1986
32. Tanaka T, Takamatsu T, Sawada T, et al: DNA contents in Wilms' tumor: A cytofluorometric study. Cancer 52:1269, 1983
33. Schmidt D, Wiedemann B, Keil W, et al: Flow cytometric analysis of nephroblastomas and related neoplasms. Cancer 58:2494, 1986
34. Rainwater LM, Hosaka Y, Farrow GM, et al: Wilms' tumor: Relationship of nuclear DNA ploidy to patient survival. J Urol (in press)
35. Blute ML, Tsushima K, Farrow GM, Lieber MM: Transitional cell carcinoma of the renal pelvis: Nuclear DNA ploidy by flow cytometry. J Urol (in press)
36. Winkler HZ, Lieber MM: Squamous cell carcinoma of the male urethra: Nuclear DNA ploidy studied by flow cytometry. J Urol (in press)
37. Tribukait B, Moberger G, Zetterberg A: Methodological aspects of rapid flow cytofluorometry for DNA analysis of human urinary bladder cells. In Pulse-Cytophotometry, part 1. Ghent, Belgium, European Press, Medicon, 1975
38. Tribukait B, Esposti PL: Comparative cytofluorometric studies in non-neoplastic and neoplastic human urothelium. Second International Symposium on Pulse Cytophotometry. Ghent, Belgium, European Press, Medicon, 1976
39. Melamed MR: Flow cytometry of the urinary bladder. In Zincke H (ed): Urologic Clinics of North America, vol 11. Philadelphia, Saunders, 1984
40. Coon JS, Schwartz D, Summers JL, et al: Flow cytometric analysis of deparaffinized nuclei in urinary bladder carcinoma: Comparison with cytogenetic analysis. Cancer 57:1594, 1986
41. Wijkstrom H, Granberg-Ohman I, Tribukait B: Chromosomal and DNA patterns in transitional cell bladder carcinoma: A comparative cytogenetic and flow-cytofluorometric DNA study. Cancer 53:1718, 1984
42. DeVonec M, Darzynkiewicz Z, Kostyrka-Claps ML, et al: Flow cytometry of low stage bladder tumors: Correlation with cytologic and cystoscopic diagnosis. Cancer 49:109, 1982
43. Fausund T, Laerum OD, Hostmark J: Ploidy distribution of normal-appearing bladder mucosa in patients with arothelial cancer: Relationship to morphology. J Urol 130:1076, 1983
44. Pritchett TR, Kanzler AW, Nichols PW, et al: A simple and practical technique

for detecting cancer cells in urine and urinary bladder washings by flow cytometry. Am J Clin Pathol 84:191, 1985

45. Murphy WM, Emerson LD, Chandler RW, et al: Flow cytometry versus urinary cytology in the evaluation of patients with bladder cancer. J Urol 136:815, 1986
46. Tribukait B, Gustafson H, Esposti PL: The significance of ploidy and proliferation in the clinical and biological evaluation of bladder tumors: A study of 100 untreated cases. Br J Urol 54:130, 1982
47. Gustafson H, Tribukait B, Esposti PL: DNA profile and tumor progression in patients with superficial bladder tumors. Urol Res 10:13, 1982
48. Gustafson H, Tribukait B: Characterization of bladder carcinomas by flow DNA analysis. Eur Urol 11:410, 1985
49. Gustafson H, Tribukait B, Esposti PL: The prognostic value of DNA analysis in primary carcinoma in situ of the urinary bladder. Scand J Urol Nephrol 16:141, 1982
50. Hosaka Y, Kakizoe T: Superficial papillary bladder carcinoma: Nuclear DNA ploidy studied by flow cytometry. J Urol (in press)
51. Bichel P, Frederiksen P, Kjaer T, et al: Flow microfluorometry and transrectal fine-needle biopsy in the classification of human prostate carcinoma. Cancer 40:1206, 1977
52. Tribukait B, Esposti PL, Ronstrom L: Tumour ploidy for characterization of prostatic carcinoma: Flow-cytoflurometric DNA studies using aspiration biopsy material. Scand J Urol Nephrol 55 (suppl):59, 1980
53. Roters M, Laemmel A, Kastendieck H, Becker H: DNA distribution pattern of prostatic lesions measured by flow cytometry. Acta Pathol Microbiol Scand [A] 274 (suppl):431, 1984
54. Pontes JE, Wajsman Z, Huben RP, et al: Prognostic factors in localized prostatic carcinomas. J Urol 134:1137, 1985
55. Benson MC, McDougal DC, Coffey DS: The use of multiparameter flow cytometry to assess tumor heterogeneity and grade prostate cancer. Prostate 5:27, 1984
56. Benson MC, Walsh PC: The application of flow cytometry to the assessment of tumor cell heterogeneity and the grading of human prostatic cancer: Preliminary results. J Urol 135:1194, 1986
57. Fordham MVP, Burdge AH, Matthews J, et al: Prostatic carcinoma cell DNA content measured by flow cytometry and its relation to clinical. Br J Surg 73:400, 1986
58. Winkler H, Rainwater LM, Myers RP, et al: Stage D1 prostatic adenocarcinoma: Significance of nuclear deoxyribonucleic acid ploidy studied by flow cytometry. Mayo Clin Proc (in press)
59. Klein FA, Kay S, Ratliff JE, et al: Flow cytometric determinations of ploidy and proliferation patterns of adrenal neoplasms: An adjunct to histological classification. J Urol 134:862, 1985
60. Klein FA, Miller NL, Hacklar RH: Flow cytometry in feminizing adrenocortical carcinoma. J Urol 134:933, 1985
61. Bowlby LS, Debault LE, Abraham SR: Flow cytometric analysis of adrenal cortical tumor DNA: Relationship between cellular DNA and histopathologic classification. Cancer 58:1499, 1986
62. Hosaka Y, Rainwater LM, Grant CS, et al: Pheochromocytoma: Nuclear deoxyribonucleic acid patterns studied by flow cytometry. Surgery 100:1003, 1986

63. Rainwater LM, Young WF Jr, Farrow GM, et al: Benign and malignant aldosterone-producing adrenal neoplasms: Flow cytometric analysis of DNA ploidy. J Urol (in press)
64. Hosaka Y, Rainwater LM, Young WF Jr, et al: Adrenal cortical carcinoma: Nuclear DNA ploidy studied by flow cytometry. Surgery (in press)
65. Watson JV, Evan G, Ritson A, et al: The clinical significance of flow cytometric c-myc oncoprotein quantitation in testicular cancer. Br J Cancer 53:331, 1986
66. Van NT, Raber M, Barrows GH, et al: Estrogen receptor analysis by flow cytometry. Science 224:876, 1984
67. Gratzner HG: Monoclonal antibody to 5-bromo and 5-iododeoxyuridine: A new reagent for detection of DNA replication. Science 218:747, 1982
68. Gonchoroff NJ, Greipp PR, Kyle RA, Katzmann JA: A monoclonal antibody reactive with 5-bromo-2-deoxyuridine that does not require DNA denaturation. Cytometry 6:506, 1985

Luteinizing Hormone-Releasing Hormone Analogues in the Treatment of Metastatic Prostate Cancer
An Alternative to Orchiectomy?

Leroy M. Nyberg, Jr.

INCREASING INCIDENCE OF PROSTATE CANCER IN THE AGING POPULATION

Prostate cancer is forecast to be the second most common cause of cancer deaths in all males in 1988.[1] It has been estimated that there will be 90,000 newly diagnosed cases of prostate cancer in 1988 making it second only in incidence to lung cancer. The relative 5-year survival rates for all cases of prostate cancer have improved from 50 percent for white males in 1963 to 72 percent in 1977 through 1982 and from 35 percent for black males in 1963 to 62 percent in 1977 through 1982. Since the treatment of metastatic prostate cancer has not changed significantly during that time interval, it must be assumed that the improved survival rate reflects an improvement in the treatment of localized prostate cancer and an increasing number of prostate cancer cases being diagnosed at a stage amenable to cure.

A more sobering view of the incidence of prostate cancer is given when one realizes that 81 percent of all prostate cancer cases occur in men aged 65 years and older and that the prostate is the leading site of cancer for males in that age group.[2] This incidence increases rapidly past age 65. The majority of these newly diagnosed patients have advanced prostate cancer at the time of presentation.[3] Statistically, 40 percent of these patients with metastatic disease may live for at least 5 years. Thus, as the over 65 aged population continues to increase, the numbers of patients with metastatic prostate cancer will increase. Urologists must care for this increasing patient population and must evaluate and prescribe the best therapy for these patients.

HORMONAL THERAPY

The basis of hormonal treatment for metastatic prostate cancer originated more than 45 years ago when the Nobel Prize winning research of Huggins and Hodges reported the partial androgen dependence of most prostatic cancers.[4] They demonstrated that the majority of patients with metastatic prostate cancer underwent an objective and subjective remission of the disease, for variable lengths of time, after ablation of testicular androgens by either orchiectomy or oral estrogen administration. These findings prompted many clinical trials which have provided the data for comparison of the alternative forms of hormonal therapy of metastatic prostate cancer.

Orchiectomy Versus Estrogens

Orchiectomy and oral estrogens produce equally favorable responses in about 70 percent of prostate cancer patients.[5] The duration of response ranges from a few months to greater than 10 years and is extremely variable and unpredictable.[6] After orchiectomy, improvement in bone pain usually occurs within 1 to 5 days, and may be evident a few hours after surgery.[7] The response may take from 5 to 15 days with oral estrogen therapy. Objectively, an elevated serum acid phosphatase starts to fall within 1 week after castration and within 2 to 3 weeks after administration of estrogen. Although treatment after initial relapse with the alternate method of hormone therapy may produce occasional periods of renewed remission of disease, these remissions are brief and purely symptomatic. No objective signs of remission have been reported.[5] The survival of the hormonally treated patient, whatever the duration of response, is not any longer than that of the untreated individual.[8] Thus, orchiectomy and estrogen therapy provide equal relief of symptoms for an indeterminate length of time to the patient with metastatic cancer, but do not prolong life.

Side Effects. Both methods of treatment incur well-documented side effects, and these must be a major consideration in the selection of therapy. Castration is a surgical procedure which is psychologically repugnant to many men because of the thoughts of emasculation. This procedure can be made more acceptable by such tissue-sparing procedures as a subcapsular orchiectomy or a simple orchiectomy without epididymectomy or by the insertion of testicular prostheses. While the psychologic side effects of surgical castration depend on the individual, impotence, mild-to-moderate gynecomastia, and hot flashes are more nearly universal. Oral estrogens produce more severe forms of gynecomastia, breast tenderness, and hot flashes, in addition to increased risk for morbidity and mortality from cardiovascular and thromboembolic disorders.[9] The post-treatment level of serum androgens may vary with oral estrogens, especially if the patient is not diligent in compliance with his medication regimen, or if he has gastrointestinal disturbances. Orchiectomy, with the advantage of consistently depressed post-treatment androgen levels and less severe side effects, is the treatment of choice for the patient with metastatic prostate cancer. The psychologic effects of castration and surgery prevent many men from choosing this preferred treatment and many physicians from recommending it.

ALTERNATE METHODS OF HORMONAL THERAPY

Progestational Agents

Other methods of hormonal therapy, which deprive the prostate and its metastatic cells from the growth-supporting source of androgens, have been investigated. Megestrol acetate, a synthetic progestational agent, produced symptomatic results equivalent to orchiectomy and did not cause gynecomastia, thromboembolic events, or salt retention.[10] However, an escape of plasma testosterone to normal occurred after 6 months of therapy.

Antiandrogens

Antiandrogens have been developed which act by direct competition with androgens at the target organ. Cyproterone acetate is the antiandrogen which has been most extensively tested. A clinical remission of metastatic disease has been demonstrated to last up to 17 months in approximately 60 percent of the 26 patients treated.[11] Gynecomastia and other estrogenic side effects developed in 38 percent of the patients. Smith et al showed a symptomatic response lasting from 1 to 36 months in 19 of 28 patients previously treated with diethylstilbestrol (DES) or orchiectomy.[12] No side effects were noted. Jacobi et al, in a randomized trial comparing cyproterone acetate with estradiol undecylate, showed no basic difference in symptomatic response between the two forms of therapy.[13] However, gynecomastia and other estrogenic side effects were minimal with cyproterone, and impotence occurred in 19 of 21 patients.

Flutamide is a nonsteroidal antiandrogen without estrogenic or other hormonal side effects. A symptomatic remission of disease, lasting from 35 to 54 months, in 77 percent of the 72 patients studied has been reported.[14] The side effects of treatment were mild gynecomastia in most of the patients and impotence in 15 percent. It was concluded from these and other smaller studies, that there was no significant difference between orchiectomy, DES, and the antiandrogens in symptomatic response of prostate cancer.[15] Objective, evaluative, tumor responses to the antiandrogens have not been reported. The antiandrogenic agents have not been widely used nor have they been investigated in any extensive clinical trials in the United States.

NONHORMONAL METHODS OF THERAPY

A major factor in the lack of development of the antiandrogens for general clinical use is that they are expensive to produce and they have a limited clinical application, i.e, the treatment of patients with metastatic prostate cancer. Drugs which are developed for applications in addition to prostate cancer therapy project a financial advantage for the pharmaceutical firm.

Aminoglutethamide

One of these drugs is aminoglutethamide which is used to treat patients with Cushing's syndrome and other adrenal disorders. It inhibits all adrenal steroidogenesis. Palliation has been reported in five of six of the metastatic prostate cancer patients treated with aminoglutethamide as primary therapy,[16] and in three of seven hormone refractory patients treated.[17] Aminoglutethamide was not extensively investigated as a method of primary hormonal therapy because the side effects of hypotension, nausea and vomiting, lassitude and depression were intolerable and cortisone and fludrocortisone had to be administered simultaneously to replace the adrenal steroid depletion.

Spironolactone

Spironolactone is a drug with a broader clinical application. It is used for the treatment of aldosteronism, cirrhosis, heart disease, and as a potassium-sparing diuretic in hypertension. This drug inhibits the synthesis of androgens. In one study, a limited clinical remission in three of seven hormone refractory patients treated with spironolactone was obtained.[18] Hyperkalemia, however, could be a significant problem in these patients, especially if they have decreased renal function.

Ketoconazole

A more unique investigation has been conducted with ketoconazole which is used in the treatment of superficial and deep fungal infections. A side effect of its mechanism of action is the reduction of adrenal and testicular androgen production in both animals and humans.[19] In one study of 14 patients with previously untreated metastatic prostate cancer, a decrease in pain occurred in all the patients within 2 weeks of therapy with ketoconazole.[20] Most had a response within 3 days of treatment. Serum testosterone dropped from 17.7 to 1.4 nmol/L in the first 24 hours of treatment.[21] The side effects were decreased libido, impotence, and gynecomastia. At 3 months of therapy, mild addisonism resulted, necessitating the addition of prednisone each day to the therapy.

Thus, although numerous agents have been investigated as an alternative to orchiectomy and oral estrogens for treatment of metastatic prostate cancer, none could offer an inexpensive, low side effect, reliable, treatment alternative.

LUTEINIZING HORMONE-RELEASING HORMONE ANALOGUES

Nobel Prize winning research again led to a new approach to the treatment of metastatic prostate cancer. Andrew Schally and his group, in the early 1970s, isolated, elucidated the structure of, and synthesized luteinizing hormone-releasing hormone (LH-RH).[22,23] The LH-RH analogues initially aroused much investigative interest because of their potential for fertility control in human and veterinary medicine. They were primarily investigated as agents to induce ovulation in women with numerous gynecologic and hormonal disorders.[24] Because of its simple decapeptide structure, LH-RH was much easier to produce than the specific gonadotrophins which had been previously used for this purpose. Many superactive analogues of LH-RH were synthesized by simple amino acid substitution on the ten amino acid chain of the LH-RH molecule. By 1978, more than 700 analogues had been synthesized.[25] The reason for the synthesis of this great number of analogues is that all peptides, including LH-RH, have very transitory effects after injection. An attempt was therefore being made to synthesize analogues which had both an increased and a prolonged activity. Since the continuous administration of these superactive analogues or agonists had the paradoxical effect of inhibiting ovulation or spermatogenesis, they were investigated as potential long-acting female and male contraceptive agents.[26]

Paradoxical Response Initiates Anticancer Therapy

When these studies demonstrated that continuous administration of a superactive analogue of LH-RH markedly reduced the sex steroids in both sexes, the investigation of the treatment of hormonally responsive tumors was begun. LH-RH analogue treatment significantly reduced the weight of the Dunning rat prostate tumor and increased the cell doubling time of the tumor from 18 to 87 days.[27,28] The serum testosterone, LH, FSH, and prolactin, in experimental animals, were reduced to barely detectable levels whereas the serum progesterone remained elevated. Preliminary studies with superactive, long-acting analogues administered, either by multiple subcutaneous injections or intranasal spray, on ten patients with prostate cancer showed objective and subjective relief of disease in approximately 80 percent of the patients.[29] These early studies initiated many clinical trials because a pharmacologic agent, with many clinical applications, had been synthesized which suppressed prostate tumor growth and serum androgen levels equivalent to those with orchiectomy.

Importance of the Mechanism of Action

Studies on the mechanism of action of LH-RH and its analogues demonstrated that the pattern of delivery was important.[30] Intermittent administration, at the physiologic frequency of gonadotropin release, stimulated pituitary gonadotropin release. Constant infusion of the analogue, paradoxically, suppressed LH and follicle-stimulating hormone (FSH) release. Thus, when the mode of delivery was being evaluated, a method which could sustain the most constant infusion of LH-RH analogue would provide the best LH and FSH suppression. The site and mechanism of action was postulated to be by "down regulation" of the LH-RH receptors of the pituitary.[31] Studies with hypophysectomized rats suggested a direct suppressive action of the LH-RH analogues on the testicular Leydig cells.[32,33] This direct action on the testes has not been demonstrated in men and studies correlating LH and FSH levels with serum testosterone levels have suggested that the direct testicular action does not occur in humans.[34] The method of administration of the drug thus became important. When it was delivered by intra-nasal insufflation, 100 times more material was required to give a result comparable to injection.[35]

Early long-term studies compared these two methods of administration of the long-acting LH-RH agonistic analogue, buserelin (HOE-766).[36] After 12 weeks of treatment, 12 of the 16 patients receiving the intra-nasal treatment had an "escape" of their suppressed plasma testosterone and dihydrotestosterone (DHT) levels to pretreatment levels. Those patients with subcutaneous injections had continued suppression of their androgen levels for up to 29 months. Thus, even with an increased dosage, intra-nasal administration could not provide optimal prolonged androgen suppression. The side effects of LH-RH agonist treatment, by either method of administration, were hot flashes in 65 to 85 percent of the patients, decreased libido, and impotency.[37] These side effects tended to decrease with duration of treatment.

Minor Side Effects

An alarming side effect became increasingly evident as studies with the LH-RH agonists progressed. In a study of nine patients, increased flank pain was noticed in two of the patients during the first week of therapy.[38] Both of these patients had radiographically demonstrated hydroureteronephrosis before treatment. The pain subsided after treatment had been continued for 1 week. A similar, more severe response was reported by Kahan et al in two patients.[39] A marked increase in pain 4 to 5 days after initiation of LH-RH therapy was noted by both patients. These patients progressed to delirium and died in 12 to 15 days after initiation of therapy. This tumor "flare" was explained by the observed initial rise in LH concentration during the first 24 hours of initiation of treatment.[40] Although an increase in LH was seen in all the treated patients, a rise in serum testosterone was seen in only 3 of the 15 patients. These three experienced a marked increase in pain coincident with their testosterone increase. Serum hormone levels, followed on a daily basis, showed that the serum LH had increased to 5.8 times the base level on day 2 after initiation of treatment.[41] The serum FSH had increased to 2.8 times the base level and the serum testosterone increased longitudinally for 2 days, plateaued for 2 days, then returned to the base level at day 6. It was at the castrate level of depression by day 15.

Tumor Flare

The tumor flare presented a severe side effect for this therapy which otherwise compared favorably to orchiectomy and DES in percentage response and duration of response. The incidence of tumor flare remains unpredictable. In one study of 30 patients treated with the LH-RH agonist, leuprolide, 3 of the 30 patients had symptoms of increased bone pain during the initial week of therapy.[42] In another study of 29 patients, no tumor exacerbation was reported,[43] while another reported that 1 of 24 patients had a flare.[44] In the largest series reporting early tumor exacerbation or flare, 17 of 32 patients experienced increased bone pain, 1 of 46 patients developed transient lymphedema, and 1 of 46 had transient increase in creatinine.[45] The other side effects of the LH-RH agonist therapy are mild pain at the injection site in 49 percent of those patients administered daily subcutaneous injections of the agonist buserelin, and mild nasal irritation in 43 percent of the patients using the intra-nasal form of buserelin.[44]

Comparison of Tumor Response to Orchiectomy, DES, and LH-RH

Comparison of the objective response of the LH-RH agonists, orchiectomy, and DES shows that castrate levels of androgens are reached in a slightly longer period of time with the LH-RH agonists as opposed to orchiectomy, 15 days versus 2 to 3 days, respectively. A more rapid decline in prostate size is also seen with orchiectomy, although at the 3-month period, the decrease in size is equal for either treatment method.[43] When the LH-RH agonist, leuprolide, was compared with DES in a prospective study of 199 patients, the objective response rate, as judged by the National Prostatic Cancer Project criteria, and the time for first progression were not significantly different (86 percent response for leuprolide, 85 percent for DES; and 60 weeks versus 61 weeks).[46] The major differences between the LH-RH agonist and the DES treatment were the side effects. Although no symptoms of tumor exacerbation were reported in the leuprolide group, the LH-RH agonist group reported significantly more troublesome hot flashes, 51 of 98 versus 11 of 101 for DES. Gynecomastia or breast tenderness was much more prevalent with DES, 49 of 100 versus 39 of 98. Nausea and vomiting, cardiovascular complications, peripheral edema, thrombosis, and phlebitis were also more prevalent with DES treatment. Suppression of gonadotropins and testosterone, for periods up to 46 months, has been shown to be equivalent for all three treatment methods.[47] The LH-RH agonists thus showed response rates equal to DES and orchiectomy, but with much less significant side effects than DES.

MODIFICATIONS IN METHOD OF ADMINISTRATION OF LH-RH AGONISTS

In most respects, then, the LH-RH analogues are equivalent to orchiectomy in subjective and objective response rates and in morbidity. They alleviate the troublesome psychologic effect of castration but introduce the problem of early tumor exacerbation or flare, which occurs in from 0 to 45 percent of the patients treated. The irritation at the site of administration, whether that be either nasal mucosa or the daily injection site, is minor. Modifications of the method of administration of the LH-RH agonists are being made to eliminate the irritation of the daily injections. A preparation of timed-release microcapsules has been developed to provide controlled release of a single injection over a 30-day period.[48] When this method was compared with daily subcutaneous injections on the Dunning prostate tumor in rats, the microcapsular injection was seen to have a significantly greater effect on the reduction of tumor weight, testis weight, and depression of serum testosterone. This is postulated to be because of the more constant levels of LH-RH agonist present in the blood with the timed-release preparation. This preparation also permits once-a-month injections with a lower total dose of the LH-RH agonist. Less severe vasomotor side effects, such as hot flashes, occur. Another form of preparation is the depot formulation, goserelin (Zoladex), made into a biodegradable implant by incorporation of the LH-RH analogue in a matrix of a lactide-glycolide copolymer similar to absorbable suture material which biodegrades into lactic and glycolic acids.[49,50] When this monthly depot injection is compared with a continuous subcutaneous infusion, or daily injection, the serum hormones are equally suppressed.[51,52] These timed-release forms of LH-RH administration provide a more constant LH and FSH suppression and a constant tumor suppression with just a monthly injection.

Side Effects

Thus, as the mode of administration becomes increasingly modified, the discomfort of daily injection is relieved. The major troublesome side effects of the early tumor exacerbation, or flare, with LH-RH analogue treatment have also been remedied. Labrie et al showed that with simultaneous administration of the antiandrogen (Anandron) the increased levels of androgen, which occur at the initiation of LH-RH agonist treatment, can be neutralized.[53] Pretreatment with oral DES for 1 week before initiation of leuprolide therapy also prevents the symptoms of tumor exacerbation and, in addition, shortens the delay for subjective improvement, even though the serum testosterone levels transiently increase, initially.[50,54] Treatment of metastatic prostate cancer with the LH-RH agonists has thus been shown to result in less mobidity than DES therapy and to eliminate the psychologic effects of castration. Tumor response is equivalent with all three forms of therapy.

Recent studies have suggested that the combination of the LH-RH agonists with either adrenal ablation or chemotherapy may prolong the response interval in metastatic prostate cancer.[55,56]

SUMMARY

No treatment presently available can cure metastatic prostate cancer. The question thus remains as to whether the psychologic effect of over-riding concern to the patient is the form of treatment or whether it is the impact of the diagnosis of incurable cancer.[57] The physician must provide personal support to the patient with the diagnosis of incurable metastatic cancer through the patient-physician relationship. If the enforced monthly physician visit for an injection of an LH-RH agonist will reassure the patient of the physician's continued observation, then that is the treatment of choice. If the permanent removal of the source of stimulation to tumor growth provides comfort to the patient, then that is the procedure of choice. The outcome of either procedure is equivalent in response and in side effects. It is up to the patient and physician to decide which is best.

REFERENCES

1. Silverberg E, Lubera J: Cancer statistics. CA 36(1):9, 1986
2. Baranovsky A, Myers MH: Cancer incidence and survival in patients 65 years of age and older. CA 36(1):26, 1986
3. Droller MJ: Adenocarcinoma of the prostate: An overview. Urol Clin North Am 7(3):579, 1980
4. Huggins C, Hodges CV: Studies of prostatic cancer. I. Effect of castration, estrogen and androgen injections on serum phosphates in metastatic carcinoma of the prostate. Cancer Res (4):293, 1941
5. Nesbit RM, Baum WC: Endocrine control of prostatic carcinoma. JAMA 143(15):1317, 1950
6. Reiner WG, Scott WW, Eggleston JC, Walsh PC: Long term survival after hormonal therapy for stage D prostatic cancer. J Urol 122(2):183, 1979
7. Whitmore, WF: Hormone therapy in prostate cancer. Am J Med 21(5):697, 1956
8. Lepor H, Ross A, Walsh PC: The influence of hormonal therapy on survival of men with advanced prostatic cancer. J Urol 128(2):335, 1982
9. The Veterans Administration Co-operative Urological Group: Treatment and survival of patients with cancer of the prostate. Surg Gynecol Obstet 124(5):1011, 1967

10. Geller J, Albert J, Samuels SCY, et al: Medical castration of males with megestrol acetate and small doses of diethylstilbestrol. J Clin Endocrinol Metab 52(3):576, 1981
11. Wein AJ, Murphy JJ: Experience in the treatment of prostatic carcinoma with cyproterone acetate. J Urol 109(1):68, 1983
12. Smith RB, Walsh PC, Goodwin WE: Cyproterone acetate in the treatment of advanced carcinoma of the prostate. J Urol 110(1):106, 1973
13. Jacobi GH, Altwein JE, Kurth KH, et al: Treatment of advanced prostatic cancer with parenteral cyproterone acetate: A phase III randomised trial. Br J Urol 52:208, 1980
14. Sogani P, Vagaiwala M, Whitmore, WF: Experience with flutamide in patients with advanced prostatic cancer without prior endocrine therapy. Cancer 54(4):744, 1984
15. Jacobo E, Schmidt JD, Weinstein SH, Flocks RH: Comparison of flutamide (SCH-13521) and diethylstilbestrol in untreated advanced prostatic cancer. Urology 8(3):231, 1976
16. Robinson MRG, Sheaver RJ, Fergusson JD: Adrenal suppression in the treatment of carcinoma of the prostate. Br J Urol 46:555, 1974
17. Sanford EJ, Drago JR, Rohner TJ, et al: Aminoglutethimide medical adrenalectomy for advanced prostatic carcinoma. J Urol 115(2):170, 1976
18. Walsh PC, Silteri PK: Suppression of plasma androgens by spironolactone in castrated men with carcinoma of the prostate. J Urol 114(2):254, 1975
19. Pont A, Williams PL, Azhar S, et al: Ketoconazole blocks testosterone synthesis. Arch Intern Med 142(11):2137, 1982
20. Trachtenberg J, Pont A: Ketoconazole therapy for advanced prostate cancer. Lancet 2(8400):433, 1984
21. Trachtenberg J: Ketoconazole therapy in advanced prostatic cancer. J Urol 132(1):61, 1984
22. Matsuo H, Baba Y, Nair RMG, et al: Structure of the porcine LH and FSH-releasing hormone. The proposed amino acid sequence. Biochem Biophys Res Commun 43(6):1334, 1971
23. Schally AV, Arimura A, Baba Y, et al: Isolation and properties of the FSH and LH-releasing hormone. Biochem Biophys Res Commun 43(2):393, 1971
24. Schally AV, Kastin AJ, Coy DH: LH-releasing hormone and its analogues: Recent basic and clinical investigations. Int J Fertil 21(1):1, 1976
25. Coy DH, Schally AV: Gonadotrophin releasing hormone analogues. Ann Clin Res 10(3):139, 1978
26. Schally AV, Arimura A, Coy DH: Recent approaches to fertility control based on derivatives of LH-RH. Vit Horm 38:258, 1980
27. Redding TW, Schally AV: Inhibition of prostate tumor growth in two rat models by chronic administration of D-Trp^6 analogue of luteinizing hormone-releasing hormone. Proc Natl Acad Sci USA 78(10):6509, 1981
28. Redding TW, Coy DH, Schally AV: Prostate carcinoma tumor size in rats decreases after administration of antagonists of luteinizing hormone-releasing hormone. Proc Natl Acad Sci USA 79(4):1273, 1982
29. Tolis G, Ackman D, Stellos A, et al: Tumor growth inhibition in patients with prostatic carcinoma treated with luteinizing hormone-releasing hormone agonists. Proc Natl Acad Sci USA 79(5):1658, 1982
30. Belchetz PE, Plant TM, Nakai Y, et al: Hypophysical responses to continuous

and intermittent delivery of hypothalamic gonadotropin-releasing hormones. Science 202(4368):631, 1978

31. Arimura A, Serafini P, Talbot S, Schally AV: Reduction of testicular luteinizing hormone/human chorionic gonadotropin receptors by [D-Trp^6]-luteinizing hormone releasing hormone in hypophysectomized rats. Biochem Biophys Res Commun 90(3):687, 1979
32. Hsueh AJW, Erickson GF: Extra-pituitary inhibition of testicular function by luteinizing hormone releasing hormone. Nature 281(5725):66, 1979
33. Sharpe RM, Fraser HM: Leydig cell receptors for luteinizing hormone releasing hormone and its agonists and their modulation by administration or deprivation of the releasing hormone. Biochem Biophys Res Commun 95(1):256, 1980
34. Swerdloff RS, Heber D, Bhasin S, Rajfer J: Effect of GnRH superative analogs (alone and combined with androgen) on testicular function in man and experimental animals. J Steroid Biochem 19(1):491, 1983
35. Coy DH, Schally AV: Gonadotropin releasing hormone analogues. Ann Clin Res 10(3):139, 1978
36. Tolis G, Faure N, Koutsilieris M, et al: Suppression of testicular steroidogenesis by the GnRH agonistic analogue buserelin (HOE-766) in patients with prostatic cancer: Studies in relation to dose and route of administration. J Steroid Biochem 19(1):995, 1983
37. Waxman JH, Wass JAH, Hendry WF, et al: Treatment with gonadotrophin releasing hormone analogue in advanced prostatic cancer. Br Med J 286(6374):1309, 1983
38. Trachtenberg J: The treatment of metastatic prostatic cancer with a potent luteinizing hormone releasing hormone analogue. J Urol 129(6):1149, 1983
39. Kahan A, Debrien F, Amar B, et al: Disease flare induced by D-Trp^6-LH-RH analogue in patients with metastatic prostatic cancer. Lancet 1(8383):971, 1984
40. Kerle D, Williams G, Ware H, Bloom SR: Failure of long term luteinising hormone releasing hormone treatment for prostatic cancer to suppress serum luteinising hormone and testosterone. Br Med J 289(6440):468, 1984
41. Roger M, Dochier J, Lahlov N, et al: Treatment of prostatic carcinoma with D-TRP-6-LHRH: Plasma hormone levels after daily subcutaneous injections and periodic administration of delayed-release preparations. Prostate 7(3):271, 1985
42. Smith JA: Androgen suppression by a gonadotropin releasing hormone analogue in patients with metastatic/carcinoma of the prostate. J Urol 131(6):1110, 1984
43. Koutsilieris M, Tolis G: Long-term follow-up of patients with advanced prostate carcinoma treated with buserelin (HOE-766) or orchiectomy: Classification of variables associated with disease outcome. Prostate 7(1):31, 1985
44. Presant CA, Soloway MS, Klioze SS, et al: Buserelin as primary therapy in advanced prostatic carcinoma. Cancer 56(10):2416, 1985
45. Waxman J, Man A, Hendry WF, et al: Importance of early tumor exacerbation in patients treated with long acting analogues of gonadotrophin releasing hormone for advanced prostatic cancer. Br Med J 291(6506):1387, 1985
46. Leuprolide Study Group: Leuprolide versus diethylstilbestrol for metastatic prostate cancer. N Engl J Med 311(20):1281, 1984
47. Glode LM, Smith JA, The Leuprolide Study Group: Long-term suppression of luteinizing hormone, follicle-stimulating hormone and testosterone by daily administration of leuprolide. J Urol 137(1):57, 1987

48. Redding TW, Schally AV, Tice TR, Meyers WE: Long acting delivery systems for peptides: Inhibition of rat prostate tumors by controlled release of [D-Trp^6] luteinizing hormone-releasing hormone from injectable microcapsules. Proc Natl Acad Sci USA 81(18):5845, 1984
49. Ahmed SR, Grant T, Shallet SM, et al: Preliminary report on use of depot formulation of LHRH analogue ICI 118630 (Zoladex) in patients with prostate cancer. Br Med J 290(6464):185, 1985
50. Van Cangh PJ, Opsomer RJ: Treatment of advanced carcinoma of the prostate with a depot luteinizing hormone-releasing hormone analogue (ICI-118630). J Urol 137(1):61, 1987
51. Thomas EJ, Jenkins J, Lenton EA, Cooke ID: Endocrine effects of goserelin, a new depot luteinizing hormone releasing hormone agonist. Br Med J 293:1407, 1986
52. Grant JBF, Ahmed SR, Shalet SM, et al: Testosterone and gonadotropin profiles in patients on daily or monthly LHRH analogue ICI 118630 (Zoladex) compared with orchiectomy. Br J Urol 58:539, 1986
53. Labrie F, Dupont A, Belanger A, et al: Simultaneous administration of pure antiandrogens, a combination necessary for the use of luteinizing hormone-releasing hormone agonists in the treatment of prostate cancer. Proc Natl Acad Sci USA 81(12):3861, 1984
54. Stein BS, Smith JA: DES lead-in to use of luteinizing hormone releasing hormone analogues in treatment of metastatic carcinoma of prostate. Urology 25(4):350, 1985
55. Williams G, Kerle DJ, Doble A, et al: Objective responses to ketoconazole therapy in patients with relapsed progressive prostate cancer. Br J Urol 58:45, 1986
56. Schally AV, Kook AI, Monje E, et al: Combination of a long-acting delivery system for luteinizing hormone-releasing hormone agonist with novatrone chemotherapy: Increased efficiency in the rat prostate cancer model. Proc Natl Acad Sci USA 83(11):8764, 1986
57. Parmer H, Lightman SL, Allen L, et al: Randomized controlled study of orchiectomy vs. long-acting D-Trp-6-LHRH microcapsules in advanced prostatic carcinoma. Lancet 2(8466):1201, 1985

Transrectal Ultrasonography of the Prostate

Martin I. Resnick

Transrectal ultrasonic imaging of the prostate is not a new diagnostic study. Within the past 2 years, however, there has been much interest and enthusiasm in attempting to define both the value and limitations of this technique in assessing patients with prostatic disease. The reasons for this wave of enthusiasm are multiple but are primarily related to the development of new and refined instrumentation and the influx of a variety of clinical investigators who have developed an interest in the technique. Many claims have been made as to the value of the technique, particularly as it relates to the evaluation of patients with carcinoma of the prostate and it is likely that, with time and the completion of carefully controlled clinical studies, the true role of this modality in the assessment of this and other diseases will become apparent. Before discussing the current status of transrectal prostatic ultrasonography, it would be useful to review the subject historically because as noted these developments have had a significant impact on the current "state of the art."

Wild and Neal,[1,2] of St. Martin's Hospital in Minneapolis, Minnesota, began their early work in ultrasonography in 1949 and in 1951 published their work which is aimed primarily at determining the possibility of using ultrasound to detect the differences in normal and diseased tissue by an A-mode display. In 1952, Wild and Reid published two-dimensional scans which included a breast carcinoma, normal kidney, and normal muscle and they noted that malignant tissue reflected more sound than normal tissue and that the tissue of nonmalignant tumors reflected less than normal tissue.[1,2] These same investigators attempted transrectal studies of the prostate during this period of time but the scans were so poor that they did not repeat their studies and did not report them. In 1963, Japanese urologists reported the use of A-mode scans of the prostate but also noted difficulties in interpretation and because of poor picture quality application of these modalities were not believed to be feasible.[3]

Interestingly, the first reports of endoscopic scanning were by Mizuno and co-workers who used specially constructed fingertip transducers to diagnose and differentiate solid and cystic tumors.[4] While A-mode studies can be very informative, time-amplitude echograms of the pelvic organs with their thousands of interfaces are much too complex for reliable interpretation. Von Micsky[5,6] initially developed a transvesical scanning approach for viewing the pelvic organs and subsequently developed a transrectal scanner which was placed through a standard sigmoidoscope. Though experimental data were reported, controlled clinical studies were never carried out. In 1968, Watanabe and associates[7,8] reported ultrasonograms of the prostate using transrectal scanning with a specially prepared concave transducer. The instrumentation used was B-mode and prostatic images were displayed on a black and white screen. The transducer was covered with a water-filled balloon which assured good contact with the rectal wall. The examinations were performed with the patient in the sitting position and the bladder was filled with water to assist in the demonstration of the prostate, seminal vesicles, and other pelvic structures. They studied a large number of patients with a variety of prostatic diseases and demonstrated consistent and reproducible prostate images. The first report of prostate imaging in the United States was by King and associates[9] in 1973 using similar equipment and another report from the same laboratory was the first to use gray scale imaging in association with transrectal prostatic ultrasonography.[10] Further studies continued over the remaining 1970s and early 1980s further documenting the application of the technique. Coordinated with these clinical studies was the development of improved gray scale instrumentation, higher frequency transducers, and also the introduction of real-time imaging, which provided enhanced visualization of the prostate and related structures. Additionally, investigations were carried out using transabdominal techniques and transurethral techniques in visualization of the prostate but most investigators concluded that transrectal imaging provided the most consistent and reproducible images of the prostate that had application in clinical practice.[11,12]

INSTRUMENTATION

As noted the original studies carried out by Watanabe were performed with B-mode imaging and, in the early 1970s, gray scale techniques were used for transrectal ultrasonography. This form of imaging has continued and has greatly improved the visualization of the prostate and subsequent interpretation of images. With newer instrumentation, real-time imaging has been developed and these techniques have been not only useful in visualizing the prostate but also have been helpful in application of biopsy techniques.

The basic technique for transrectal ultrasonography as developed by Watanabe and associates[7,8] consists of a transrectal transducer, radial scanner and imaging screen (Fig. 1). Originally performed with the patient in the sitting position in a special chair allowing for placement of the probe, examinations have also been carried out with placement of the probe while

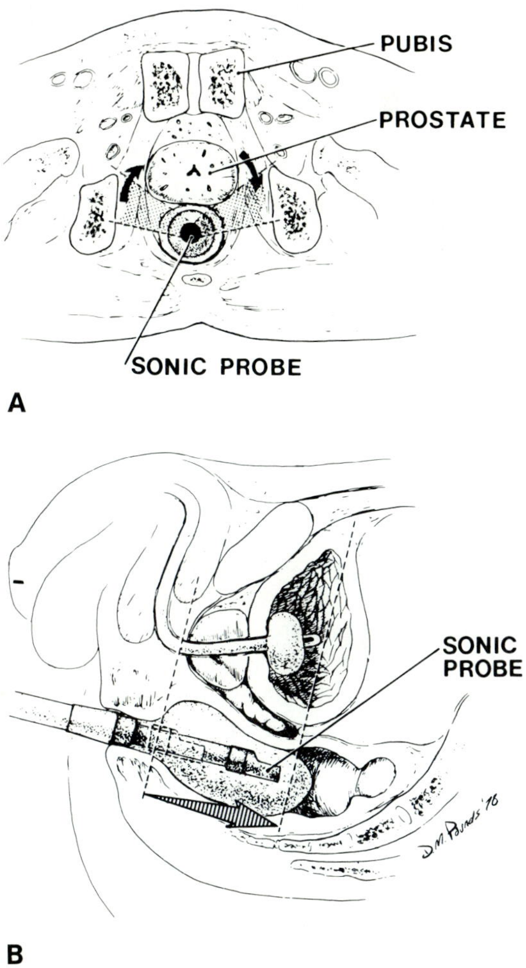

Figure 1. Diagram demonstrating basic technique of transrectal radial scanning of prostate. **A.** Cross-section. **B.** Sagittal section. Linear array scanning produces images in sagittal section (see text).

the patient is in the lithotomy position, the knee-chest position, and the decubitus lateral position.

Present instrumentation consists of a two part probe: an outer stationery unit and a freely movable inner assembly. The outer stationery unit provides inflow and outflow ports for the fluid interface and a condom or rubber balloon covering the transducer allows for contact with the distended rectal wall. The inner assembly is free to move in longitudinal and rotational directions. Longitudinal movement provides an infinite number of serial sections of the prostate and bladder and the rotational movement provides sonograms of the sections. An ultrasonic beam is emitted at right angles to the probe and the transducer receives the echos and transmits them to the gray scale unit. The frequency of most early transducers was 3.5 MHz, however, transducers of higher frequency have been used recently; 7.0-MHz transducers have provided increased resolution but it has yet to be determined that those higher frequency transducers allow for improved diagnostic capabilities.

Advances have also occurred with the development of the linear array scanner. These have consisted primarily of 3.5- and 5.0-MHz transducers and allow for visualization of the prostate in the sagittal plane.[13,14] Linear array scanners have also been helpful in performing prostate biopsy, although biopsy under ultrasound guidance has also been carried out with the radial scanner.[15–17]

IMAGE CHARACTERISTICS

Normal Prostate

The normal prostate on radial scanning appears ultrasonically as a symmetric, triangular elipsoid structure that is delineated circumferentially by a continuous prostatic capsule (Fig. 2). The capsule is usually free of distortion and is also symmetric. The posterior portion of the prostate appears concave because of the distortion produced by the inflated balloon during the course of the examination. As the probe is moved in a cephalad-caudad direction, the apex of the prostate can be regularly delineated as can the midsection of the prostate and its base. Towards the base, however, the prostate gland may be difficult to differentiate from portions of the bladder neck, particularly if a prominent median lobe is present. In this region, the seminal vesicles are typically visualized as symmetrically paired structures that may vary somewhat in shape but are typically present when free of congenital anomalies or malignancy. As the probe is moved along the base of the bladder, the seminal vesicles typically extend laterally from the midline and will tend to parallel the distended rectal wall. The internal characteristics of the prostate are such that multiple diffuse echoes are produced but generally the echoes produced are of lower intensity than those ob-

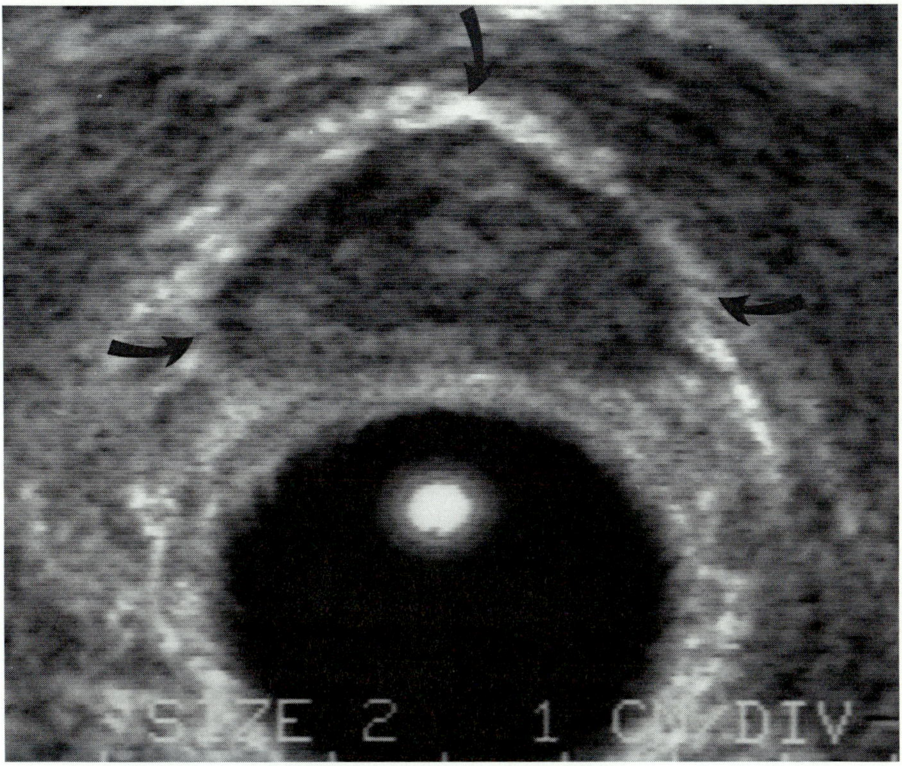

Figure 2. Radial scan with 4.5-MHz transducer. Normal prostate. Note the symmetry of the gland and the triangular appearance of the normal prostate. The capsule is well delineated circumferentially (*arrows*).

served in a variety of pathologic conditions, including benign prostatic hyperplasia and prostatic carcinoma.

The linear array scanner visualizes the prostate in a longitudinal direction and the section seen is in the saggital plane. The accoustic characteristics of the prostate are similar to those seen with radial scanning; however, because of the plane of examination the prostate appears round or ovoid in the midline. When the lateral margins of the gland are visualized, further rounding of, or a circular pattern of, the capsule is seen. When the midportion of the prostate is seen, the anterior pubic symphysis is delineated as is the space of Retzius with its fat and venous tissue. The apex of the prostate is well delineated as is the base and the urinary bladder. The seminal vesicles appear as areas of reduced echogenicity as they do on the radial scan and their relationship to the posterior wall of the bladder is usually easily delineated.

Benign Prostatic Hyperplasia

Benign enlargement of the prostate is one of the most common neoplasms seen in men and is recognized to occur in approximately 80 percent of men over 40 years of age. It has been estimated that 95 percent of men will have histologic evidence of benign prostatic hyperplasia by age 70 years. Ultrasonically the true capsule of the prostate is clearly delineated and the capsule may actually be thickened because of the inability of the technique to differentiate the true prostatic tissue that is compressed by the enlarging adenoma from the true capsule of the gland (Fig. 3). The gland tends to be diffusely enlarged and the most notable change usually occurs along the anterior-posterior diameter. The interior portion of the gland is characterized by the presence of multiple fine homogeneous echoes believed to be created by the multiple small adenomas, fibrous tissue located between glandular elements and multiple interfaces created by dilated prostatic

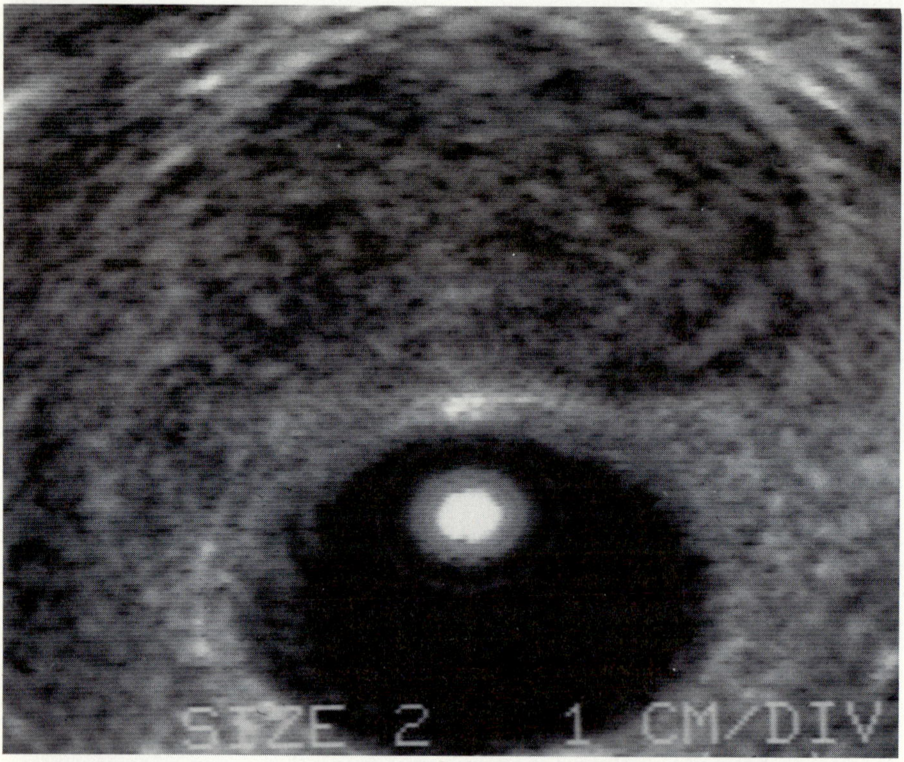

Figure 3. Radial scan with 4.5-MHz transducer. Benign prostatic hyperplasia. The gland assumes a more round appearance with an increase in the anterior-posterior diameter in addition to the width. Multiple areas of low echogenicity are present which represent areas of nodular hyperplasia and prostatic secretions. The gland remains symmetric and relatively homogenous.

ducts containing viscous secretions termed corpora amalacea and microcalculi. At times the adenomatous tissue can be differentiated from the compressed true prostatic tissue and, though a symmetric pattern exists, the general echogenicity of the central tissue tends to be of lower intensity than the peripheral tissue. Areas of increased or decrased echogenicity can be associated with the hyperplastic tissue which is likely related to the configuration of the adenomatous tissue, presence or absence of calculi, and inflammatory changes. It is important to emphasize that the capsule of the prostate in association with benign hyperplasia is generally well delineated and is free of any disruption or evidence of invasive disease.

Linear array or longitudinal scanning reveals the prostate associated with benign hyperplasia to be crescent or triangular shaped and is associated with rounding or a semicircular appearance of the gland with marked enlargement (Fig. 4). As the gland grows, it tends to assume a more round appearance. As noted, the echogenicity of the benign gland tends to be symmetric, however, areas of increased or reduced echogenicity are not infrequently seen. In association with benign prostatic hyperplasia, it is not uncommon to observe prostatic calculi, inflammatory changes, and the development of secretions within the prostatic ducts. All of these processes, in addition to the nodular characteristic of the growth process itself, result in these changes. Because of these diffuse changes, it is difficult if not impossible to draw strict conclusions as to the significance of a hyperechoic or a hypoechoic region. Rifkin and colleagues have noted that many focal

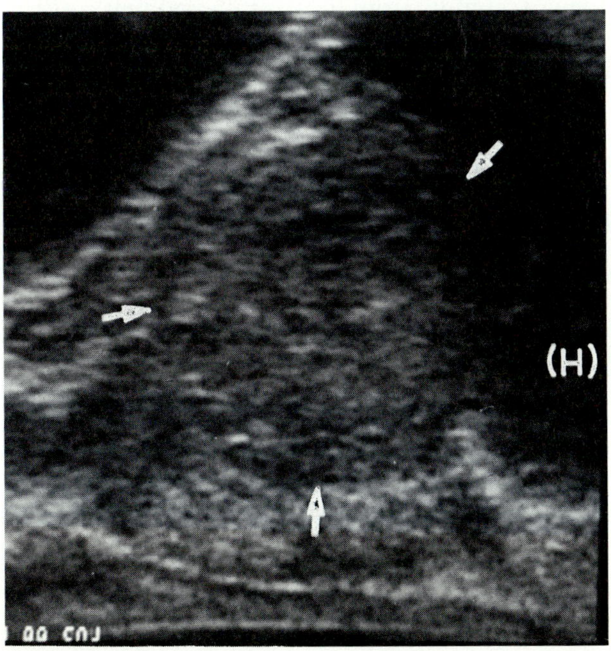

Figure 4. Linear array scan with 5.0-MHz transducer. Benign prostatic hyperplasia. The gland is triangular in appearance in the sagittal plane and the area of adenomatous growth is apparent (*arrows*). H = head. (*Courtesy of Matthew D. Rifkin, M.D., Thomas Jefferson University Hospital, Philadelphia, PA.*)

benign lesions will appear as hyperechoic regions compared to the surrounding normal prostatic tissue.[18,19] They subdivided the echoes into grades based on thickness and noted that the majority of benign lesions have echoes that are 3 mm or greater in thickness and tend to be more reflective than the surrounding prostatic capsule. Only about 25 percent of echoes are 1 to 2 mm in thickness and are only slightly more hyperechoic than normal prostatic tissue. It is believed that the thicker echoes are caused by calcifications and the lower intensity and smaller echoes which often do not shadow are related to corpora amylacea.

Prostatitis

Inflammatory changes of the prostate can either be acute or chronic. Transrectal ultrasonography is infrequently performed on patients with acute prostatitis because palpation of the prostate either digitally or with a rectal probe is usually not necessary to establish a diagnosis and also is usually not recommended because of the possibility of associated dissemination of the infection and resultant sepsis. The gland will, however, appear diffusely enlarged with decreased echogenicity because of the diffuse inflammation secondary to the infection. Isolated infections of the prostate, particularly small abscesses, are generally uncommon but when they occur the abscess cavity is usually well delineated.

Chronic inflammation of the prostate usually results in a diffuse change but at times these can be difficult to differentiate from other pathologic processes, particularly malignancy. The dense echoes of prostatitis are typically symmetric and extend laterally from the urethra and never distort or obscure the prostatic capsule (Fig. 5). It is important to recognize that other clinical parameters should also be assessed in patients with chronic inflammatory changes of the prostate. Typically these patients have symptoms of lower urinary tract irritability (frequency, urgency, and nocturia) and the prostate is often tender and soft on physical examination. Finally, the diagnosis would be highly suspected by the microscopic identification of clumps of white blood cells in the expressed prostatic secretions.

Prostatic Calculi

Prostatic calculi appear as clearly defined echo dense areas that are well delineated both on radial and linear array scanners. They typically are asymmetric areas which produce sonic shadowing anteriorly because of the ability of the calculi to impair the transmission of sonic impulses (Fig. 6). When associated with benign prostatic hyperplasia, they are typically posterior and it is well known that they are located anatomically in the plane between the enlarged hyperplastic adenomatous benign tissue and the compressed true prostatic capsule. Calculi do not cause distortion of the prostatic capsule and their position can be confirmed with careful radiographic studies. Rifkin has shown that prostatic calculi which at times can be con-

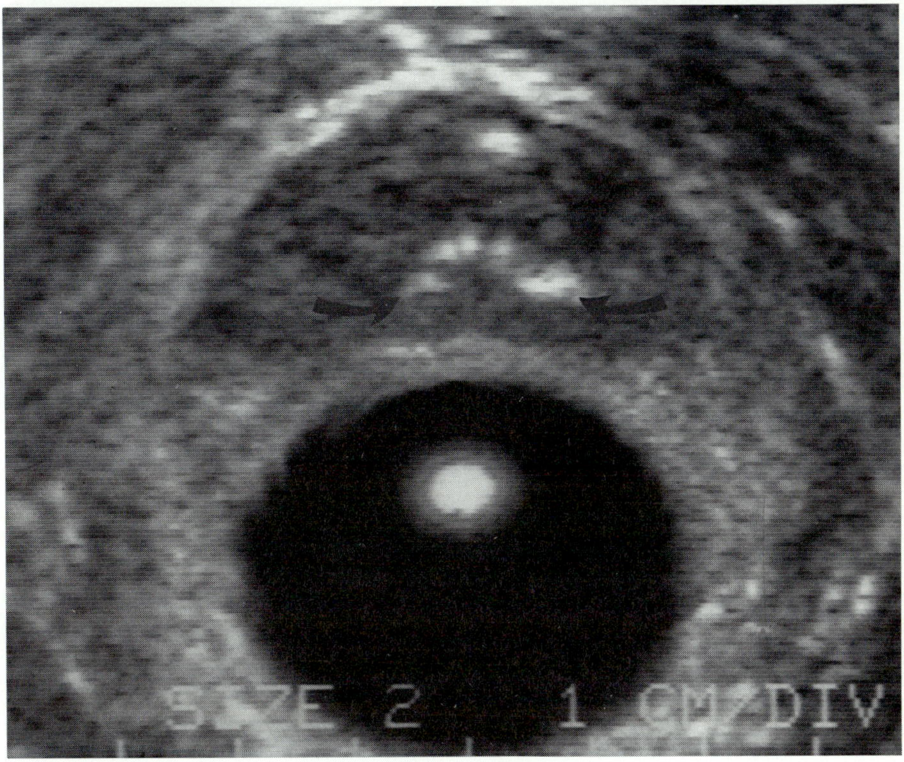

Figure 5. Radial scan with 4.5-MHz transducer. Chronic prostatitis. Note echogenic area in region of urethra (*arrows*). These are typically symmetric and can also be associated with calcification.

fused with other abnormalities in the prostate can be more accurately identified with linear array scanners than their radial counterparts.[14]

Carcinoma of the Prostate

It has been estimated that carcinoma of the prostate and carcinoma of the lung will be the most commonly diagnosed malignancies in the American male population in 1988. It is estimated that 96,000 new cases will be diagnosed during this year and 27,000 patients will die of the disease.[20] Ultrasonography of the prostate has received its greatest attention in this disease and has been applied to early diagnosis of the disease, staging of the disease, monitoring response to therapy, and assisting in biopsy. Though much has been written in the past several years, there has not been a unanimity of opinion as to the most appropriate applications of this technology.

Transrectal ultrasonography has been used in the assessment of patients with carcinoma of the prostate. It has been shown to be helpful in staging the disease and also in documenting a response to therapy, particu-

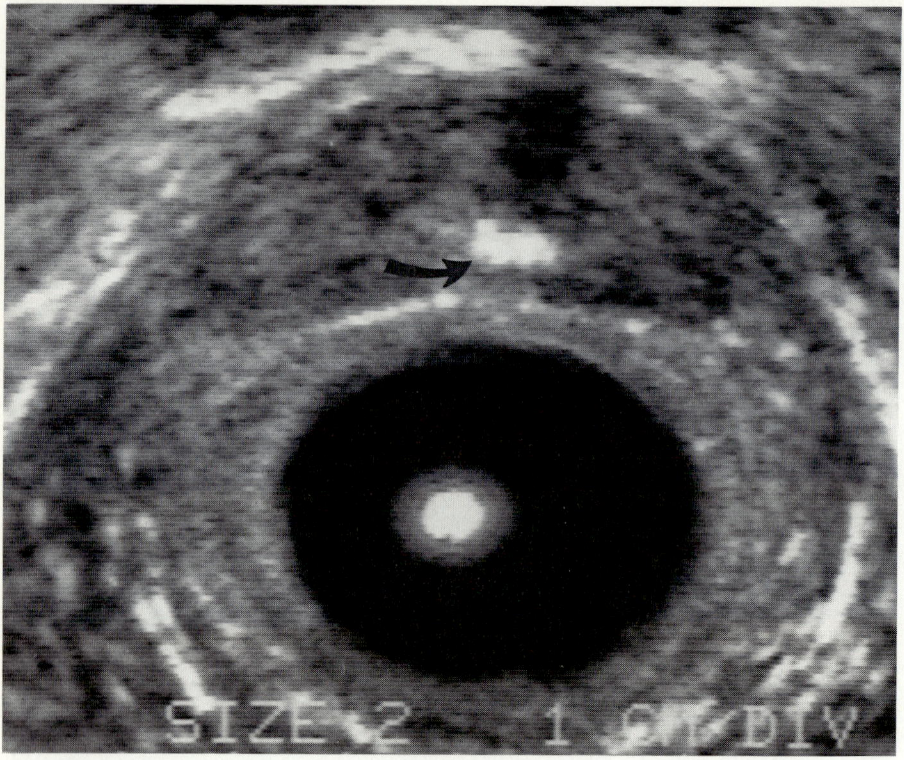

Figure 6. Radial scan with 4.5-MHz transducer. Prostatic calculi. Calculi typically are highly echogenic and produce sonic shadowing (*arrow*) because of the ability of the calculi to impair the transmission of sonic impulses.

larly endocrine therapy. Not only has transrectal ultrasonography been used to assist in biopsy but also it has been reported that interstitial radiation therapy can be administered with this technique.[21] Perhaps the most controversial area of transrectal ultrasonography relates to its role in early detection and screening for carcinoma of the prostate.

The ultrasonic characteristics of carcinoma of the prostate are varied. Early study particularly with B-mode and initial gray scale evaluation reported that carcinomas appeared as echo dense or hyperechoic areas.[7–10,22,23] With improvement in instrumentation and use of higher frequency transducers, it became evident that not all tumors had this appearance (Figs. 7 through 9). Some investigators have demonstrated that prostatic malignancies only appear as hypoechoic areas while others have shown that the tumors can appear as hyperechoic, hypoechoic, isoechoic, or of mixed echogenicity.[19,24–26] Experience seems to indicate that early carcinomas tend to be of lower echogenicity; however, as the tumor grows and invades other areas of the prostate, increased echogenicity that is likely secondary to the development of increased tissue interface results. For this reason, many of

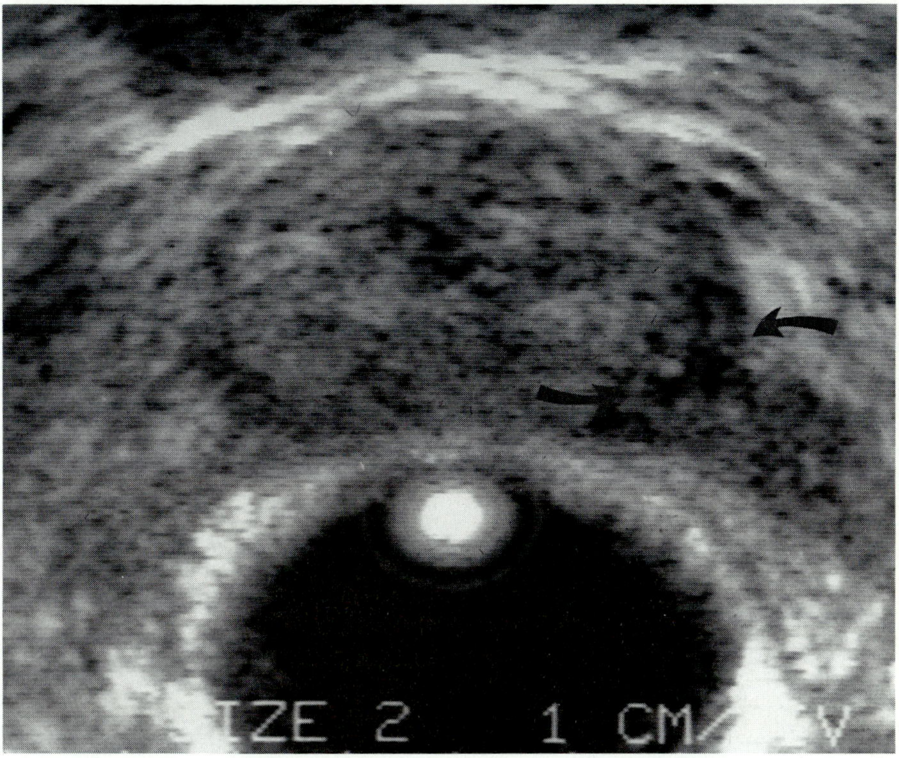

Figure 7. Radial scan with 4.5-MHz transducer. Carcinoma of the prostate. Area of low or hypoechogenicity (*arrows*) in patient with localized carcinoma of the prostate. Multiple scans demonstrated the prostatic capsule to be intact which was confirmed histologically following radical prostatectomy.

the larger tumors tend to be either of mixed or of hyperechogenicity. Additionally, it is important to emphasize that not all tumors can be detected with ultrasonography. It has been well demonstrated that patients with confirmed carcinoma will have normal prostate ultrasound examinations. Typically these patients have undergone simple prostatectomy for seemingly benign disease and stage A2 or diffuse carcinomas were detected on histologic examination of the removed tissue.[27] It is also important to realize that, with the increased resolution that has accompanied the development of new machines and the recognition that many prostatic malignancies appear as hypoechogenic areas, other benign conditions within the prostate also have similar ultrasonic characteristics. There have been no reports to date to indicate that the sensitivity and specificity of the examination has changed in association with the altered ultrasonic characteristics of these multiple abnormalities within the prostate.

Another important consideration in evaluating patients with carci-

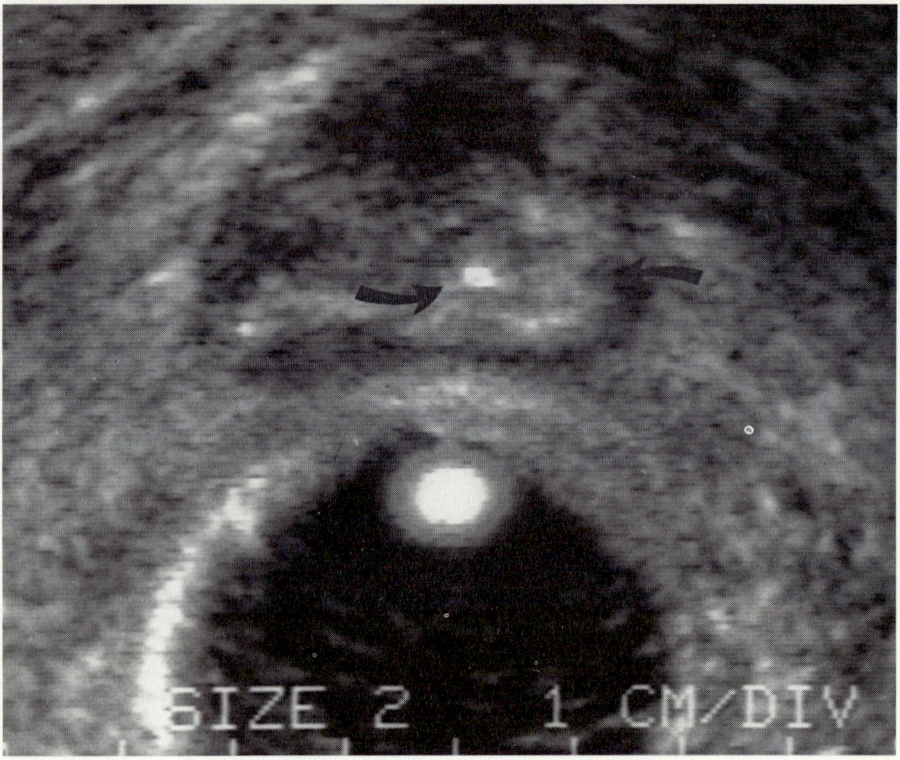

Figure 8. Radial scan with 4.5-MHz transducer. Carcinoma of the prostate. Area of increased echogenicity with distortion of the capsule (*arrows*) in patient with locally invasive adenocarcinoma of the prostate.

noma of the prostate is the configuration of the prostatic capsule and seminal vesicles. In patients with confined disease, the capsule is seen circumferentially and no distortion or disruption of the capsule is noted. In patients with invasion of the prostatic capsule, however, deformity occurs. This finding is a reliable technique for documenting involvement of the capsule with invading tumor and with more extensive disease documenting the presence of seminal vesical involvement (Fig. 10). When only microscopic involvement occurs, however, ultrasonography is generally not useful in making this determination.[28-30] The study by Pontes and associates[29] indicated that preoperative transrectal ultrasonography was sensitive in detecting capsular and seminal vesical involvement 89 and 100 percent of the time respectively. The specificity of the method, however, was low for capsular involvement (50 percent) likely because of the inability of this method to detect microscopic disease.

Ultrasonography can be used to document gland volume.[31,32] This information may be of help in planning specific surgery in patients with pros-

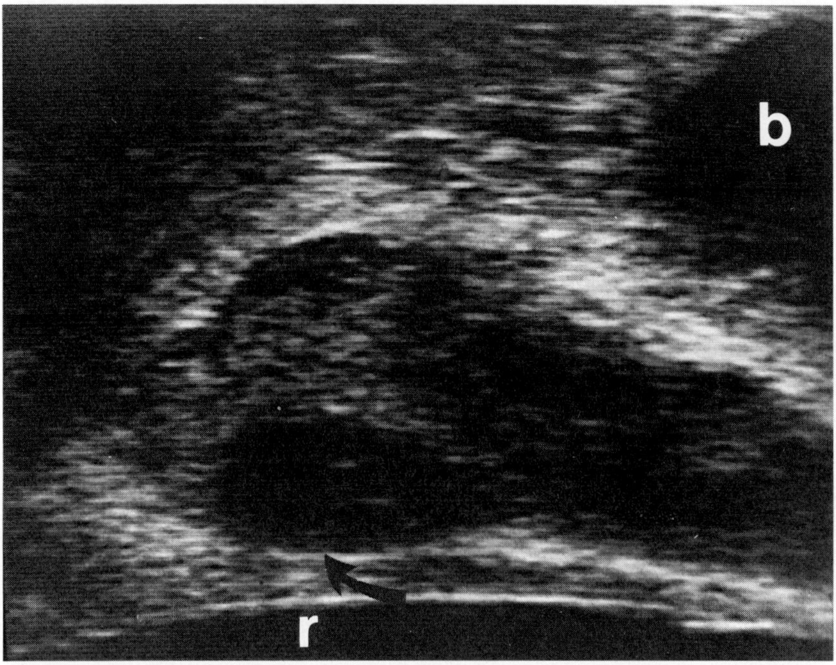

Figure 9. Linear array scan with 5.0-MHz transducer. Note hypoechogenic area along posterior aspect of prostate (arrow). b = bladder; r = rectum. *(Courtesy of Matthew D. Rifkin, M.D., Thomas Jefferson University Hospital, Philadelphia, PA.)*

tatic disease or more importantly for documenting response to therapy in the treatment of patients with carcinoma. Studies have indicated that ultrasonography can be reliably used to document reduction in prostatic size following administration of endocrine therapy for managing patients with diffuse disease.[27,33] Experience indicates that within 3 months following either orchiectomy or administration of estrogen therapy, a reduction of prostatic volume of approximately 30 percent can be documented. It has also been documented that in those individuals who develop progressive disease within 1 year after castration that the reduction in prostatic size was significantly less than the remaining patients who have had a more sustained response. Carpentier and associates[33] noted that in those patients whose prostatic volume decreased to at least 50 percent of pretreatment volume after 3 months, none developed distant progression within 1 year. Of those whose prostatic volume did not decrease to at least 70 percent of pretreatment volume after 3 months, however, 78 percent developed distant progression before or after 1 year.

Fujano and Scardino also used prostatic ultrasonography to document response to radiotherapy and chemotherapy.[34] After definitive radiation

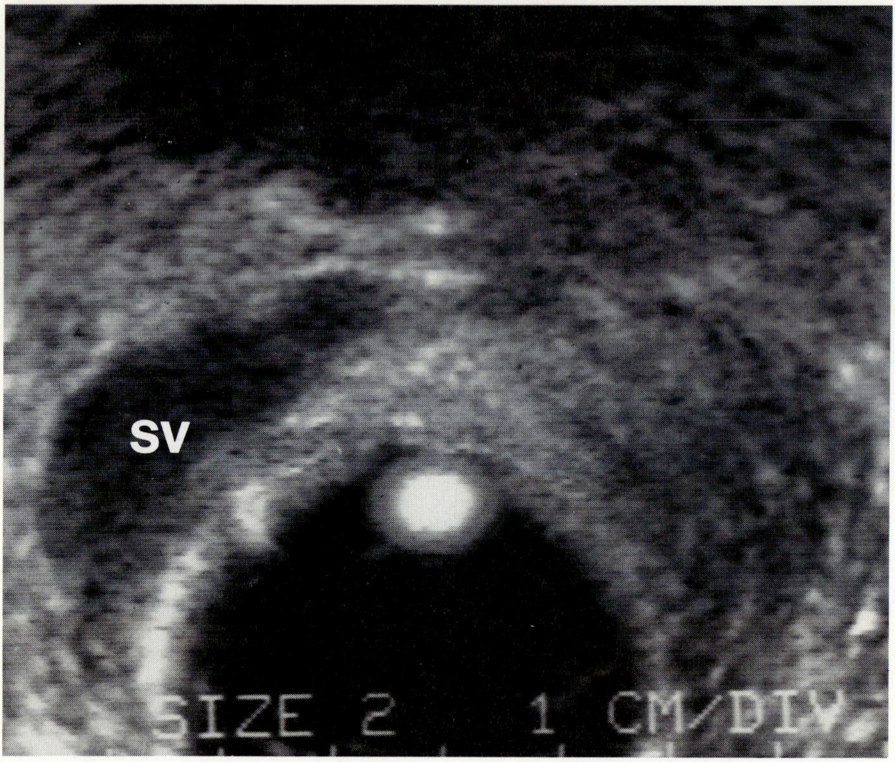

Figure 10. Radial scan with 4.5-MHz transducer. Carcinoma of the prostate with seminal vesicle invasion. The right seminal vesicle (SV) is normal and is viewed as an oblong structure of low echogenicity. The left seminal vesicle is absent due to tumor invasion.

therapy, those patients having a satisfactory response experienced a decrease in size of the prostate and it resumed a more normal symmetric pattern with reconstitution of the prostatic capsule that was often distorted because of extensive disease. Finally they noted that the seminal vesicles also resumed a more normal appearance following satisfactory response to radiation therapy. They also noted that in those patients responding to chemotherapy that reduction in prostatic size of up to 30 percent occurred within 3 months following initiation of treatment.

Prostate ultrasonography has also been used in assisting in prostatic biopsy.[15–17,35] These studies have definitely shown that transrectal ultrasonography with use of the radial scanner and the linear array scanner is useful in accurate placement of the needle within the prostate (Figs. 11 through 13). Though one study demonstrates the superiority of this technique over digitally directed biopsies in patients with prostatic nodules, another shows the two methods of biopsy as being comparable.[35,36] In one

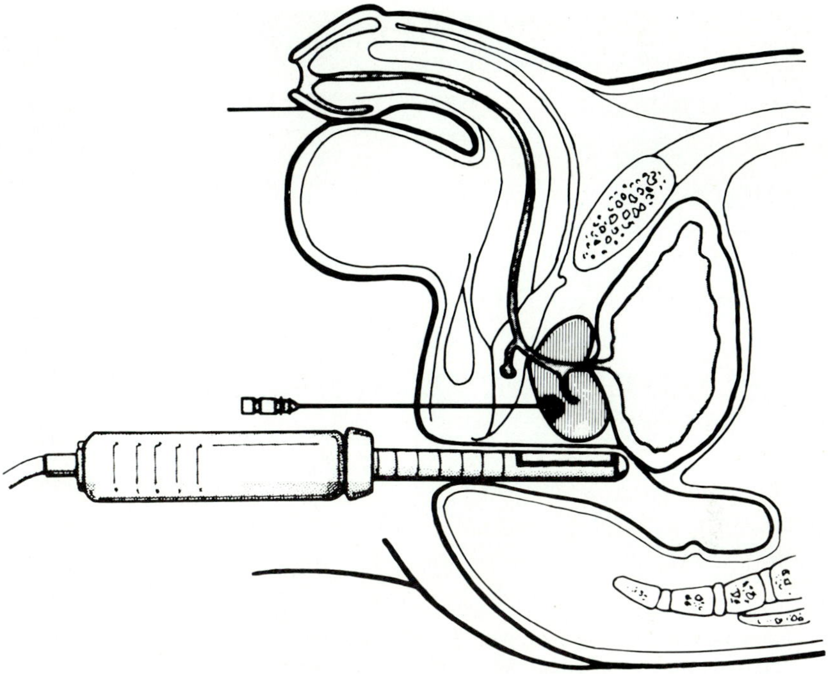

Figure 11. Diagram demonstrating basic technique of transrectal ultrasound guided perineal needle biopsy of prostate. Diagram is of linear array scanner. *(Courtesy of Matthew D. Rifkin, M.D., Thomas Jefferson University Hospital, Philadelphia, PA.)*

study of 15 patients with prostatic carcinoma, 9 were diagnosed correctly with perineal digital biopsy and all 15 were diagnosed correctly with ultrasound guided biopsy. Another study included 45 patients who presented with prostatic nodules and of these 14 were subsequently found to have carcinoma. Of this group the two techniques were in concordance in 11 patients. Of the remaining three patients, two were positive only with digitally directed biopsy and one was positive only with the ultrasound-guided biopsy suggesting that ultrasound-guided biopsy was not necessary as a routine procedure when a distinct nodule is palpable. It is also important to recognize that it has been demonstrated that transrectal aspiration biopsy is more accurate than digitally directed perineal biopsy and, if this former technique is used routinely, the need for ultrasound-guided biopsy becomes even less significant in those patients with palpable nodules.[37,38]

It is important to recognize that ultrasound-guided biopsy does have a role in the evaluation of patients with suspected prostatic malignancies. If an ultrasound examination was performed and a nonpalpable abnormality was detected, indeed the ultrasound-guided biopsy would be of value. Additionally, in those patients presenting with metastatic disease of unknown

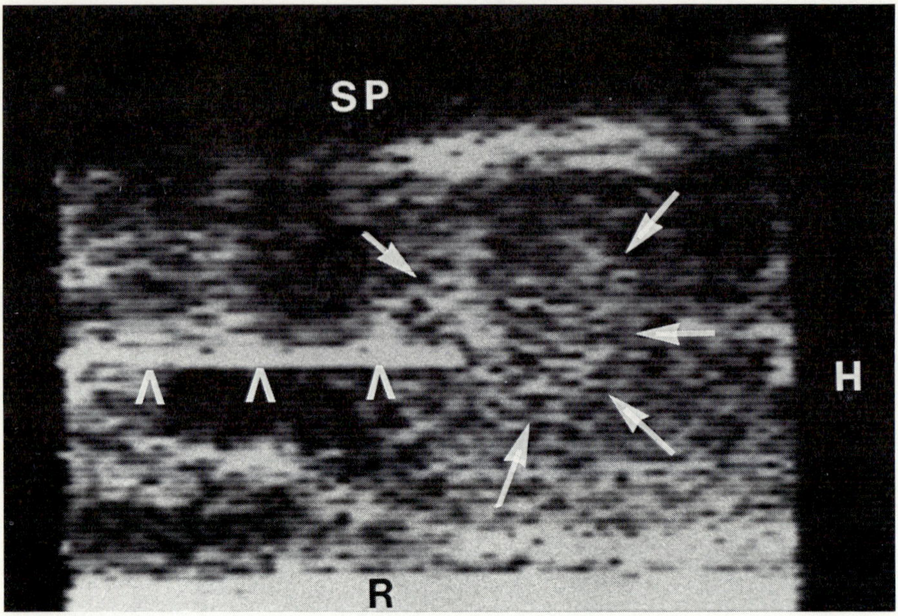

Figure 12. Linear array scan with 5.0-MHz transducer. Biopsy needle (ΛΛΛΛ) is guided into area of suspected malignancy (*arrows*). *(Courtesy of Matthew D. Rifkin, M.D., Thomas Jefferson University Hospital, Philadelphia, PA.)*

etiology with suspicious ultrasound examination and a normal digital rectal examination, guided biopsies of suspicious areas may assist in establishing the diagnosis so that appropriate therapy can be instituted.

Probably the most controversial area related to the use of transrectal ultrasonography is in its application and use as a screening study for carcinoma of the prostate. Watanabe and associates have been proponents of its use in this manner but others have not advocated its use in this regard.[39,40] The problem with the use of transrectal ultrasonography for screening purposes is that its low sensitivity and specificity is an impediment to its generalized use. There are very little data accurately comparing the ultrasound examination with the intraprostatic histologic findings. Studies indicate that stage A2 carcinomas cannot be imaged with reliability and many benign conditions such as prostatic calculi, benign prostatic hyperplasia, and chronic prostatitis will mimic the echo changes observed in carcinoma.[18,22,27] Studies have indicated that, because of the inability of transrectal ultrasonography to differentiate these conditions, its use as a screening modality is not of benefit because of the low predictive values.[41,42] Statistical analyses reveal that the positive predictive values of transrectal ultrasonography is not significantly higher than digital rectal examination and, based on these calculations, it appears that the added gain from screening a population with transrectal ultrasonography is not worth the time and expense because

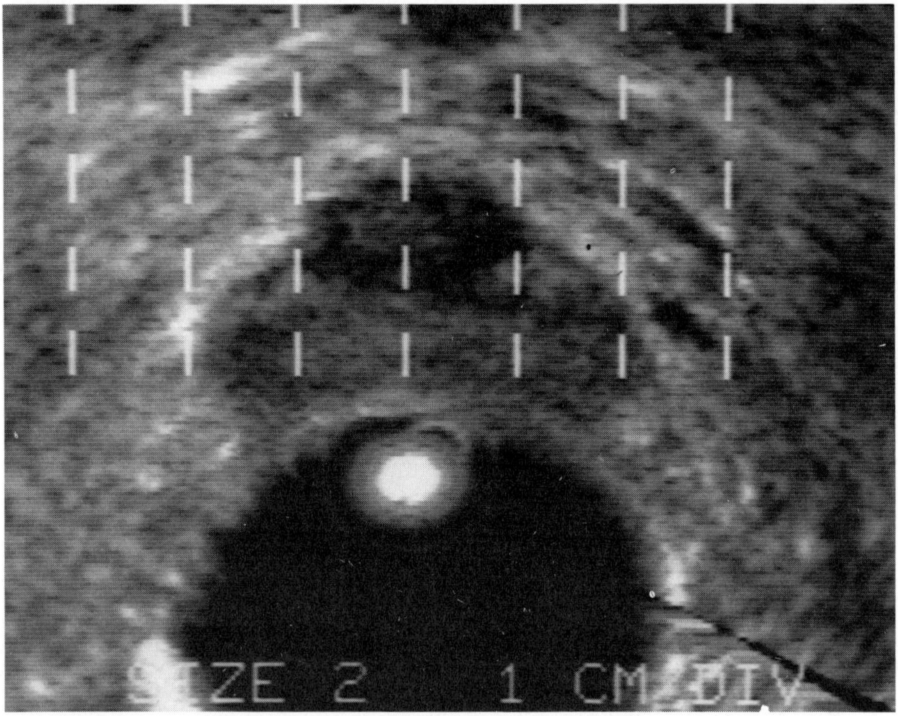

Figure 13. Radial scan with 4.5-MHz transducer. Biopsy grade corresponds to template placed on perineum. Needles can be directed into specific areas of the prostate and appear as hyperechoic areas on the screen. A similar technique is utilized for placement of interstitial seeds for radiation therapy.

the additional useful information would be minimal to nonexistent. Approximately 25 percent of patients with palpable prostatic nodules would prove to have carcinoma, a statistic not dissimilar from individuals having a positive ultrasound examination. Conversely a negative rectal examination or ultrasound examination excludes the presence of carcinoma in only 90 to 95 percent of patients (negative predictive values). These false-positive and false-negative examinations are what negate the use of this examination as a screening study in an asymptomatic population. Many patients with false-positive examinations would be subjected to further studies and expense, which would result in much anxiety to the family and patient even though the chance of the individual having the disease would be remote. It must also be remembered that a significant number of patients would have had positive rectal examinations that would suggest the presence of carcinoma and the ultrasound examination would not then detect malignancies in all these instances. Though evidence exists that it is important to detect the malignancy early so as to effect cure, it has yet to be determined that routine transrectal ultrasonography in an asymptomatic population can accomplish this goal.[43] Only after well-controlled, carefully performed clinical studies are completed will the answer to the question as to the efficacy of this technique as a screening modality be answered.

Transrectal ultrasonic imaging of the prostate is a diagnostic tool much like computerized tomography, magnetic resonance imaging, and a variety of other studies and tests that are readily available in many clinical settings. Analogous with the wave of enthusiasm associated with the introduction of a new drug, with time most new developments and breakthroughs find their niche in clinical practice. Transrectal ultrasound has not as yet fully arrived at this point. With time, further clinical studies, and experience, its true role in the assessment of prostatic disease will become apparent.

REFERENCES

1. Wild JJ, Neal D: Use of high frequency ultrasonic waves for detecting changes in texture in living tissues. Lancet 2:655, 1951
2. Wild JJ, Reid JM: Application of echo-ranging techniques to the determination of structure of biological tissues. Science 115:226, 1951
3. Takahashi H, Ouchi T: The ultrasonic diagnosis in the field of biology. In Japanese Medicine and Ultrasonics The First Report, 7, 1963; The Second Report, 35, 1964
4. Mizuno S, et al: Diagnostic application of ultrasound in obstetrics and gynecology. In Grossman CC (ed): Diagnostic Ultrasound. New York, Plenum, 1966, pp 452–464
5. von Micsky LI: Transvesical pelveosonography: A new theoretical and experimental approach to the investigation of gynecological cancer. Obstet Gynecol 27:597, 1966
6. von Micsky LI: Gynecologic ultrasonography. In King DL (ed): Diagnostic Ultrasound. St. Louis, Mosby, 1974, pp 207–241
7. Watanabe H, Katoh H, Katoh T, et al: Diagnostic application of the ultrasonography for the prostate. J Urol 59:279, 1968
8. Watanabe H, Igari D, Tanahasi Y, et al: Development and application of new equipment for transrectal ultrasonography. J Clin Ultrasound 2:91, 1974
9. King WW, Wilkiemeyer RM, Boyce WH, McKinney WM: Current status of prostatic echography. JAMA 266:444, 1973
10. Boyce WH, McKinney WM, Resnick MI, Willard JW: Ultrasonography as an aid in the diagnosis and management of surgical disease of the pelvis: Special emphasis on the genitourinary system. Ann Surg 184:477, 1976
11. Henneberry M, Carter MF, Neiman HL: Estimation of prostate size by suprapubic ultrasonography. J Urol 121:615, 1979
12. Holm HH, Northeved A: A transurethral ultrasonic scanner. J Urol 111:238, 1974
13. Shapeero LG, Friedland GW, Perkash I: Transrectal ultrasonic voiding cystourethrography: Studies in neuromuscular bladder dysfunction. AJR 141:83, 1983
14. Rifkin MD: Transrectal prostatic ultrasonography: Comparison of linear array and radial scanners. J Ultrasound Med 4:1, 1985

15. Holm HH, Gammelgaard J: Ultrasonically guided precise needle placement in the prostate and seminal vesicles. J Urol 125:385, 1981
16. Rifkin MD, Kurtz AB, Goldberg BB: Prostate biopsy utilizing transrectal ultrasound guidance: Diagnosis of non-palpable cancers. J Ultrasound Med 2:165, 1983
17. Rifkin MD, Kurtz AB, Goldberg BB: Sonographically guided transperineal prostatic biopsy: Preliminary experience with a longitudinal linear array transducer. AJR 140:745, 1983
18. Rifkin MD: The prostate and seminal vesicles. In Diagnostic Imaging of the Lower Genitourinary Tract. New York, Raven Press, 1985, pp 121–207
19. Rifkin MD, Friedland GW, Shortliffe L: Prostatic evaluation by transrectal endosonography: Detection of carcinoma. Radiology 158:85, 1986
20. Cancer Statistics, 1987: Ca—A Cancer Journal for Clinicians. Jan/Feb 1987, Vol. 37, pp 2–19
21. Holm HH, Juul N, Pedersen JF, et al: Transperineal ^{125}Iodine seed implantation in prostatic cancer guided by transrectal ultrasonography. J Urol 130:283, 1983
22. Resnick MI, Willard JW, Boyce WH: Recent progress in ultrasonography of the bladder and prostate. J Urol 117:444, 1977
23. Resnick MI, Willard JW, Boyce WH: Transrectal ultrasonography in the evaluation of patients with prostatic carcinoma. J Urol 124:482, 1980
24. Lee F, Gray JM, McLeary RD, et al: Prostatic evaluation by transrectal sonography: Criteria for diagnosis of early carcinoma. Radiology 158:91, 1986
25. Lee F, Gray JM, McLeary RD, et al: Transrectal ultrasound in the diagnosis of prostatic cancer: Location, echogenicity, histopathology and staging. Prostate 7:117, 1985
26. Dahnert WF, Hamper UM, Eggleston JC, et al: Prostatic evaluation by transrectal sonography with histopathologic correlation: The echogenic appearance of early carcinoma. Radiology 158:97, 1986
27. Resnick MI: Evaluation of prostatic carcinoma: Non-invasive and preoperative techniques. Prostate 1:311, 1980
28. Cohen JM, Resnick MI: The use of transrectal ultrasonography in the diagnosis of stage A prostatic carcinoma. World J Urol 1:12, 1983
29. Pontes JE, Eisenkraft S, Watanabe H, et al: Preoperative evaluation of localized prostatic carcinoma by transrectal ultrasonography. J Urol 134:289, 1985
30. Egender G, Furtschegger A, Schachtner W, et al: Transrectal ultrasonography in diagnosis and staging of prostatic cancer. World J Urol 4:163, 1986
31. Bartsch G, Egender G, Hubscher H, Rohr H: Sonometrics of the prostate. J Urol 127:1119, 1982
32. Gastak SM, Gammelgaard J, Holm HH: Transrectal ultrasonic volume determination of the prostate: A pre-operative and post-operative study. J Urol 127:1115, 1982
33. Carpentier PJ, Schroeder FH, Schmitz PIM: Transrectal ultrasonometry of the prostate: The prognostic relevance of volume changes under endocrine management. World J Urol 4:159, 1986
34. Fujimo A, Scardino PT: Transrectal ultrasonography for prostatic cancer: Its value in staging and monitoring the response to radiotherapy and chemotherapy. J Urol 133:806, 1985
35. Liddell HT, McDougal WS, Burks DD, Fleischer AC: Ultrasound versus digitally directed prostatic needle biopsy. J Urol 135:716, 1986

36. Resnick MI: Transrectal ultrasound guided versus digitally directed prostate biopsy: A comparative study. Proc Am Urol Assoc Ann Meet, Anaheim, California, 1987
37. Ljung BM, Cherrie R, Kaufman JJ: Fine needle aspiration biopsy of the prostate gland: A study of 103 cases with histological follow-up. J Urol 135:955, 1986
38. Carter HB, Riehle RA Jr, Koizumi JH, et al: Fine needle aspiration of the abnormal prostate: A cytohistological correlation. J Urol 135:294, 1986
39. Watanabe H, Ohe H, Inabe T, et al: A mobile mass screening unit for prostatic disease. Prostate 5:559, 1984
40. Resnick MI: Use of transrectal ultrasound in evaluating prostatic cancer. J Urol 134:314, 1985
41. Resnick MI: Editorial comments—Methods of detecting prostatic tumors. In Ratliff TL, Catalona WC (eds): Urologic Oncology vol III. The Netherlands, Martinus Nijhoff, 1987
42. Chodak GW, Wald V, Parmer E, et al: Comparison of digital examination and transrectal ultrasonography for the diagnosis of prostatic cancer. J Urol 135:951, 1986
43. McNeal JE, Kindrachuk RA, Freiha FS, et al: Patterns of progression in prostate cancer. Lancet 1:60, 1986

Piezoelectric Extracorporeal Lithotripsy by Ultra Short Waves with the EDAP LT 01

G. Vallancien, J. Dory, P.H. Thibault, and J.M. Brisset

INTRODUCTION

Extracorporeal shock wave lithotripsy has demonstrated its capacity to treat 80 percent of all renal stones.[1,2] The published results reveal that complete elimination of the stones is achieved in an average of about 75 percent of cases at 3 months. The best success rates have been obtained in cases of single renal pelvic stones less than 25 mm in diameter.[3–5] Virtually all of the published data and clinical use to date have been based upon the Dornier Lithotriptor, a machine that generates hydroelectric shock waves.

Unfortunately, lithotripsy by hydroelectric shock waves requires a complicated infrastructure and equipment with a very high initial investment and extremely high operating costs. Primarily for these economic reasons, multiple efforts to produce alternative types of lithotriptors have been underway for several years.

One of these efforts has resulted in a piezoelectric extracorporeal litho-

Editor's Note: The Editor went to Paris in February, 1987 to see the EDAP machine in operation and was impressed enough with it that he asked Dr. Guy Vallancien, the principal urologist associated with the development and testing of the EDAP lithotriptor, to write the chapter printed here. The Editor is quite convinced that the piezoelectric type of lithotriptor, using ultrasound localization, is the "wave of the future" for all of the various reasons noted in this chapter. Both EDAP and Wolf are making piezoelectric lithotriptors at the present time and both machines have had extensive human trials in Europe. By the time that this volume is published, both of these machines should be in the United States undergoing clinical trials in order to secure Food and Drug Administration approval to market them here.

triptor, LT 01, which requires no specific infrastructure and virtually no running costs, and has been developed in collaboration with the EDAP company (France). Following a phase to demonstrate the safety and efficacy of the machine,[6] preliminary clinical trials using a prototype were conducted in 1985 in 74 patients and demonstrated encouraging results with a global fragmentation rate of 60 percent.[7]

This review presents the analysis of 433 consecutive treatments performed between January 1986 and January 1987 by the same team, using the lithotriptor developed from the prototype.

BASIS OF THE PIEZOELECTRIC SYSTEM

Disintegration Mechanism (Fig. 1)

A solid substance breaks when a stress greater than the limit known as the critical load is applied.

Fracture may take place at stress values below this limit if an alternating load is applied. There is nevertheless a minimal stress below which the substance will never break, regardless of the number of cycles imposed. This value is known as the fatigue limit and must of course be exceeded in lithotripsy although in this case it is not necessary to attain critical load. Indeed, experience has shown that excess power results in coarser disintegration. It must be added that stress may be either positive (compression) or negative (tension). It is easy to apply stress to a substance if all sides thereof are directly accessible. In this case, any prehensile power device is perfectly suitable.

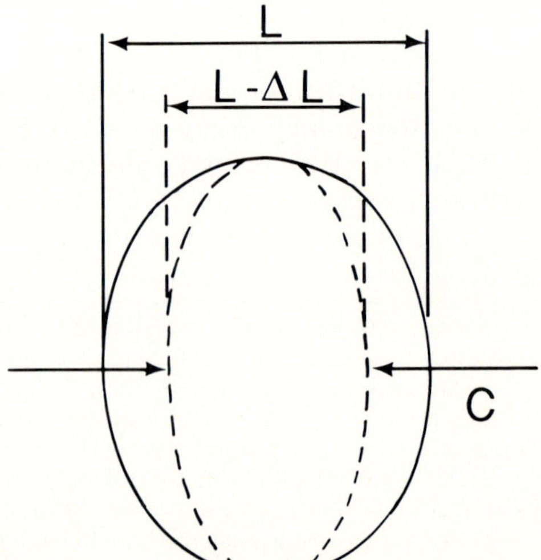

Figure 1. A stress "C" applied to a structure is accompanied by a distortion ΔL/L.

A stress "C" is always accompanied by a relative distortion ΔL/L and vice versa. These two values are linked in the relation

$$C = E \times \Delta L/L$$

where E is the material's elastic modulus.

Problem of Remote Disintegration

Things become more complex, because it is not possible to have direct access to the substance to be destroyed, as would be the case with renal calculi. Stress must then be transmitted from a distance to the substance to be destroyed. Since transmission implies waves, the only solution is to use what are known as "elastic waves."

Elastic Waves (Fig. 2)

Any change in pressure or any elementary movement initiated at a point in a substance is propagated from this point in the form of elastic waves. These waves may propagate in gases, liquids, and solids but not in a vacuum. As opposed to electromagnetic waves, they require a material medium.

Propagation speed depends on the type of ambient medium—approximately 300 m/s in gases, 1500 m/s in liquids, and 3000 to 10,000 m/s in solids. These waves are given different names depending on their shape and frequency, e.g., acoustic waves, sounds, ultrasounds, shock waves. Nevertheless, all these varieties of elastic waves obey the same propagation principles and are governed by the same equations.

Shock waves are somewhat more specific since they appear when a body in motion in a fluid travels faster than the speed of sound in that fluid. The most prominent example of this is the well-known sonic boom caused by supersonic aircraft. This phenomenon is due to the sudden increase in pressure at the front of the moving body when it catches up to the wave

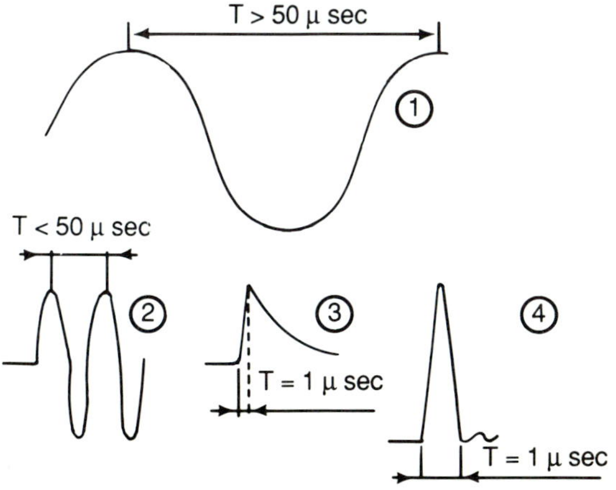

Figure 2. Different kinds of elastic waves: acoustic waves (1); ultrasonic waves (2); shock waves (3); and impulse waves (for lithotripsy) (4). T = time period of oscillation.

produced by it in its movement. This wave has a very steep wave front followed by a gradual tailing off. It is exceptional for waves to be generated in liquids in this fashion and lithotriptor "shock waves" are produced by more conventional means.

Choosing the Type of Elastic Wave for Lithotripsy (Fig. 3)

Several phenomena occur in the surrounding medium in which an elastic wave is propagated:

1. *Relative distortion,* accompanied by the corresponding stress. These two parameters depend only on the wave's specific power (intensity).
2. *Global displacement* around the quiescent point. This displacement is proportional to the square root of the signal's intensity as well as to its duration.

A stress, and therefore a minimum intensity, must be attained to destroy a calculus. Calculations show that the intensity (I) in a calculus, rated in watts/cm^2, is equal to:

$$I\ (W/cm^2) \simeq 0.6 \times C^2(kg/cm^2)$$

This is given here as an average value since the 0.6 coefficient may depend on the type of calculus.

If one wishes to attain a stress of 500 kg/cm^2, enough to destroy most calculi, the intensity needed is therefore equal to I = 150,000 W/cm^2. However, as a result of phenomena related to reflections at the interfaces, scarcely one fifth of incident energy penetrates into the calculus. In fact, an intensity of some 75 kW/cm^2 must therefore be created at the focal point. This intensity is actually far greater if one takes into account losses caused

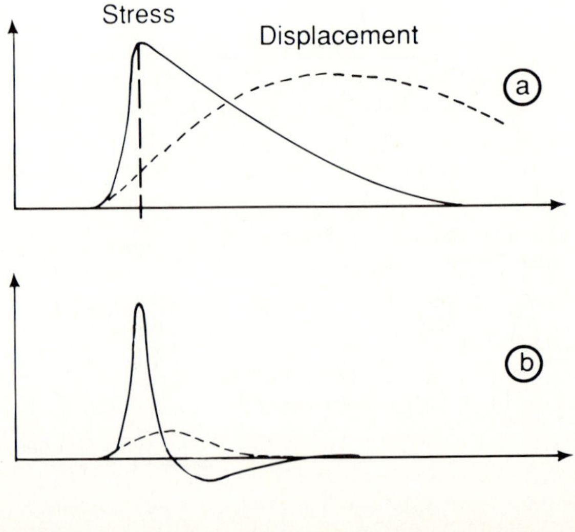

Figure 3. Stress and displacement of a structure submitted to an elastic wave: shock wave (electrohydraulic generator) (a); short impulse (piezoelectric generator) (b).

by forces such as absorption and diffraction. This is true *regardless of the wave form used.*

One may therefore be led to believe that any elastic wave form is suitable for destroying a calculus, provided that its intensity is sufficient. One must, however, take a certain number of factors into consideration:

- *Average power must be low* so as to avoid overheating tissues. This precludes the use of continuous waves and imposes the need to work with short pulses.
- *The amplitude of displacements must be as small as possible* so as to reduce risk of injury to biologic tissues. This implies the use of short pulses. The situation is particularly critical at gas interfaces as displacements may quickly attain dangerous amplitudes there if pulse duration is excessive.
- *It must be possible to focus the wave* so as to center energy on the calculus and in the smallest possible zone. According to theory, the shorter the signal the more efficient is focusing.

The foregoing considerations show that all factors point to the choice of elastic waves with pulses of very short duration, easy to focus, and capable of disintegrating calculi without displacing or damaging tissues. One is nevertheless limited in this area by the absorption factor, which is all the more important as pulse duration is shorter, as it prevents wave propagation. A good compromise is reached by choosing pulses with a duration of some 1 μsec. This type of pulse allows for excellent focusing and little of it is absorbed by biologic tissues through which it passes without causing any damage. This, then, represents the ideal wave form for lithotripsy. The question is how to generate it and how to obtain sufficient intensity to achieve stresses of some 500 kg/cm^2 (approximately 500 bars or 5×10^7 Pas) at the focal point. Total peak power is important. Considering safety margins, one must allow for 150 kW/cm^2 at the focal point. It is therefore advisable to have a small focal point so as to limit global power requirements.

Elastic Wave Generation and Focusing (Fig. 4)

Two types of generators may be used:

1. *Point source generators:* The elastic pulse is generated at a point with the smallest possible volume. Spherical divergent waves thus produced are refocused by mirrors or lenses.
2. *Dispersed source generators:* Pulses are emitted from a surface where all points vibrate in phase (coherent source). The wave produced may be focused merely by giving a spherical shape to the emitting surface. Lenses may also be used.

Point source generators were the first to be used, probably because they were the only generators available at the time of the first experiments. The best known and practically the only generator operated uses a very

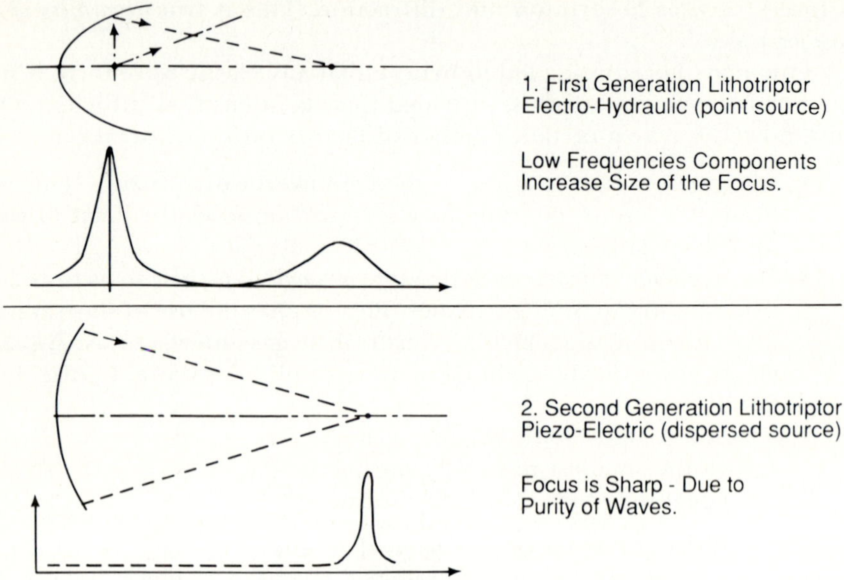

Figure 4. Variation of acoustic pressure along the axis.

powerful electric field to induce, in water, an explosive steam generation. This method should have no more than an historic interest due to a large number of shortcomings:

- Extremely rapid consumption of electrodes on account of the enormous concentration of energy at the source
- Unstable focal point position, especially with consumed electrodes
- Impossibility of controlling the form of the signal produced which is accompanied by an interference drag increasing its duration, thus causing the appearance of a large number of undesirable components dangerous for tissues through which it must pass

Moreover, this type of pulse may provoke heart beat disturbances and therefore necessitates a synchronization of discharges with the refractory period of the cardiac pulse and this is monitored with an ECG.

All of these shortcomings are avoided by employing dispersed source generators which are much more recent. It would seem that the most efficient and reliable of such generators use the piezoelectricity phenomenon (deformation of a special material when subjected to an electric field). The form of the wave emitted reproduces that of the exciting electric signal and, under these circumstances, it is possible to obtain a pulse whose shape is very close to the ideal form allowed for in the theoretical study. Optimum performance is obtained by using an electronic generator to produce the exciting electric signal, thus enabling perfect control of wave form and amplitude. Experience has shown that this type of generator is very efficient and remarkably untraumatic, to such an extent that treatments can be conducted without any form of anesthesia.

Localizing the Calculus

It must be possible to localize the focal point on the calculus with accuracy. This necessitates a localization device.

Two methods may be used:

1. *X-ray system:* To obtain the position of the calculus, two views taken from different angles must be observed. The operation is greatly facilitated if two brilliancy amplifiers are available.

   This method is relatively easy to use but exposes the patient to considerable radiation and does not allow localization of radiolucent calculi or permanent observation of the lithiasis. Furthermore, since the type of wave used for localization is totally different from that used for treatment, it is not possible to verify actual transmission possibility and thus choose the best discharge "window." For instance, a gas interface is an insurmountable obstacle for elastic waves while being perfectly permeable to x-rays.
2. *Ultrasound scanning:* Ultrasound scans provide tomographic type cross-section views. A single view suffices therefore to perfectly localize the calculus. The images are a bit more difficult to interpret but this technique is very quickly learned.

   An elastic wave is used this time and is therefore the same type of wave as that used for treatment. This makes it possible to choose the best discharge position and to avoid any obstacles, provided of course that the localization probe is properly placed in relation to the treatment head.

   The absence of any ionizing radiation enables, on well-designed devices, constant monitoring of the calculus during discharges. Any stone movement is immediately detected and the position of the head can be readjusted. Discharges may even be stopped automatically in the event of a position error.

THE LITHOTRIPTOR

The instrument consists of a processing head, composed of an ultrasonographic system for localization of the stone and a piezoelectric destruction system (Fig. 5).

The localization system is composed of a real-time 5 MHz sector ultrasound transducer situated in the center of a spherical cup oriented in the axis of the pressure focus. This is a rotating transducer which is able to provide longitudinal and transverse images and all oblique views.

The destruction system results from the convergence of a series of ul-

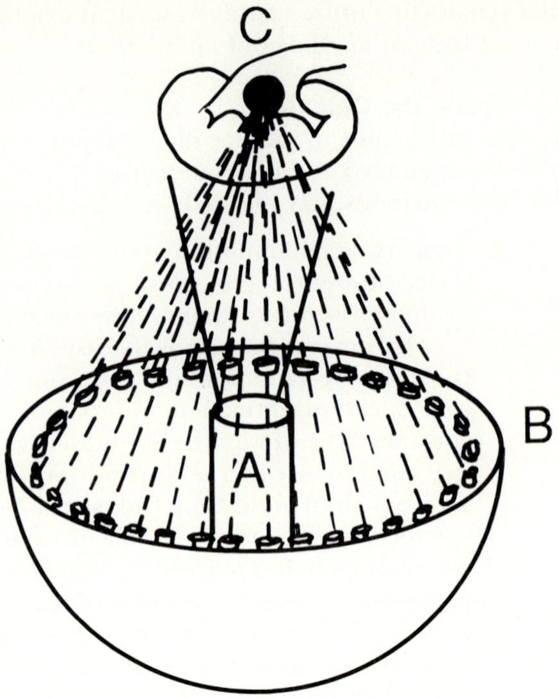

Figure 5. Diagram of the moving treatment head: central 5 MHz adjustable real-time ultrasound localization probe (a); piezoelectric elements focused at point C which is to be brought up to the stone by maneuvering the moving head (b).

trashort impulses generated by 320 ceramics activated by the piezoelectric effect. The ceramics are distributed over the surface of the spherical cup around the detection transducer.

The acoustic waves generated for the detection and destruction of the stone are transmitted through a non-degased water pouch of variable height adjusted by means of a reservoir. The elastic membrane of the water pouch impregnated with jelly is placed in contact with the patient's lumbar fossa.

All of the processing head can be oriented in every direction, allowing selection of the best firing axis. The energy delivered can be adjusted by means of a potentiometer and reaches a maximum of about 900 bars in vitro. The rate of firing varies between 1.25 and 160 per second. The elastic wave generated has extremely steep sides, reaching its maximum within one millionth of a second. It falls as rapidly as it rises and does not possess any significant negative components. The pressure focus is about 5 mm wide and 15 mm high.

An adapted bed allows a plain x-ray or fluoroscopic image to be performed by horizontal rotation. This bed is fitted with two leg pieces allowing endoscopic manipulations such as placement of a double-J ureteral stent concomitant with the extracorporeal lithotripsy.

PATIENTS

Four hundred thirty-three lithotripsies have been performed in 386 patients, consisting of 253 men, 129 women, and 4 children.

The mean age was 45.5 years (minimum: 8, maximum: 81); mean weight was 75.4 kg (range: 28 to 115 kg); 174 patients (45 percent) had a past history of calculi and 104 (27 percent) had undergone at least one operation for renal stones; 50 patients (13 percent) also presented with asymptomatic urinary tract infection; 336 (87 percent) had sterile urine before treatment.

All of the patients referred to us in the Department of Urology with an indication for lithotripsy were treated by the same lithotriptor (Fig. 6) without any prior selection of the cases. The contraindications were patients with symptomatic urinary tract infection, patients with major blood dyscrasias or severe hypertension, and those with an obstructive anomaly of the lower urinary tract or a nonfunctioning kidney.

Patients with cardiac arrhythmias were able to be treated in the same way as the others. A systematic study of 200 cases with continuous cardiac recordings and a study of 50 patients by Holter monitoring demonstrated the total absence of arrhythmias related to the short wave emission.

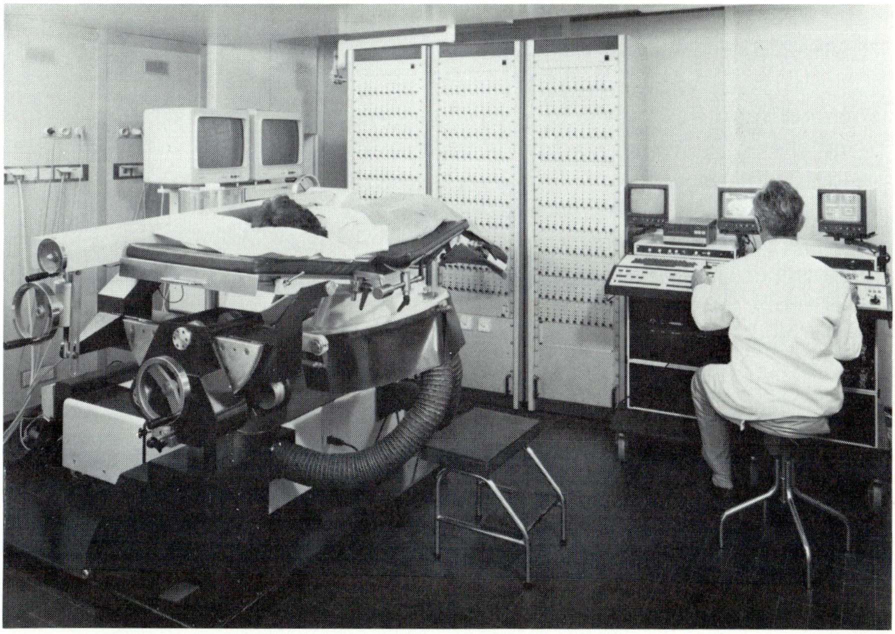

Figure 6. Entire lithotriptor unit in operation as a patient is being treated.

TABLE 1. SITE OF THE RENAL STONES

	Single Stone		Multiple Stones	
	No.	%	*No.*	%
Renal pelvis	104	30	17	5
Superior calyx	10	3	—	—
Middle calyx	10	3	3	1
Inferior calyx	175	51	23	7
Total	299	87	43	13

RENAL STONES

The features of the stones treated are summarized in Tables 1 and 2. The mean dimension of the stones was 13.2 mm with a range of 3 to 50 mm.

Seven stones in solitary kidneys and five cases of bilateral stones were treated. The stones were composed of calcium oxalate in 89 percent of cases, struvite in 9.5 percent of cases, uric acid in 1 percent of cases, and cystine in 0.5 percent of cases.

TECHNIQUE

The operation was commenced by ultrasonographic detection of the stones by means of a manual 3.5- or 5-MHz transducer with the patient sitting on a stool. This preliminary detection enabled the operator to rapidly determine the correct axes of inclination of the mobile head.

The patient gets onto the bed and the firing head is mobilized to bring the focus of the lithotriptor in contact with the stone. The treatment is followed continuously on the ultrasound screen until fragmentation of the stone. The signs of good fragmentation of the stone are linear appearance

TABLE 2. DIMENSIONS OF THE RENAL STONES

	No.	%
<1 cm	168	49
1–2 cm	153	44
2–3 cm	20	6
>3 cm	3	1

Mean dimension = 13.2 mm

of the interface of the stone and widening of the conical acoustic shadow (Figs. 7 and 8).

We have always compared these ultrasonographic findings to those obtained on pre- and postlithotripsy fluoroscopy. The mean duration of treatment was 35 minutes at low frequency, with a range of 10 minutes to 1 hour. The mean number of shocks was 2700 at 1.25 shocks/sec.

The mean postoperative hospital stay was 2.5 days when anesthesia was necessary.

ANESTHESIA

One hundred sixty-one patients were treated under anesthesia at a rate of 120 impacts/sec and the rate was then gradually reduced until, at a rate of 1.25/sec, it was found possible to perform the treatment without any anesthesia, i.e., no premedication, no local anesthesia, no general or regional anesthesia, and no sedation. The brief ascending slope of the wave without a pressure tail appears to be the origin for the possibility of this treatment without anesthesia, as there is barely enough time for pain to be experienced by the patient. At rates higher than 5 per second, analgesia is re-

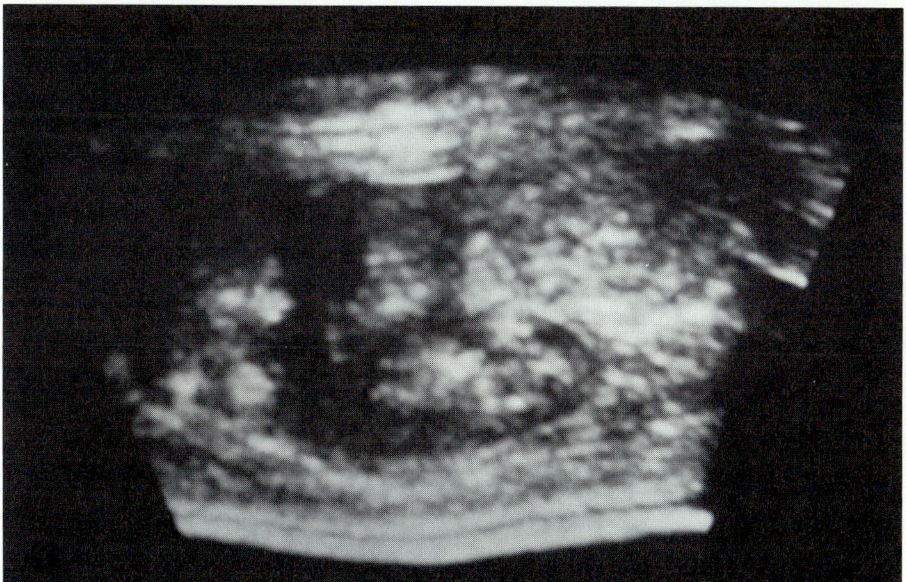

Figure 7. Ultrasound image of the pelvic stone at the beginning of discharges. The calculus is in the middle of the kidney and the characteristic "umbra" or shadow is seen directly above the calculus and running directly in a superior direction.

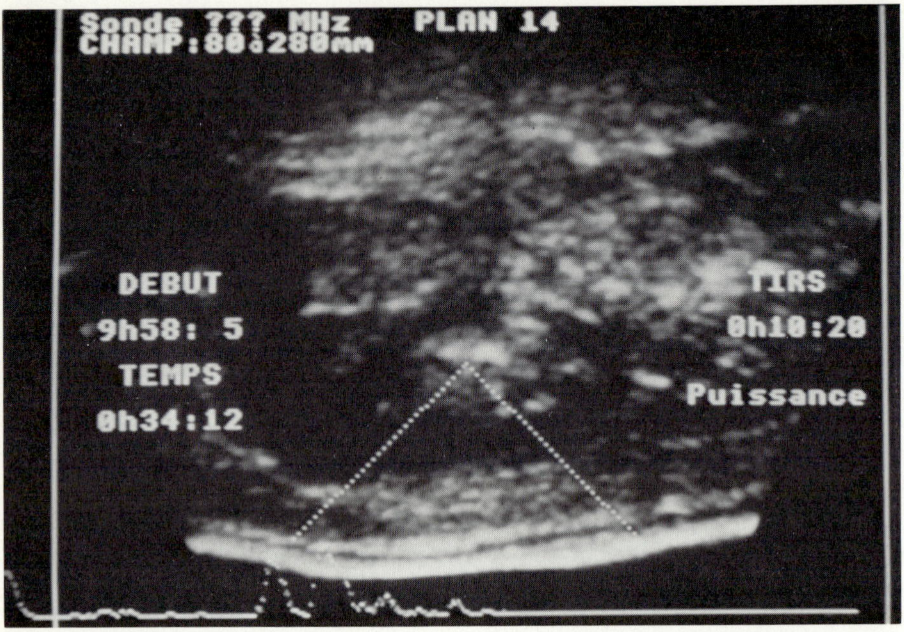

A

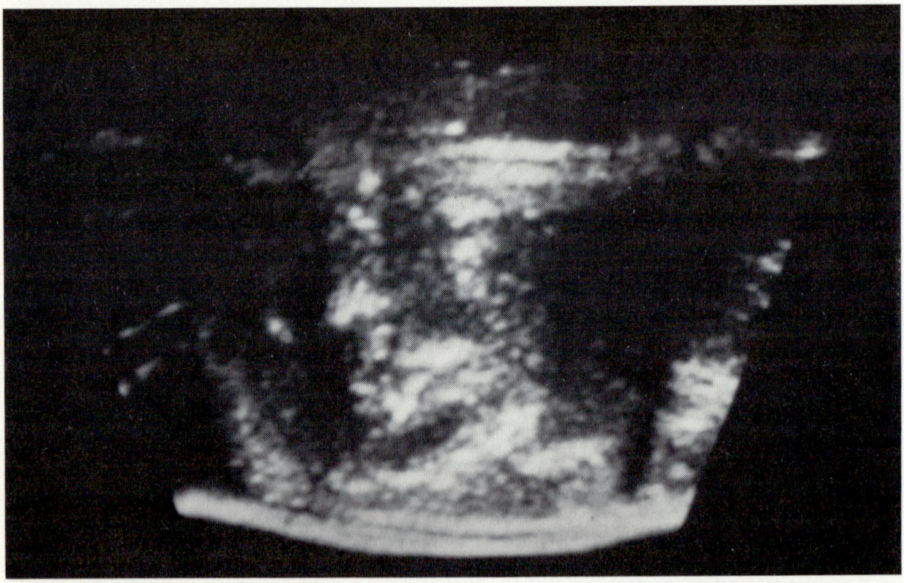

B

Figure 8. A. Ultrasound image of the same calculus seen longitudinally and disintegrated at the end of discharges. The conic image of the stone interface has become linear and the umbra has widened. **B.** Same aspect at the end of discharges in a transversal view.

quired. The reduction in the firing rate increases the operating time by about 30 percent.

At the present time, we treat one patient per hour. Overall, general anesthesia was used in 42 cases, including 20 cases that were combined with endoscopic procedures for flushing of ureteric stones, and neurolept-analgesia was used in 181 cases. Since August 1986, 210 patients have been treated without any analgesia, sedation, or anesthesia. In 8 percent of cases, a transient vagal reaction, e.g., nausea, vomiting, sweating, was observed but did not require any particular treatment.

ADMISSION TO HOSPITAL

One hundred three patients with renal stones less than 20 mm in diameter were treated on an outpatient basis. In order to perform this outpatient treatment, we selected patients in good general health under the age of 70 years and with no signs of associated urinary tract infection. The patients came to the center, underwent lithotripsy, and left half an hour after the procedure. Written explanations were given to these patients concerning the possible incidents likely to occur after the procedure. Only four patients had to be admitted to hospital for renal colic or fever.

The development of outpatient extracorporeal lithotripsy has further modified the indications for the technique. Small, asymptomatic caliceal stones can obviously now be treated by outpatient piezoelectric lithotripsy. Only two patients in this group of patients treated on an outpatient basis requested a certificate for absence from work. The economic benefit of this form of extracorporeal lithotripsy without admission to hospital, which is currently under evaluation, already appears to be extremely important.

TRAINING

Urologists from other centers currently using the EDAP lithotriptor have come to the Department of Urology for training periods of 1 or 2 weeks. Although ultrasound-guided extracorporeal lithotripsy is a new technique, it can be learned relatively quickly and requires above all a good understanding of volume and planes in space.

RESULTS

The destruction of the stone was evaluated on plain x-ray films and on ultrasonograms performed during the 48 hours following treatment and then after 1 month and after 3 months. The evaluation of the safety of the technique was based on clinical data, ultrasonography, and intravenous pyelography performed after 1 month. In addition, 50 computed tomography (CT) scans and 45 complete laboratory surveys were also performed in patients receiving high frequency (120 per second) and low frequency (1.5 to 5 per second) lithotripsy, in the context of a standardization protocol. Four groups of patients were distinguished:

1. *Group I:* 148 patients with renal stones (calyx and/or renal pelvis), treated by a single session between January and July 1986, during which time the lithotriptor derived from the prototype was still undergoing improvements—modifications of the bed, modification of the ultrasound detection transducer, and increase in the power of the elastic waves. As a result of these modifications, the fragmentation rate at 48 hours increased from 19 of 29 cases in January (66 percent of cases) to 35 of 39 cases in July (90 percent of cases).

   One hundred twenty-four patients were reviewed after 3 months; 78 (63 percent) had completely eliminated the stones (no residual fragments visible on the plain film); 26 cases (21 percent) had persistent fragments in the renal cavities which, in 15 cases, were smaller than 5 mm in diameter and, in 11 cases, more than 5 mm in diameter; 20 cases (16 percent) had to be considered to be failures.
2. *Group II:* 184 patients had renal stones and were treated at a single session between August 1986 and January 1987. These patients were treated with the machine following the improvements described above. Effective fragmentation was obtained by 48 hours in 169 cases (92 percent); 15 cases (8 percent) were considered to be failures. These failures, like those in group I, generally corresponded to patients with a stone situated more than 10 cm from the skin, tightly wedged stones, or stones in extrarenal pelvises.

   At 3 months, 126 patients in this group had a sufficient follow-up and 93 patients had been completely reviewed; 62 of them (67 percent) had no residual fragments, 20 (22 percent) had stone fragments which could be eliminated, and 9 (10 percent) were considered to be failures.
3. *Group III:* 42 patients with renal calculi were treated by two sessions (37 cases) or three sessions (5 cases). This group included patients who were considered to be failures or partial successes at the time of treatment with the prototype or before the improvements were made to the second machine.

   At the 48th hour, fragmentation was achieved in 34 patients (81 percent). This success rate is good in view of the fact that the stones were more refractory in these cases; 29 patients were reviewed after 3 months: a complete success was obtained in 20 cases (69 percent).

   Global results: Overall, in the 217 patients in these three groups of renal stones reviewed after 3 months, 156 (72 percent) were con-

TABLE 3. RESULTS OBTAINED AFTER 3 MONTHS IN THE 217 PATIENTS REVIEWED (KIDNEY STONES)

Complete Success		Partial Success		Failures		2 Sessions	
No.	%	*No.*	%	*No.*	%	No.	%
156	72	35	16	27	12	30	14

sidered to be complete successes; 27 of these patients (12 percent) had to undergo two or three treatment sessions (Table 3).

4. *Group IV:* 54 patients had a stone in the ureter or bladder; 31 patients had a stone in the lumbar ureter (mean dimension: 9 mm); 7 of them underwent lithotripsy in situ: 3 failures, 4 successes. In 21 cases, the stone was pushed back into the renal pelvis or calices by means of a ureteric catheter inserted on the lithotriptor itself: 21 successes (95 percent) and 1 failure; 3 cases were treated with a contact catheter: 2 successes (67 percent).

   Fifteen stones of the pelvic ureter (mean dimension: 7 mm), situated in the last 3 centimeters, were treated with the patient in the abdominal position without ureteric catheter and without anesthesia. The stone was completely or partially fragmented in seven cases and was totally eliminated within the first month.

   Eight cases were considered to be failures. These failures can be attributed to problems of localization of the stone and to the depth of the pelvic ureter (frequently more than 9 cm from the skin).

   Eight bladder stones were treated: four successes, four failures. In every case, the failures occurred in the presence of hard large stones with a diameter of more than 3 cm.

MORBIDITY

Morbidity is summarized in Table 4. There were no deaths and no nephrectomies. Obstructive complications were rare (Table 5): nine extractions (2 percent) by dormia basket or ureteroscopy. Two repeat lithotripsies were successfully performed for fragments obstructing the lumbar ureter. Percutaneous nephrolithotomy was only performed in failures of complete fragmentation in 14 cases. When percutaneous nephrolithotomy was performed early after extracorporeal lithotripsy (within 3 days), no particular damage of the cavities was observed on endoscopy. In three cases, the stone had started to fragment and it is possible that a simple prolongation of the extracorporeal lithotripsy may have avoided the need for the percutaneous procedure.

TABLE 4. COMPLICATIONS

	No.	%
Subcapsular hematomas	8	1.6
Trauma to adjacent organ	0	
Ureteric obstruction	11	2.5
Renal colic	73	17
Fever	19	4.5
Bacteremia	2	
Renal failure	0	
Nephrectomy	0	
Death	0	
Cardiac arrest (anesthetic shock)	1 recovered	

In three cases, percutaneous nephrolithotomy was performed before lithotripsy in order to decrease the volume of the stone (complex pyelocaliceal stones).

In 73 cases (17 percent), renal colic occurred after the procedure and was relieved by usual analgesics.

Nineteen patients (5 percent) developed a fever higher than 38°C, which resolved with antibiotics; two of them had bacteremia.

Thirteen patients developed posterior cutaneous petechiae when the firing rate was 120/sec. No subcutaneous hematomas or petechiae have been observed since the introduction of slower firing rates.

All of the patients developed moderate hematuria which, with slow firing rates, resolved after one or two micturitions. With the earlier treatment at rapid frequencies, seven subcapsular hematomas (1.5 percent) were detected on ultrasonography or on CT scan. None of them required surgical reoperation or blood transfusion.[7]

Since the use of slow firing rates, 1 small hematoma (5 × 10 mm) has been detected in the 125 patients followed (0.8 percent).

CT almost always reveals moderate perirenal edema with thickening

TABLE 5. CONCOMITANT OPERATIONS

Ureteric endoscopy	9
Flush and lithotripsy	2
Ureterotomy	1
Pyelotomy	2
Secondary percutaneous lithotripsy	14
Scheduled percutaneous lithotripsy	3

TABLE 6. ALTERATIONS IN LABORATORY PARAMETERS

	24 hr Before (mmol)	24 hr After (mmol)
Creatinine	101	102
LDH	202	240
CPK	118	158
Amylase	41.3	32.7
Platelets	320,000	300,000
Leukocytes	7,800	8,200
Hematocrit	42	42
Hemoglobin	11.3	11.5

of the retrorenal fascia at the 24th hour. With low frequencies we have never observed images of parenchymal trauma as previously described.[6,7] No lesions of adjacent organs were detected. In particular, we did not observe any pulmonary lesions when extracorporeal lithotripsy was performed for superior caliceal stones.

No cases of renal failure were observed in our series, even in the seven cases with a single kidney. The results of the laboratory tests before and after treatment are presented in Table 6; none of the modifications of the parameters measured were significant. Studies of the medium-term and long-term effects on renal function are currently underway.

DISCUSSION

Since the preliminary clinical results reported in 1980 by Chaussy et al,[8] lithotripsy has become the technique most frequently used to treat renal stones. It has gradually been extended to the treatment of stones in the lumbar ureter and the pelvic ureter.

Since the beginning of our experience in September 1985, the use of a lithotriptor generating ultra short wave impulses by a piezoelectric effect with ultrasonographic detection of the stone has proved to be a technique of the future which requires a number of comments.

Detection

One of the most controversial points is the accuracy of the ultrasonographic localization of the renal stones.

During our preliminary studies with the prototype,[7] 10 percent of the stones could not be detected, 20 percent were difficult to detect, and 70 percent were easily detected. In the last 184 cases of renal stones treated, the stones could not be detected in 5 cases (2.7 percent), and, in 18 cases (10 percent), they were considered by the operators to be difficult to detect.

This progress is essentially due to the improvement in the equipment and also to the greater experience of the operators.

The localization of small caliceal stones less than 5 mm in diameter is only occasionally difficult (the acoustic shadow is almost always obvious and we have only had two failures of detection in these cases).

On the other hand, the localization of larger stones, particularly when they are situated in an extrasinusal pelvis close to the spine or in an obese patient, may be difficult. Certain technical things, such as positioning of the head of the lithotriptor and the operator's experience, play a definite role in the success of these cases.

The ribs do not constitute a real obstacle because of the mobility of the firing head which enables them to be avoided. However, the ribs may interfere with detection of the stones in 7 percent of cases.

Considerable progress has been made in ultrasonographic imaging over recent years and further improvements will be made in the future.

Other teams also use ultrasound to locate stones during extracorporeal lithotripsy with satisfactory results.[9,10]

Fragmentation

In vitro, the elastic wave generated by ceramics has a constant form and pressure. There is no wear-and-tear effect on the generators which could attenuate the efficacy of the wave.

The small dimension of the pressure focus demands excellent visualization of the stone to ensure permanent control of the lithotripsy on the ultrasonography screen. When the patients are not anesthetized, respiration causes movements of the kidneys over a distance of 5 to 20 mm, allowing spontaneous distribution of the pressure wave over all of the stone. At the beginning of the session, we show the ultrasonography screen, the pressure focus, and the image of the stone to the patient and we ask him or her to adapt his or her respiratory movements in order to maintain the stone within the pressure focus.

Continuous radio–ultrasonographic comparison has enabled us to demonstrate the signs of good fragmentation, i.e., transformation of the interface of the stone, which is intially curved, into a straight line and enlargement of the acoustic shadow. However, these images are not constant: in particular, in cases in which the stones are situated in narrow renal cavities, and x-ray control immediately after the procedure still seems to be necessary at the present time.

We estimate the failure or partial success rate due to an excessively short fire to be 60 percent and experience has taught us to increase the treatment time by 10 minutes after the stone appears to be well fragmented.

The failures of fragmentation which we continue to observe are related to the long focal distance of the stone (more than 10 cm from the skin), to the impacted nature of the stone, to its hardness (nonhydrated calcium oxalate, uric acid, or cystine), or to its volume (more than 3 cc). Three recent cases of impacted stones have been drained preoperatively by a double J stent which definitely seems to facilitate the fragmentation, creating an expansion chamber and limiting the pelvic or ureteric edema.[11]

Friable stones (struvite) are a good indication for piezoelectric lithotripsy and staghorn stones can be treated by cutting a first part of the calculus with the small focus of pressure and by waiting for the elimination of fragments before a second session on the remaining pieces.

Elimination

We consider that extracorporeal lithotripsy is the best treatment for nonimpacted stones of the renal pelvis measuring less the 20 mm, small mobile caliceal stones, and stones of the upper ureter provided a flushing technique or a contact catheter is used.[11]

The least satisfactory results are obtained with inferior caliceal stones situated in calculous pockets or in caliceal diverticuli with a narrow neck. Intermediate results are obtained in inferior caliceal stones without any significant expansion chamber. These results are similar to those obtained in the American multicenter study.[3] It is important to emphasize that in our study, 65 percent of stones were caliceal and we have consistently refused to pre-select or exclude certain patients so as to put ourselves in the same situation as every other department of urology. Above all, we wanted to know the exact possibilities of the piezoelectric system instead of just trying to obtain a very high success rate by a strict selection of the cases.

Functioning of the Lithotriptor

The piezoelectric lithotriptor presents a certain number of advantages: the absence of immersion, no need for a specific operating room, the mobility of the apparatus, the possibility of locating radiolucent or faintly opaque stones, moderate purchase and maintenance costs, and the almost complete lack of use of consumable material, apart from ultrasonography jelly. One urologist helped by one technician is enough for the procedure.

Over the first year of use of this new machine, we had to change the rubber membrane of the water bag because of rupture four times (changing time: 15 minutes) and we had to change the detection transducer of the lithotriptor (changing time: 15 minutes) once. None of the procedures were cancelled because of equipment failure.

CONCLUSION

The results of this series confirm the value of piezoelectric extracorporeal lithotripsy with ultrasonographic detection of the stone: the visualization of the stone is good and the fragmentation is effective.

These results reflect the progress accomplished since the development of the prototype and we continue to improve the instrument.

Today, the total absence of anesthesia in 95 percent of cases (only patients undergoing a concomitant endoscopic manipulation are anesthetized) and now the possibility of treating patients without admission to hospital in more than two thirds of cases constitute real therapeutic and economic advances.

Ultrasound, which has become an essential part of diagnosis in urology, is now revealing an extremely large field of therapeutic applications. It is essential for the urologist to realize the importance of mastering this technique, the first aspect of which we can refer to as "telesurgery."[12]

REFERENCES

1. Chaussy C, Schiedt E, Jocham D, et al: Extra corporeal shock wave lithotripsy (ESWL) for treatment of urolithiasis. Urology 23:59, 1984
2. Alken P, Hardeman S, Wilbert D, et al: Extra corporeal shock wave lithotripsy (ESWL): Alternatives and adjuvant procedures. Wld J Urol 3:48, 1985
3. Drach GW, Dretler S, Fair W, et al: Report of the United States cooperative study of extra corporeal shock wave lithotripsy. J Urol 135:1127, 1986
4. Lingeman J, Newman D, Mertz JO, et al: Extra corporeal shock wave lithotripsy: The Methodist Hospital of Indiana experience. J Urol 135:1134, 1986
5. Fuchs G, Miller K, Rassweiter J, Eisenberger F: Extra corporeal shock wave lithotripsy: One year experience with the Dornier lithotriptor. Eur Urol 11:145, 1985
6. Thibault PH, Dory J, Cotard JP, et al: Lithotripsie à impulsions ultra-courtes. Etude expérimentale sur une lithiase rénale du chien. Ann Urol 20:20, 1986
7. Thibault PH, Vallancien G, Brisset JM: Lithotripsie corporelle à impulsions ultra-courtes. Premières applications cliniques du lithotripteur. Press Med 15:1283, 1986
8. Chaussy C, Brendel W, Schmiedt E: Extra corporeally induced destruction of kidney stones by shock waves. Lancet 2:1265, 1980
9. Martin X, Mestas JL, Cathignol D, et al: Ultrasound stone localization for extra corporeal shock wave lithotripsy. Br J Urol 58:349, 1986
10. Ziegler M, Kopper B, Riedlinger R, et al: Die Zertrümmerung von Nierensteinen mit einem piezoelektrischen Geräte-system. Urologe (A) 25:193, 1986
11. Mueller SC, Wilbert D, Thueroff JW, Alken P: Extra corporeal shock wave lithotripsy of ureteral stones: Clinical experience and experimental findings. J Urol 135:831, 1986
12. Vallancien G: La télé-chirurgie. Press Med 15:2184, 1986

Current Management of Erectile Dysfunction

John J. Mulcahy

During the past decade, urologists have become the primary physicians in the treatment of impotence. With the arrival of the prototype models of our current penile prostheses, there is now a definitive way of treating almost any type of impotence problem. This has stimulated in-depth research into the anatomy and physiology of erections, an area which has long been neglected because of the attitudes of society towards this problem. Discussions about impotence are now occurring regularly on television talk shows and in newspaper columns and in all major cities in the country support groups are springing up to provide information for people who are faced with this unfortunate problem who would otherwise have nowhere to turn. In past years, a patient would consult his clergyman or turn to his family doctor for help when erectile dysfunction began. All too often, either of these sources would communicate a feeling of embarrassment or lack the knowledge or ability to definitively solve the problem. The patient always broaches the subject with some trepidation, and if he turns to his pastor or physician as the first source of help and receives a message of embarrassment or hesitation from this person, the patient may become reticent and may remain silent, never to speak about his problem again. Many physicians are more concerned with other parts of the body and consider erectile function more recreational than life threatening. They fail to realize, however, how psychologically devastating the lost erectile ability can be to a patient. Patients who become severely depressed because of their inability to perform as men often are noncompliant with medical regimens and their bodily functions deteriorate further. Alcoholism, absenteeism, decreased productivity, and irritability are traits not uncommonly seen in this group. It falls to urologists then, who are interested in this problem, to direct the evaluation and refer the patient to other appropriate sources of help when needed. Urologists should possess the necessary diagnostic acumen, have available to them the appropriate tests to make the diagnosis, and also institute the common treatments to bring about a successful resolution of the problem.

An erection occurs in response to neurologic input to the vascular supply of the penis as the arterioles within the spongy erectile tissue are opened thus flooding the venous sinusoids of the corpora cavernosa with blood.[1] The walls of the sinusoids relax allowing blood to flow in readily. As the sinusoids fill with blood, they pinch off or constrict the efferent venules which course between adjacent sinusoids. As the sinusoids fill, the pressure inside the corpora cavernosa rises and penile tumescence and rigidity develop.

Impotence, defined as the inability to achieve an erection suitable for satisfactory intercourse, can be classified into two basic types: psychologic or situational, and organic which is related to a number of disease states, medications, or physical injuries. In the late 1940s, Dr. Alfred Kinsey chronicalized the sexual habits of Americans and believed that the vast majority of cases of impotence were classified as psychologic.[2] As people are coming more to physicians seeking help, clinicians have studied this problem more accurately and with more precise diagnostic modalities, and they have found that well over one-half of the cases of impotence presenting to physicians are of the organic type. The initiating event of psychologic impotence is an episode of erectile failure. This may be due to one of a number of causes: fatigue, depression, obsessive/compulsive behavior, hostility towards the partner, a painful or awkward sexual encounter in the inexperienced male, or any episode resulting in a poor performance. The psychologic or situational type of impotence is then perpetuated by performance anxiety. At the next opportunity for sexual activity, the person remembers his previous failure. This generates anxiety and fear that a poor performance will be repeated in the current situation. This anxiety and fear reinforce the person's inability to perform. When these repeated episodes of failure occur, reinforced by this anxiety, the problem becomes more deep seated and we have the vicious cycle of anxiety reinforcing inability to perform time after time.

Table 1 lists a number of common disease entities, traumatic injuries, and surgical procedures which have been associated with loss of erectile function. Even though one of these entities may be present in a person with erectile dysfunction, one should not automatically assume that this is the cause of the problem. A very adequate history and whatever diagnostic evaluation is necessary should be peformed to elucidate the cause. It should also be kept in mind that men with organic impotence all have some anxiety regarding their inability to perform and, although the basic problem is or-

TABLE 1. DISEASE STATES ASSOCIATED WITH IMPOTENCE

Endocrine
Diabetes mellitus
Hyperprolactinemia
Gonadal dysfunction with androgen deficiency
Numerous endocrinopathies with hormonal imbalance
Vascular disease
Hypertension
Aorto-iliac occlusive disease
Neurologic diseases
Spinal cord injury
Multiple sclerosis
Parkinsonism
Epilepsy—especially temporal lobe epilepsy
Postsurgical
Aorto-iliac bypass graft
Radical cystoprostatectomy
Abdominal perineal resection
Penile
Priapism
Peyronie's disease
Penile trauma
Renal failure

ganic, there is almost always a psychologic or anxiety-related component involved. By far the most common type of organic impotence is of a vascular nature, whether associated with the microangiopathy of diabetes mellitus, the accelerated atherosclerosis of hypertension, or the progressive hardening of the arteries of the aging American male. Medical schools teach extensively about decreased blood flow to the heart with ensuing myocardial infarction and decreased blood flow to the brain with resultant cerebrovascular accident, but little is said about decreased blood flow to the penis with concomitant impotence. The pathophysiology in these three situations is similar. In cases of diabetes mellitus, the debate continues as to whether it is mainly a microangiopathy or a neuropathy, and evidence suggests that both conditions are involved.[3,4] About one half of juvenile onset diabetics will become impotent by their mid-40s. Hypertensive patients present in increasing numbers in their 50s with erectile difficulties, perhaps a decade sooner than their normotensive peers. When Peyronie's disease causes erectile difficulties, the characteristic erectile disturbance is a normal turgor at the base of the penis with softening distal to the site of the plaque. Erectile dysfunction in Peyronie's disease is variable with many patients who exhibit this penile plaque formation maintaining normal erectile ability, while others demonstrate such pain with erection or embarrassment and repulsion at the deformed penis that a strong psychologic proscription to proper performance prevails.

Radical prostatectomy almost universally was associated with erectile failure postoperatively, but recently a nerve-sparing technique of performing this procedure has been introduced with up to 80 percent of patients maintaining usable erections at 1 year following surgery.[5] The most useful element in the workup in differentiating organic from psychologic impotence is the history. Good performance with one partner, poor performance with another, abrupt onset without obvious injury, or the presence of strong erections upon arising in the morning would all suggest a situational type of impotence problem. The gradual loss of the strength of the erections over a period of months to years, coupled with the decrease in the length of time that erections remain functional, are the hallmarks of an organic type of impotence whether it be due to, for example, diabetes mellitus, hypertension, or Peyronie's disease. Table 2 lists a number of questions and problems to focus on when eliciting a history regarding erectile dysfunction. With experience, the interviewer can blend each of these elements to fit his or her own style and, when the answers are complete, the interviewer should have a pretty good idea of which type of dysfunction is prominent and the degree of disability that is present. Certainly a pelvic injury, surgical procedure, or the beginning of a new medication associated with the onset of impotence would also be helpful in pinpointing the cause. Table 3 lists some of the medications commonly associated with erectile dysfunction. This list highlights the more prominent and common medications and is

TABLE 2. ELEMENTS IN THE HISTORY OF ERECTILE DYSFUNCTION

Pattern of onset	
Duration of erections	
Turgor—ability to penetrate	
Ejaculation	
Presence of nocturnal and AM erections	
Other partners	
Effect of fatigue	
Presence of pain	
Emotional overlay especially:	
Anxiety	Guilt
Depression	Fear
Obsession	Anger
Common diseases affecting erections	
Surgical procedures or trauma affecting erections	
Effect of alcohol on erections	
Use of tobacco	
Use of street drugs	

TABLE 3. MEDICATIONS KNOWN TO ALTER MALE SEXUAL FUNCTION

Alcohol
Anticholinergics
Antidepressants
Antihypertensives
Aldactone
Aldomet
Catapres
Inderal
Ismelin
Minipress
Reserpine
Barbiturates
Cimetidine
Estrogens
Marijuana
Narcotics
Sympatholytic agents
Tranquilizers

not at all intended to be comprehensive. If a medication is causing impotence, one should consider discontinuing the drug or reducing the dosage. Few medications are so essential that an alternative could not be found with a less adverse effect on erections.

The physical examination should focus on the blood pressure, peripheral pulses, retinal examination, and specific examination of the genitalia and penis, checking for the presence of Peyronie's plaques and the presence or absence of sensitivity to pin prick in the S 2-3-4 dermatomes, i.e., the saddle area. In the vast majority of organic impotence cases, however, physical examination of the genitalia is normal.

When there is a question as to whether the type of impotence in question is situational or organic, the best test to differentiate between the two is nocturnal penile tumescence monitoring. In the mid-1960s, Karacan[6] and Fisher et al,[7] working independently, characterized the association of erectile activity with the period of rapid eye movement (REM) sleep. All males will have erections during this period of sleep if the erectile mechanism is physically intact. These episodes are usually four to five in number per night, and last between 20 and 25 minutes each. The total tumescence time represents about 25 percent of sleep time. This total tumescence time is maximal during the teen years and decreases gradually to the eighth decade. These erections can be quantitated and, if good penile expansion and rigidity are demonstrated, a situational or psychologic impotence problem is most likely present. This nocturnal penile tumescence monitoring is a valid and reliable index of the potential awake erectile capacity of the individual, since the physiology of erection does not change in proportion to the level of consciousness. The original devices used to measure penile expansion during REM sleep were the mercury-filled strain gauges.[8] A loop was placed at the base of the penis and one at the tip and, as the penis was stretched, the mercury column was narrowed giving increased electrical resistance. This was quantitated and changed into mechanical energy by a strain gauge and a tracing of the expansion and relaxation of the penis could be recorded. Barry and colleagues attempted to simplify penile tumescence monitoring by using a circumferential ring of postage stamps.[9] With the expansion of the penis during sleep, the perforations between each of the stamps would separate and if the connections between two stamps were broken, it was presumptive evidence that a good erection occurred. They found that this correlated 90 percent with the results of the mercury-filled strain gauge tumescence-monitoring technique. An adaptation of this is the use of the Snap-Gauge which is an expansion measuring device strapped around the penis and held in place by a Velcro band.[10] There are three successive plastic bridges which will break with increasing pressure and expansion of the penis developing. The first bridge is designed to break, supposedly, at 10 ounces of pressure, the second at 15, and the third at 20. This is a relatively crude measurement, but has the advantage of simplicity and low cost. Because of these features, it is currently the most widely used method of measuring nocturnal penile tumescence. None of these three types of devices give an accurate measurement of the rigidity which develops during erections, and it is well known that expansion of the penis can occur without the concomitant presence of adequate rigidity to support an erection for intercourse. This problem has been obviated by the recent introduction of the Rigiscan, which is a computerized tumescence-monitoring device which quantitates both penile base and tip expansion and rigidity.[11] Base and tip expansion are recorded in centimeters, and the percent of rigidity is given compared with a piece of wood as 100 percent. The device itself is fairly expensive and requires an IBM or compatible computer for interpretation. Although expansion and rigidity can be measured, the question still arises as to whether REM sleep has actually been experienced by the patient. This can be obviated by having an observer document the hours at which the patient had experienced restful sleep during the evening, by the concomitant use of an electroencephalogram, or by performing three successive nights of nocturnal penile tumescence monitoring. It is impossible for a patient to go for three successive nights without experiencing REM sleep.

Elevation of serum prolactin or deficiency of testosterone has been associated with the loss of erectile ability.[12] The common denominator with each of these hormonal aberrations has been loss of libido. When questioning patients regarding libido, it is important to consider the age. Certainly the sex drive is prominent in the teens and 20s, and it does start to temper in the late 30s, and certainly in the 40s, 50s, and beyond. Questions, which are helpful to determine if true loss of libido is present, are frequency of intercourse for the patient and who is the initiator. One should also ascertain whether he has a stimulating partner and whether the patient is aroused by masturbation, fantasy, or by the presence of visual sexual stimuli. When loss of libido is present or when there is doubt about the cause of impotence, especially in the younger patient, prolactin and testosterone levels should be measured. Most problems with loss of libido, however, are situational, such as the aging process, depression, or obsessive-compulsive behavior, and in these circumstances the prolactin and testosterone levels will be normal. When there is a deficiency of testosterone and it is replaced by intramuscular injection, return to aggressive sexual behavior may occur, but usually only a slight increase in libido is achieved. When elevated prolactin levels are found, evaluation for pituitary tumor is mandatory as half of these men will have such a neoplasm present.[13] Treatment with bromocriptine, a prolactin inhibitor, or hypophysectomy has been dramatic in restoring sexual desire and function in these cases as well.

Psychologic screening tests, such as the Minnesota Multiphasic Personality Inventory (MMPI)[14] and the Derogatis Sexual Functioning Index (DSFI)[15] may be helpful in categorizing the personality traits of the individual and perhaps helping sex therapists with a place to start. However, they have not been helpful in differentiating a psychologic from an organic type of impotence.

Quantitative measurements of penile blood pressure and flow have been advocated as useful in the diagnosis and treatment of erectile problems.[16] A digital blood pressure cuff placed around the base of the penis and a Doppler stethoscope positioned over the deep penile arteries can be used to obtain the penile blood pressure. It can be compared with that in the brachial artery and the penobrachial index (PBI), the ratio of the penile systolic pressure to brachial systolic pressure, recorded. A figure of 0.75 or less is considered abnormal. Plethysmograph studies delineating the pulse volume recording and the attenuation of the dichrotic notch are also helpful in determining abnormalities in the penile vasculature. Aberrations of the PBI and plethysmography are more common when large vessel occlusive disease is present rather than with small vessel blockage. The value of these studies is enhanced by the performance of the pelvic steal test.[17] Base line parameters of PBI and plethysmography are obtained, and the lower extremities are exercised by jogging in place or walking on a tread mill. As blood is shunted to the gluteal and lower extremity muscles, latent or borderline cases of large vessel occlusion now show a prominent decrease in penile systolic pressure and attenuation of the plethysmography parameters.

Intracavernous injection of the vasodilator, papaverine, is now being used diagnostically to suggest various causes of impotence.[18] When papaverine is injected intracorporeally, the patient with normal erectile function or with psychologic impotence will respond by obtaining an erection. In the patient with vasculogenic impotence, a relatively higher dose of papaverine is necessary to achieve this result, or no erection at all may ensue. In the neurogenically impotent patient, such as the paraplegic, a relatively small amount of vasodilator injected into the corpus cavernosum is necessary to bring forth penile turgor and tumescence. Individual variation is great and this test is not, at the present time, standardized.

In instances of perineal trauma resulting in erectile loss or in persons with primary impotence, a situation where a good quality erection has never occurred, internal iliac and pudendal arteriography may be indicated. This may elucidate blocked arteries to the penis or the presence of arteriovenous (AV) shunts which prevent the development of good turgor to the erections. Two common symptoms of erectile dysfunction are premature loss of erectile turgor and the inability to achieve complete penile rigidity. These may be the symptoms of a venous leak, i.e., the rapid loss of blood from the erectile body to the degree that a complete erection is not achieved or sustained.[19] This may be detected by the use of dynamic infusion cavernosography.[20] Twenty mg of papaverine is injected into the corpora cavernosa after the penis has been locally anesthetized. A tourniquet maintained at the base of penis for about 1 minute will help to keep the vasodilator medication within the corpora cavernosa where it may act to cause sinusoidal relaxation. Radiographic contrast material is then infused at a rate of between 60 and 100 cc/minute. In the normal situation, an erection is achieved and maintained at this rate, but is not sustained in situations of venous leak or rapid runoff of the infused fluid. This infusion range of 60 to 100 cc is relatively broad, and the exact rate of infusion is not that critical and can be readily accomplished by hand infusion with a large syringe. In normal situations, the erection is maintained at infusion rates somewhat below 60 cc/min. When a true venous leak occurs, infusions at greater than 100 cc/min will still not be able to sustain the erection. Ligation of the deep dorsal penile vein, at the neck of the penis, has shown some early success at ameliorating this problem in about 60 percent of patients.[21] Deep dorsal vein arterialization, a technique where the inferior epigastric artery is anastomosed directly to the deep dorsal vein or where a saphenous graft is used to shunt blood from the femoral artery to the deep dorsal vein, has given comparable results.[22]

Many times the problems of situational impotence are self-limiting. For the hard working executive who is too tired to perform at night, a weekend in peaceful, undisturbed surroundings appreciating his partner's finer points may be all that is necessary to restore confidence and proper sexual performance. For the young male who may have had a painful or unpleasant first sexual encounter, a man-to-man talk highlighting that such an episode is the exception rather than the rule, may be all it takes to overcome the problem. A fairly well-established case of psychogenic impotence may require sex therapy to help break the vicious cycle of anxiety reinforcing inability to perform. Therapists usually prescribe exercises that the patient and his partner can perform which will encourage foreplay and the appreciation of each other's bodies. Intercourse or vaginal penetration is prohibited, thus taking away the anxiety of having to perform. While enjoying each other without the pressure of performance, the patient soon appreciates that his erection is returning and that he can once again function properly. The more deep-seated and longer lasting cases of psychogenic impotence do not respond as easily to this technique.

In cases of organic impotence, correcting the basic disease process will frequently not restore erectile capabilities. Diabetes can be curtailed by the proper use of insulin or other medications and diet, but the neuropathy and microangiopathy cannot be reversed. Altering medications, such as antihypertensives, may improve erectile abilities, but rarely will this restore a total lack of erectile ability to a fully functional state. If there is one group of medications which tend to promote or enhance erections, it is the vasodilators. Some patients who are taking sublingual or transdermal nitroglycerin for angina have reported improved erections while on this medication. The closer to the area of the penis that the transdermal patches are applied, the better the quality of the erection seems to be. Nitroglycerin paste rubbed into the penis has had some limited success. This compound is actively absorbed by the vagina, however, and protection against this occurrence should be used as wives have reported headaches from the cerebral vasodilator effects of this medication. Oral vasodilator-type medications have been used successfully in a very limited number of cases.[23] These have included Peritrate, Vasodilan, and Yohimbin. They may work perhaps 20 percent of the time where there is a situation of true vascular impotence such as the impotence of aging or impotence associated with hypertension. They will usually improve an erection that is about 50 percent of former turgor to perhaps 70 percent of turgor. The patient can function better at the augmented turgor and duration, but usually this therapy is short lived, lasting only a matter of months.

Injections of papaverine, and the alpha-blocking agent, phentolamine, directly into the corpus cavernosum have gained widespread usage, therapeutically as well as diagnostically, since the vivid demonstration of the success of these compounds in bringing on an erection by Dr. Giles Brindley at the National AUA meeting in 1983.[24] With a thorough history, one should be able to ascertain the degree of impairment of function that exists in the particular patient. If neurogenic or psychogenic impotence is suspected, a relatively low dose of papaverine alone, perhaps in the range of 10 to 15 mg, should be used initially. If the patient has a relatively severe impairment of erectile function or no erections at all for a prolonged period of time, one may start in the higher ranges such as 30 to 60 mg of papaverine combined with 1 mg of phentolamine.[25] A test dose should always be given in the office before the patient is sent home with prefilled syringes to be used before intercourse. The patient is taught to inject the medication in the midshaft area, in the upper outer quadrant, of either erectile body. Since there is cross-communication between the corpora cavernosa, injection into only one corporal body is necessary. A 3-cc disposable syringe with a 30-gauge needle is ideal to use for injection. A tourniquet effect is maintained at the base of the penis for approximately 1 minute to allow the medication to mix throughout each corporal body. Within 10 minutes, a reasonable degree of penile turgor and tumescence should be achieved if the injected medication is going to work effectively. Total maximal turgor is usually not achieved in the office and, if it is, certainly a lesser dose should be used. As the patient returns to the privacy of his bedroom and commences to use foreplay following the injection, the effects of the erotic stimulation will add to the effects of the injected vasodilator medication bringing about a fuller and more firm erection. The effect of the injection should last from ½ to 2 hours, and certainly if penile tumescence is prolonged beyond 4 to 5 hours, especially if painful, an antidote should be injected to reverse the penile rigidity. The situation of priapism has resulted in perhaps 5 to 10 percent of cases where the injections have been used. Reversal may be accomplished by intracorporeal injections of a very dilute epinephrine solution. This solution in the concentration of 1:100,000 is readily mixed by taking .3 cc of epinephrine from the 1:1000 vial available in all emergency rooms, and mixing in a 30-cc vial of sterile saline for injection. About 5 to 10 cc of blood is then aspirated from the corpus cavernosum and an equal volume of the diluted epinephrine solution is injected. This procedure of aspiration and injection may be repeated until detumescence has occurred. Neither papaverine nor phentolamine has been approved by the Food and Drug Administration (FDA) for injection into the penis to achieve erections and the patient should be so informed. Other side effects and complications to be aware of are postural hypotension, headache, fibrosis from repeated injections into the same location in the penis, and infection. If papaverine is injected subcutaneously rather than intracorporeally, sloughing of the skin at the site of the extravasation may occur. This technique has been particularly useful in two situations. The psychogenically impotent patient may be helped by intracorporeal injections of small dosages of papaverine. This will readily bring on a good erection and help to relieve the performance anxiety which is present from previous repeated failures to achieve erections at the time of attempted sexual activity. After a number of successes with the intracorporeal injections, the patient regains his confidence and may be able to function properly in the future without the injected medication. In cases of long-standing chronic impotence in which the patient has not had usable erectile activity for a number of years, use of pharmacologic injections may obviate the need for insertion of a penile prosthesis. The attrition rate for the use of pharmacologic penile injections is relatively high. Over one-half of the patients will drop out within a matter of months. A percentage of these will opt for the insertion of a penile prosthesis, and a very small percentage, perhaps in the range of 20 percent, who begin the pharmacologic injection technique will continue using this past 1 year.

Counseling the patient to stop smoking has often made a significant difference in improvement of his erections. The nicotine in cigarettes is vasoconstrictive. In cases of a positive penile vascular study where a pelvic arteriogram has demonstrated large vessel occlusive disease, balloon dilation of the hypogastric arteries has improved erectile function.[26] This procedure has been done on a limited basis and may prove to be more useful in the future. The long-term tendency, however, is for vascular reocclusion to occur. Penile revascularization by numerous methods has been tried on a limited basis in this country but is more widely used in Europe.[27] Success rates for the usual cases of organic impotence in the older patients have been in the range of 20 to 30 percent. In the young traumatically impotent patient, the success has been better, approaching 50 percent or more in some series. Procedures which have been tried include anastomosing the inferior epigastric artery to the corpus cavernosum, to the deep penile arteries, or to the deep dorsal vein. These operations are more extensive, require greater surgical skills, and are far less reliable in restoring erectile function than insertion of a penile prosthesis.

Penile implants have come into vogue in the last 13 years with the introduction in 1973 of the prototype inflatable and small-carrion sponge filled semirigid rod types.[28,29] The inflatable prosthesis is a hydraulic system consisting of two inflatable inner tube-like cylinders which are placed one in each corpus cavernosum (Fig. 1). These are connected to a pump located in the scrotum which in turn is connected to a spherical fluid reservoir positioned next to the urinary bladder. Pumping through the scrotal wall moves fluid from the reservoir into the cylinders and the penis becomes erect. Pressing a release valve on the pump allows fluid to pass from the cylinders back into the reservoir thus returning the penis to the flaccid state. The original inflatable models were prone to develop mechanical problems, such as tubing kinks and fluid leaks, as well as penile deformities, and repairs were running in the range of 20 percent at 3 to 5 years after insertion.[30,31] The manufacturer has improved the product considerably over the years by eliminating the causes of wear or reinforcing areas which were prone to wear, as well as by providing cylinders which now expand uniformly without aneurysms, thus eliminating many of the penile deformities which were seen in the past. The incidence of problems developing in the current model of the inflatable device is very low and the repair rate is well under 5 percent since this generation was introduced in 1983.

In the semirigid rod category, malleable rods of silver or stainless steel covered by silicone have become more popular than the original sponge-filled types.[32] These malleable rods can be bent in whatever position is desired, and the most desirable feature is the simplicity of operation. They do, however, give permanent stiffness to the penis which may interfere with

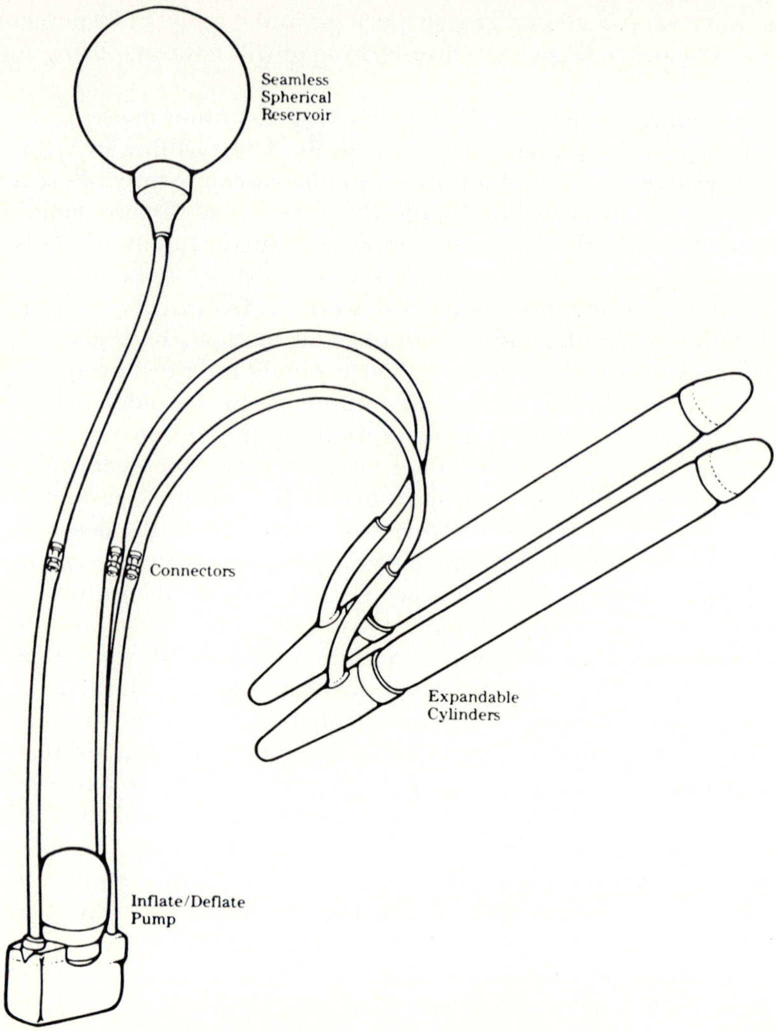

Figure 1. AMS 700 inflatable penile prosthesis.

the life style of many patients. Recently two hydraulic devices, the Hydroflex[33] (Fig. 2) and the FlexiFlate[34] (Fig. 3) have been introduced. Each consists of paired cylinders totally contained within each corpus cavernosum. By pumping behind the head of the penis, fluid is transferred from the rear, or outer portion of the device, to the midshaft area and the cylinder becomes turgid thus producing a firm penis. In the Hydroflex type, the fluid is returned to the rear reservoir through a side channel by pressing the release valve located behind the pump. The FlexiFlate is rendered flaccid by simply bending the penis 45 degrees. This exerts pressure on the spring of the relief valve assembly, a trap door-like mechanism, which allows fluid

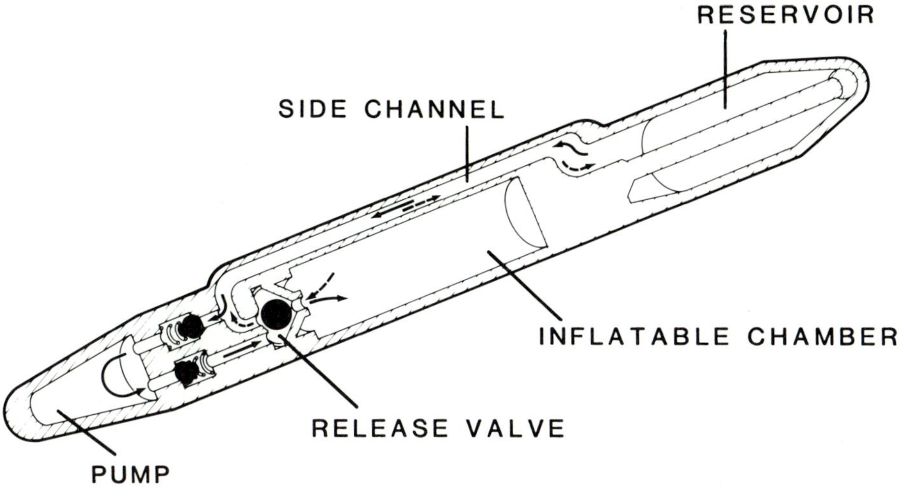

Figure 2. Hydroflex penile prosthesis.

to return to the outer chamber. These self-contained hydraulic devices give a very satisfactory erection when properly sized and good flaccidity is achieved in the deflated state. Neither give increased girth beyond the 11- or 13-mm width sizes as the Dacron sleeve imbedded in the wall of each cylinder prohibits expansion beyond these limits. Patients with a very broad or very narrow penis are not as suitable candidates for these devices as those with an average width penis. In the former case, the cylinder cannot adequately fill the erectile bodies and an unstable erection with diminished axial rigidity results. In the latter category, there is not sufficient room in the erectile cavity to cram in a cylinder, and a semierect penis in the deflated state would result. Patients who have had an old inflatable-type prosthesis with an extrapenile pump and reservoir almost universally prefer the old inflatable to the self-contained inflatable. They miss the almost pipe-like rigidity and girth expansion which the old inflatable affords. The vast majority of patients with the self-contained inflatables are very satisfied with

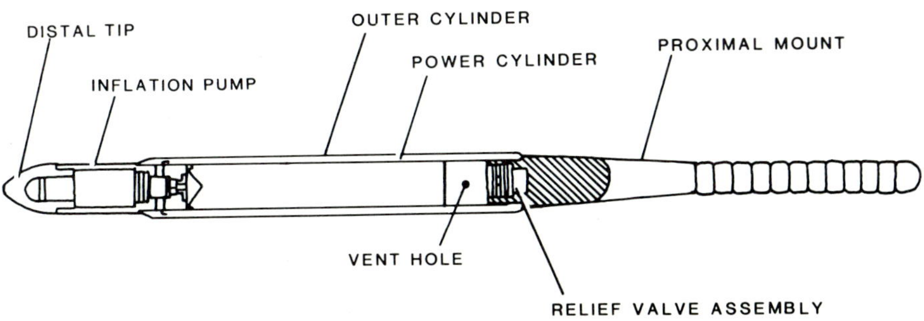

Figure 3. FlexiFlate penile prosthesis.

the results and the quality of the erections which these devices provide. The advantages include ease of insertion, mechanical reliability, and ease of repair when necessary.

Another concept in prostheses, recently introduced, is the Omni-Phase.[35] This is a mechanical rather than hydraulic system with a pair of cylinders contained within the corpora cavernosa. This type consists of a series of plastic balls and sockets through which courses a central cable (Fig. 4). An activator mechanism lengthens or shortens the cable and, with the cable taut, the balls are pulled into the sockets and the cylinder becomes rigid and can be bent as a goose neck lamp. With the cable loose, the balls fall away from the sockets and the cylinders become flaccid. The mechanisms for activating and deactivating the device is the same, i.e., pushing the device 120 degrees from the horizontal position into the scrotum analogous to protruding and retracting a ball point pen. The advantage of this type is its simplicity of operation, and it is well suited for the patient with impaired manual dexterity who wishes alternate flaccidity and rigidity to his penis.

The criteria for implantation of a penile prosthesis are varied. The patient must be motivated to continue sexual activity and determination of a stable sexual relationship is usually critical. The partner should be included in discussions preoperatively to be completely informed as to what

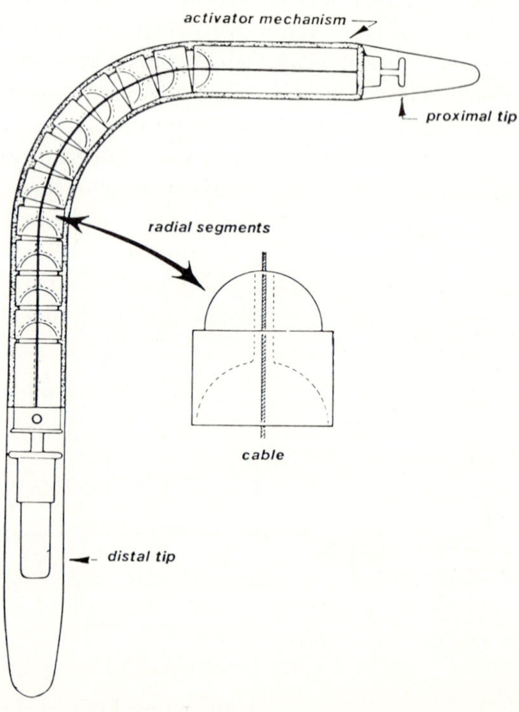

Figure 4. An OmniPhase penile prosthesis.

to expect postoperatively. The sole function of these devices is to give a firm penis. The size of the erection with a prosthesis is usually slightly smaller than the patient's original erection, and ejaculation and penile sensation are not changed by the operation. Some patients expect that a penile prosthesis will totally reorient an unsatisfactory love life or make a penis beautiful, and are sadly disappointed when only a firm penis is present postoperatively. Although choice of the type of prosthesis ultimately rests with the patient, he should be guided by the advice of the implanting urologist. Patients with limited manual dexterity, such as the neurologically impaired, those with severe arthritis, parkisonism, or those with very calloused fingers should be advised against the self-contained inflatables or possibly even the old inflatable, depending upon the degree of disability. Semirigid rods or the OmniPhase would be a more appropriate choice for this group. Those with a very active life style would do better with the hydraulic prostheses or OmniPhase than with the semirigid rods.

Psychologic impotence can frequently be treated by counseling and sex therapy. Papaverine injection into the erectile bodies has also been very useful in this group of patients in restoring the erection and thus relieving the anxiety associated with the inability to perform. In some patients with psychologic impotence who are refractory to sex therapy, and who are not candidates for penile injections, a penile prosthesis has given gratifying results.

In situations of organic impotence, the two effective treatments are currently the penile injections and the penile implant. Some patients may find the injections psychologically abhorrent and would therefore opt for the prosthesis. Other patients may initially choose the injections and later opt for the prosthesis when they find these inconvenient or painful or when problems such as priapism or fibrosis at the site of injection occur. Patients with long-standing impotence may be given a trial of the vasodilator injections to ascertain whether they will enjoy returning to erectile activity or whether they will even use their erections.

When the appropriate interpersonal relationships exist, the proper placement of a penile prosthesis gives a good functional result. The patient's outlook on life improves and although the initial implantation is somewhat painful, by 6 months he hardly knows the device is present when it is not in use. To quote a recently implanted patient, "I feel sorry for all those guys out there who don't have one."

REFERENCES

1. Lue TF, Zeineh SJ, Schmidt RA, et al: Physiology of penile erection. World J Urol 1(4):197, 1983
2. Kinsey A, Pomeroy W, Martin E: Sexual Behavior in the Human Male. Philadelphia, Saunders, 1948

3. Lehman T, Jacobs JA: Etiology of diabetic impotence. J Urol 129:291, 1983
4. Saenez de Tejada I: Mechanism for impotence in diabetes mellitus. J Urol 131:525, 1984
5. Walsh PC, Donker PJ: Impotence following radical prostatectomy: Insight into etiology and prevention. J Urol 128:491, 1982
6. Karacan I: Clinical value of nocturnal erections in the prognosis and diagnosis of impotence. Med Asp Human Sex 4:27, 1970
7. Fisher C, Gross J, Zuch J: Cycle of penile erection synchronous with dreaming (REM) sleep. Arch Gen Psychiatry 12:29, 1965
8. Karacan I: A simple and inexpensive transducer for quantitative measurements of penile erection during sleep. Behav Res Meth Instru 1:251, 1969
9. Barry JM, Blank B, Boileau N: Nocturnal penile tumescence monitoring with stamps. Urology 15:171, 1980
10. Ek A, Bradley WE, Krane RJ: Nocturnal penile rigidity measured by the Snap Gauge band. J Urol 129:964, 1983
11. Bradley WE, Timm GW, Gallagher JM, Johnson BK: New method for continuous measurement of nocturnal penile tumescence and rigidity. Urology 26:64, 1985
12. Penyman RL, Thorner MO: The effects of hyperprolactinemia on sexual and reproductive function in men. J Androl 5:233, 1981
13. Carter JN, Tyson JE, Tolis G, et al: Prolactin-secreting tumors and hypogonadism in 22 men. N Engl J Med 299:847, 1978
14. Beutler LE, Scott FB, Karacan I: Psychological screening of impotent men. J Urol 116:193, 1976
15. Derogatis LR, Meyer JK, Dupkin CN: Discrimination of organic versus psychogenic impotence with the DSFI. J Sex Marital Ther 2:229, 1976
16. Velcek D: Penile flow index utilizing a Doppler wave analysis to indentify penile vascular insufficiency. J Urol 123:669, 1980
17. Goldstein I, Siroky MB, Nath RL, et al: Vasculogenic impotence role of the pelvic steal test. J Urol 128:300, 1982
18. Virag R, Frydman D, Legman M, Virag H: Intracavernous injection of papaverine as a diagnostic and therapeutic method in erectile failure. Angiology 35:79, 1984
19. Fitzpatrick TJ, Cooper JF: A cavernosogram study on the vascular competence of the human deep dorsal vein. J Urol 113:497, 1975
20. Prost H, Altwein JE, Bach D: Dynamic cavernosography: Venous outflow studies of cavernous bodies. J Urol 134:276, 1985
21. Wespes E, Schulman CC: Venous leakage: Surgical treatment of a curable cause of impotence. J Urol 133:796, 1985
22. Balko A, Maalhotra CM, Wincze JP, et al: Deep penile vein arterialization for arterial and venous impotence. Arch Surg 121:774, 1986
23. Elist J, Jarman WD, Edson M: Evaluating medical treatment of impotence. Urology 23:374, 1984
24. Brindley GS: Cavernosal alpha-blockade: A new technique for investigating and treating erectile dysfunction. Br J Psychiatry 143:3323, 1983
25. Zorgniotti AW, Le Fleur RS: Auto-injection of the corpus cavernosum with a vasoactive drug combination for vasculogenic impotence. J Urol 133:39, 1985
26. Castaneda WR, Smith A, Kaye K, et al: Transluminal angioplasty for treatment of vasculogenic impotence. AJR 139:371, 1982

27. Zorgniotti AW, Rossie G, Padula G, Malsovsky RD: Diagnosis and therapy of vasculogenic impotence. J Urol 123:674, 1980
28. Scott FB, Bradley WE, Timm GW: Management of erectile impotence: Use of implantable inflatable prosthesis. Urology 2:80, 1973
29. Small MP, Carrion HN: A new penile prosthesis for treating impotence. Contemp Surg 7:29, 1975
30. Kessler R: Surgical experience with the inflatable penile prosthesis. J Urol 124:611, 1980
31. Fishman IJ, Scott FB, Light JK: Experience with the inflatable penis prosthesis. Urology 23:86, 1984
32. Krane RJ, Freedberg PS, Siroky MB: Jonas silicone—silver prosthesis—initial experience in America. J Urol 126:475, 1981
33. Fishman IJ: Experience with the Hydroflex penile prosthesis. Semin Urol 4:239, 1986
34. Finney RP: FlexiFlate penile prosthesis. Semin Urol 4:244, 1986
35. Krane RJ: OmniPhase penile prosthesis. Semin Urol 4:247, 1986

Artificial Urinary Sphincters

David M. Barrett, William L. Furlow, and Benad Goldwasser

Control of sphincteric urinary incontinence with implantable prosthetic devices has evolved rapidly during the past 15 years.[1–3] Clearly, the most significant contribution to the treatment of urinary incontinence was the introduction of a totally implantable artificial urinary sphincter by Scott et al in 1973.[4] This hydraulic device, composed of silicone elastomer, allowed for the placement of an inflatable cuff around the bladder neck in male and female patients of all ages or around the bulbous urethra in men.[4,5] With the original device, the AS 721, the patient controlled the sphincter by small pumps placed in the subcutaneous tissue of each hemiscrotum or labia. Unidirectional valves within the system directed the fluid from a reservoir to and from the inflatable cuff (Fig. 1). Pressure in the cuff was regulated by a bleedoff valve (V4) in the outflow tract.

An alternative prosthesis, the Rosen incontinence device, was introduced in 1976.[6] This device provided for patient control of micturition by a fluid transfer system that involves a perineally placed occlusion balloon that on activation compressed the bulbous urethra. This device allowed the patient to titrate the degree of urethral closing pressure by pumping into the compression pillow only the minimal amount of fluid required to maintain continence. Unfortunately, many patients overinflated the device, and

This article is based on Barrett DM, Furlow WL, Goldwasser B: Artificial urinary sphincter. In Yalla SV, McGuire EJ, Blaivas JG, Elbadawi A (eds): Urodynamics and Neurourology: Principles and Practice. New York, Macmillan, 1988, with permission.

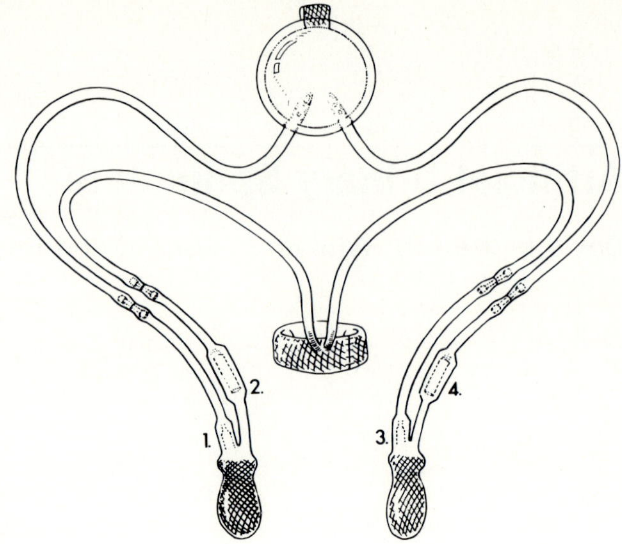

Figure 1. AS 721 artificial urinary sphincter. *(From Barrett DM, Furlow WL, Goldwasser B: Artificial urinary sphincter. In Yalla SV, McGuire EJ, Blaivas JG, Elbadawi A (eds): Urodynamics and Neurourology: Principles and Practice. New York, Macmillan, 1988, with permission.)*

the unnecessarily high urethral closing pressure resulted in erosion of the urethra. Only limited clinical experience was gained with the Rosen device, and no modifications of the device have evolved recently. Current clinical use in the United States is negligible.

The injection of polytef (Teflon) periurethrally to increase urethral resistance and thereby control urine flow was described by Politano,[7] who recently reported his 16-year experience. In select patients, the technique is reported to be safe, simple, and effective for producing good overall results in 75 percent of patients receiving injections. Some patients require repeat injections because of persistent incontinence. Although this seems to be an effective way of treating incontinence of certain causes, at the time of this report the use of polytef paste has not been approved specifically for the treatment of urinary incontinence by periurethral injection by the Food and Drug Administration.

DEVELOPMENTAL CONSIDERATIONS

The initial device developed by Scott et al[4] became commercially available in 1974 and was called the AS 721 sphincter. This device produced mixed results in patients with various types of sphincteric incontinence. Although many patients benefited from the device, the mechanical reliability and rate of erosion were unacceptably high.

In 1977, in conjunction with the manufacturer, a study group of implanting urologists began to work with a new sphincter design. The AS 742 and AS 761 devices were subtly different in design. Both used an elastic pressure-balloon reservoir to ensure constant, predetermined pressure within the hydraulic system of the sphincter. These balloon reservoirs, by virtue of the elasticity inherent in their construction, exerted a given amount of intraluminal pressure, depending on the volume of fluid in the balloon. The pressure–volume relationship was linear only to a given volume, and then it became very predictable within a very narrow range (Fig. 2). Balloon reservoirs were manufactured to deliver a range of preset pressures (51 to 60, 61 to 70, 71 to 80, and 81 to 90 cm H_2O). The implanting urologist could select a pressure to fit the clinical situation and site of cuff placement. When pressurized, the cuff provided continuous closing pressure to the underlying urethra or bladder neck. The cuff was opened by compressing the pump until all the cuff fluid was forced through a unidirectional valve into the balloon reservoir. Inherently, the fluid was directed back toward the cuff. Its rate of refilling, however, was regulated by a flow resistor that allowed the patient 3 to 5 minutes to urinate before repressurization was complete.

Because of the initial implanting success with the pressure-balloon res-

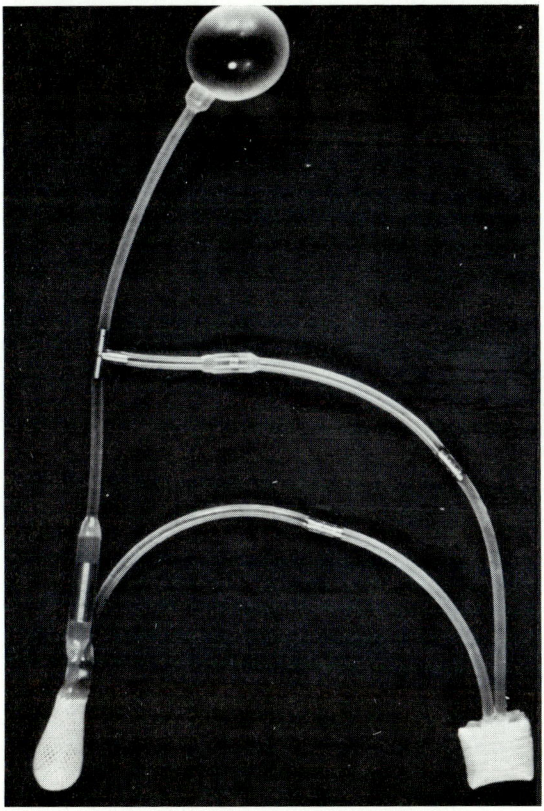

Figure 2. AS 742 artificial urinary sphincter. *(From Furlow WL: Artificial sphincter. In Stanton SL, Tanagho EA (eds): Surgery of Female Incontinence. Berlin, Springer-Verlag, 1980, pp 119–134, with permission.)*

ervoir concept, in 1979 the sphincter study group evaluated a modification of the AS 742 device—the AS 791/792.[8] Incorporating changes in the pump, cuff, and control assembly, the AS 791/792 sphincter proved to be far more mechanically reliable and afforded continence in most patients (Fig. 3). Several clinical series attested to the attributes of the device and its versatility. A distinct limitation, however, was lack of an external "on" and "off" capability. Once the sphincter had been implanted, constant pressure was delivered to the inflatable cuff, except during the short period when the cuff was emptied to allow for voiding. This function of the device, although easy to manage from the patient's standpoint, created several limiting and potentially complicated problems, as follows:

1. Cuff closing pressure began at the time of implantation without regard to the quality of the underlying tissues. Patients with previous urethral or bladder neck operations or pelvic radiation therapy or who had induced surgical trauma were at risk for vascular ischemia and cuff erosion. The inability to limit this pressure during the early postoperative healing period led to the concept of primary deactivation.[9] This technique allowed for implantation of the sphincter cuff, balloon, and pump at one operation and a second procedure 2 to 3 months later to insert the control assembly and "activate" the sphincter mechanism.[9,10]

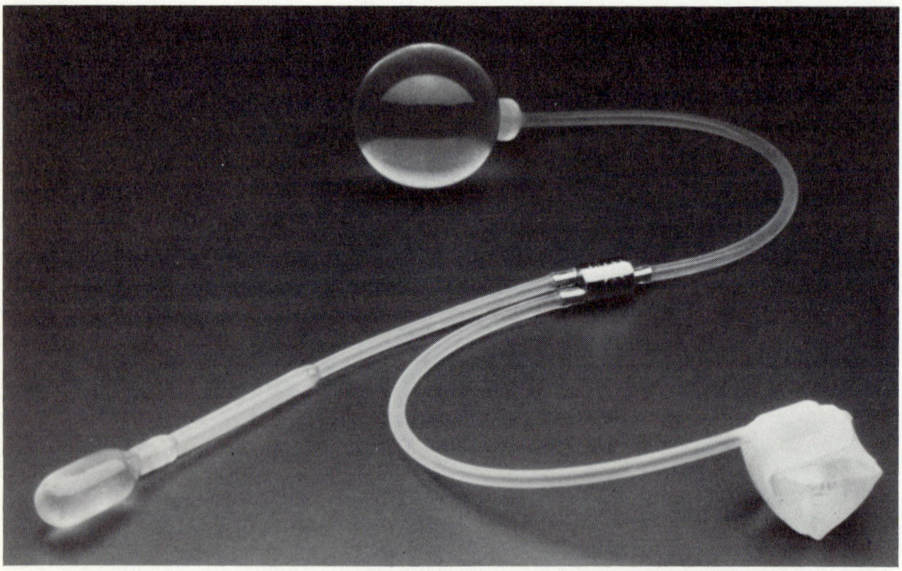

Figure 3. AS 791/792 artificial urinary sphincter. (*Figures 3 through 5 from Barrett DM, Furlow WL, Goldwasser B: Artificial urinary sphincter. In Yalla SV, McGuire EJ, Blaivas JG, Elbadawi A (eds): Urodynamics and Neurourology: Principles and Practice. New York, Macmillan, 1988, with permission.)*

2. In many patients, the implanted pump in the labia or scrotum caused extreme tenderness and edema in the overlying tissues during the early postoperative period. This problem prohibited cuff decompression for voiding and thus made necessary the use of a small caliber catheter for bladder drainage until the swelling and tenderness resolved.
3. Long-term catheterization or instrumentation of the urethra or bladder was occasionally necessary in patients who had implantation. The inability to deactivate the cuff for prolonged periods predisposed the patient to cuff erosion because the inserted tube or instrument would compress the underlying tissues.
4. Many incontinent patients are wet only when upright or during physical activity. Ideally, cuff compression is necessary only during the "at risk" times. With the AS 791/792 concept, patients endured cuff compression continuously even if they did not require the protection. Urethral or bladder neck tissues were therefore at risk for erosion and atrophic deterioration more than was necessary.

In late 1982 and early 1983, work began on a design alteration that provided for externally controlled cuff on and off capability. The result became commercially available in April 1983 and is known as the AS 800 artificial urinary sphincter (Fig. 4). The AS 800 control assembly contains the unidirectional valves, flow reservoir, on and off button, and deflate pump (Fig. 5). It allows for nonsurgical delayed activation and complete control by the physician and patient during periods of cuff compression.[11]

Also included in the currently used AS 800 device is an improved surface-treated cuff that, although it looks similar to its predecessors, has been constructed of silicone elastomer that is extremely resistant to excess wear and leakage.

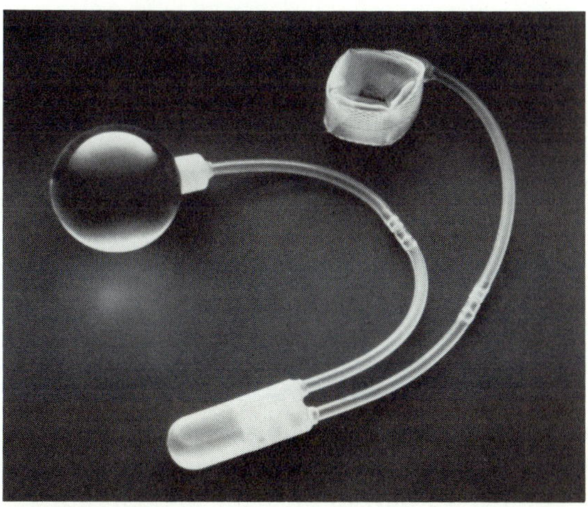

Figure 4. AS 800 artificial urinary sphincter.

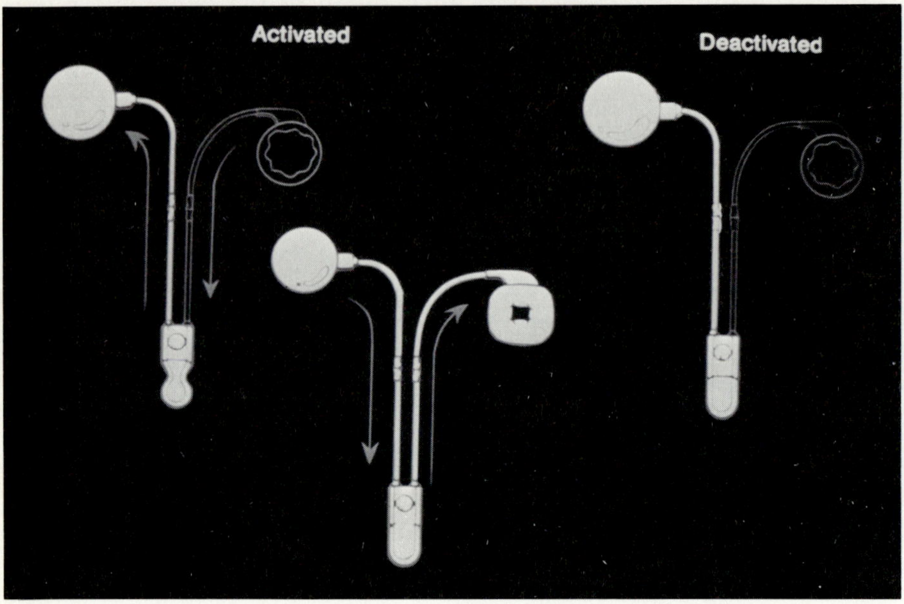

Figure 5. Functions of AS 800 artificial urinary sphincter.

SELECTION AND EVALUATION OF PATIENTS

Incontinence may be the result of a detrusor abnormality, a sphincteric abnormality, or a combination of detrusor and sphincteric abnormalities. Ideally, the artificial sphincter is most appropriate for persons with pure sphincteric incompetency who have normal detrusor function. Patients with low volume detrusor hyperreflexia are poor candidates for sphincter implantation. In these patients, contractile pressures will override sphincteric resistance pressures or a dyssynergic pattern is created that induces risk to the upper tracts. Also at risk are candidates with decreased compliance and small functional bladder capacity. A combination of pharmacologic therapy may render such patients suitable candidates; however, most often they are best managed by either neurologic blockade or augmentation cystoplasty to decrease contractility or increase compliance and functional bladder capacity.

Persons with sphincteric incompetency and decreased detrusor contractility were formerly excluded from sphincter implantation because their residual volumes were too high to risk increasing outlet resistance for fear of potentiating urosepsis and frank retention. Since the acceptance of combined sphincter implantation and intermittent, clean self-catheterization, we now consider this group of patients good candidates. As an alternative to intermittent catheterization, sphincterotomy in the male patient or bladder flap urethroplasty in the female patient may facilitate bladder emptying.

Table 1 lists the indications for implantation of the AS 800 sphincter in 221 patients at our institution through January 1986. Radical prostatectomy, which is associated with a 5 percent rate of significant incontinence, remains the main reason patients must undergo implantation. Considering the number of transurethral prostatectomies performed annually nationwide, the associated incontinence rate is very low; however, we still encounter patients with incontinence after transurethral prostatectomy who qualify for implantation of the artificial urinary sphincter.

Patients with incontinence associated with congenital abnormalities such as myelomeningocele, exstrophy-epispadias, and sacral agenesis are good candidates for an artificial urinary sphincter.[12,13] Many of these patients do not completely empty their bladders, and additional measures must be taken after the sphincter is implanted to ensure regular, complete voiding.

Select patients with acquired injuries such as spinal cord trauma, pelvic fracture, or neurogenic bladder compose a large group of candidates for implantation. In this group, care must be taken to assess bladder contractility and compliance adequately before and after implantation because some authors have suggested that deterioration in the upper tracts results from a change in detrusor function after implantation.

Patients with various other causes of incontinence may also benefit from implantation of the artificial urinary sphincter. Noteworthy is our limited experience with female patients who have undergone implantation.[14–16]

TABLE 1. CAUSE OF INCONTINENCE IN 221 PATIENTS RECEIVING THE AS 800 ARTIFICIAL URINARY SPHINCTER

Cause of Incontinence	No. of Patients
Radical prostatectomy	95
Transurethral prostatectomy	45
Myelomeningocele, sacral agenesis	42
Spinal cord injury	11
Neurogenic bladder	5
Stress incontinence	5
Urethral surgery	5
Exstrophy-epispadias	4
Pelvic fracture	2
Other causes	7
Total	221

(From Barrett DM, Furlow WL, Goldwasser B: Artificial urinary sphincter. In Yalla SV, McGuire EJ, Blaivas JG, Elbadawi A (eds): Urodynamics and Neurourology: Principles and Practice. New York, Macmillan, 1988, with permission.)

We believe that female stress incontinence is best managed by conventional methods to modify vesicourethral incompetency.[17,18] Even techniques that create relative outlet obstruction such as the sling procedure may be better options than the artificial urinary sphincter. Female patients with neurologic deficits, such as those related to myelomeningocele, who respond poorly to conventional surgical procedures are good candidates for the artificial urinary sphincter and optimal results can be expected.

Recently, McGuire et al[19] described a technique of performing a pubovaginal sling in girls with myelodysplasia. Although this approach totally obstructs the urethra, intermittent self-catheterization may be applied safely.

Evaluation of candidates for artificial urinary sphincters should be designed to quantitate voiding function, usually through a combination of radiographic, endoscopic, and urodynamic tests. Even patients with an outwardly apparent cause for incontinence such as previous radical prostatectomy should be evaluated to exclude coincident abnormalities that may preclude success of an implanted sphincter.

An excretory urogram and voiding cystourethrogram are indicated to exclude upper tract or bladder structural abnormalities that would require repair before or during sphincter implantation. Vesicoureteral reflux, for example, may not be a problem for a totally incontinent patient, because intravesical pressures do not usually exceed a critical level. With implantation of the artificial urinary sphincter, continuous low intravesical pressures and resting and voiding pressures are likely to increase and thus to potentiate the problems inherent in vesicoureteral incompetency. Our policy has been to correct reflux of grade 2 or more either before or during sphincter implantation. Cystourethroscopy is recommended to exclude urethral or bladder defects such as false passages, strictures, diverticulum, contracture, and foreign body. All such abnormalities should be appropriately managed and considered stable before implantation. The location of urethral defects is also important. A stricture in the midbulbous portion of the urethra may prevent implantation of the occlusive cuff at this level, and an alternate site should be chosen.

A urodynamic evaluation should be conducted in every patient before implantation of an artificial urinary sphincter. Hyperreflexia, especially of high pressure, should be excluded and, if present, treated before implantation. Reduced compliance is common in patients who have been incontinent for some time. The reason for this is unclear. However, it tends to disappear with time after implantation. It is essential, however, to make sure that the reduced compliance, especially if associated with low functional capacity, is not a result of a neurologic disease or other inflammatory disease of the bladder wall such as tuberculosis or interstitial cystitis.

Before a patient is considered an optimal candidate for implantation of the AS 800 device, technical feasibility must be considered. The surgeon's ability to implant the inflatable cuff around the bulbous urethra or bladder neck is the key issue. Patients who have had multiple previous bladder neck or urethral procedures, pelvic trauma, or pelvic radiation therapy are difficult surgical challenges and must be considered high risks.

In men, a cuff site that will enhance the ease of implantation and provide the best chance of continence is selected. Ideally, the bladder neck is the most physiologic location for cuff placement. In patients who have undergone a radical prostatectomy, however, it is nearly impossible to dissect the bladder neck circumferentially without damaging the rectum or bladder.[20] Thus, it becomes necessary to choose the bulbous urethra for cuff placement. In children and women, the bladder neck is the only site for cuff placement.[21] Previous bladder neck tubularization makes bladder neck dissection more difficult, but success can be achieved if the tubularization technique did not encroach on the vesicovaginal or vesicorectal plane.[22] Patients who have had previous vesicovaginal fistula repair and rectal pull-through procedures should be cautioned that cuff placement may not be technically possible.

Aside from the physical characteristics of the incontinence, the patient's expectations and motivation should be assessed. Occasionally, a patient has unrealistic expectations about the artificial urinary sphincter. Such patients must be informed about the mechanical features of the device and the likelihood of occasional stress incontinence. They must accept the fact that additional surgical procedures may be necessary in the future to make adjustments or repairs and that the components of the device will have to be removed if the prosthesis becomes infected.

PREOPERATIVE CONSIDERATIONS

Patients with urinary tract infection must be adequately treated preoperatively, and all should be given broad-spectrum parenteral antibiotics for prophylaxis. The bacterium that has been most often associated with infected prostheses is *Staphylococcus epidermidis,* and prophylaxis should be designed to include this organism. Cephalosporins or aminoglycosides are the most often used antimicrobials. Administration of antibiotics is continued for at least 4 days after implantation.

For patients with chronic urinary incontinence who have various degrees of ammonia dermatitis on the lower abdomen and pelvis, it is best to insert a Foley catheter several days in advance of implantation to reduce the bacterial counts on the skin and promote healing.

Most patients who are expected to have uncomplicated bulbous urethral cuff implantation are admitted to the hospital on the morning of the surgical procedure, and those who are to undergo implantation in the bladder neck are admitted the evening before for a limited lower bowel preparation. All hair removal is done just before operation to avoid bacterial colonization of the small scratches and nicks that may accompany shaving.

When placed on the operating table, patients having bulbous urethral cuff implantation are in the lithotomy position and those having bladder neck cuff procedures are supine with their legs slightly spread.

Iodophors are preferred for skin preparation, and a full 10-minute scrubbing is used. All female patients undergo a vaginal preparation. A soft rectal tube is placed in male patients and children who will have bladder neck cuff placement. Draping is performed in such a way that there is access to the lower anterior abdominal wall and perineum. Urethral catheters are inserted after skin preparation and draping.

An antibiotic solution should be prepared and used frequently for irrigation during the procedure. It is also best to irrigate the bladder with the solution before dissection of the urethra or bladder neck. Our formula consists of neomycin, 0.1 percent, and bacitracin, 50,000 units in 1 L of 0.9 percent sodium chloride solution.

Because of the infection risks in patients undergoing prosthetic implantation, all operating room personnel must wear hoods to ensure limited "fallout" in the operative field. Traffic in and out of the operating room is strictly limited.

OPERATIVE TECHNIQUE

Bladder Neck Cuff

A Foley catheter is passed that is appropriate in size to the age and sex of the patient. Large Foley catheters (20 to 24 Fr) are used in female patients to assess the urethral margins of the bladder neck more adequately, and small catheters (10 to 14 Fr) are used in children and male patients. A lower abdominal midline or transverse incision is used for bladder neck cuff implantation. There is no need to open the peritoneal cavity, and dissection is limited to the retroperitoneal space.

With a catheter in the bladder, the demarcation of the bladder neck and proximal portion of the urethra can be palpated. Care is taken during circumferential dissection of the bladder neck to avoid opening the endopelvic fascia. The plane between the posterior aspect of the bladder neck and the anterior surface of the underlying vagina or rectum must be established. A pack in the vagina assists in the delineation of this area. Because of the difficulty of dissecting around the bladder neck in female patients, some authorities prefer to open the bladder before beginning the dissection. This technique provides for easier orientation during the dissection between the bladder neck and vaginal wall and thus the chance of perforating any of these organs is decreased. The opening in the bladder should be made far above the bladder neck to prevent placement of the cuff over the suture line, which would increase the risk of erosion. Dissecting the plane between the bladder neck and the vagina through a vaginal approach was found to be associated with a high rate of infection; therefore, we do not recommend that approach. In the male patient, a rectal tube will assist in demarcating the plane between the rectum and the bladder neck. The point of dissection is superior to the endopelvic fascia; however, it is far enough distally to avoid the areas where the ureters penetrate the posterior aspect of the bladder and trigone. Usually, a combination of blunt and sharp dissection affords complete circumferential dissection.

Once the area has been completely opened, the width of the plane should be approximately 2 cm so that the cuff will fit without crimping. A tape is passed around the bladder neck, and the bladder is filled with antibiotic solution to detect small openings that may have been created during the dissection. If an opening is found, it can be closed with 3-0 or 4-0 absorbable suture.

If a vaginal injury is created, it also may be closed primarily. Unfortunately, if a rectal injury is created, we advise closing the rectal injury primarily and abandoning the procedure until another date.

The bladder neck is circumferentially measured with the calibrated measuring strap. The catheter remains indwelling except for cases in which a large caliber catheter has been used. In these cases it is removed before measurement of the bladder neck area. Once the appropriate-sized cuff has been passed underneath the bladder neck and snapped in place, the tubing from this sphincter component is passed through the belly of one rectus muscle and through the anterior abdominal wall fascia on the side of the patient where the pump will be placed. This tubing should penetrate the rectus muscle and fascia approximately 3 to 4 inches above the pubic symphysis.

The pressure of the balloon reservoir is chosen on the basis of the quality of tissue and the size of cuff used. In most of our patients with bladder neck cuffs, a 71- to 80-cm H_2O pressure-balloon reservoir is chosen. In patients who have tissues of substandard quality, a 61- to 70-cm H_2O pressure-balloon reservoir is commonly used. In general, the larger the cuff, the higher the pressure of the balloon reservoir.

Cuff sizes range up to 11 cm for placement around the bladder neck. In most children and women, a 6- to 8-cm inflatable cuff is chosen and, in men, an 8- to 14-cm cuff may be necessary.

The pressure-balloon reservoir is placed in the prevesical space, and its tubing penetrates the rectus muscle next to the tubing of the cuff. Before the balloon is filled, the prevesical space is drained and the anterior abdominal wall fascia is closed with absorbable suture. Once the closure is complete, the balloon is filled with 22 ml of isosmotic contrast medium and the cuff is pressurized. Once pressurized, the balloon is refilled to a maximum of 20 ml of fluid.[23]

The cuff accommodates from 0.5 to 1.5 ml of fluid, depending on the length of the cuff. The AS 800 control assembly is placed in a deep subcutaneous pocket in the scrotum or labia. Connections between the control assembly and balloon and the control assembly and cuff are established with straight connectors tied in place with polypropylene (Prolene) suture (Fig. 6).

The cuff is left in a deactivated configuration for 6 to 8 weeks. The patient's indwelling Foley catheter is removed the day after operation, and bladder emptying is augmented with intermittent catheterization if necessary.

Bulbous Urethral Cuff

A 12- or 14-Fr Foley catheter is passed, and the bladder is emptied. Two incisions are made, one on the perineum in the midline over the bulbous urethra and another transversely on the lower anterior abdominal wall, either to the right or to the left of the midline, depending on the site of pump placement. Through the perineal incision, the bulbocavernosus muscle is identified. If possible, dissection should be carried out around the bulbocavernosus muscle and a plane established between it and the tunica albuginea of the corporal bodies. The plane of dissection is about 2 cm wide and is as close as possible to the underlying tunica albuginea of the corporal bodies. This technique allows placement of the cuff around the bulbocavernosus and not directly on the bulb of the urethra and thus the risk of erosion is reduced. Care must be taken to avoid injury to the thin urethral

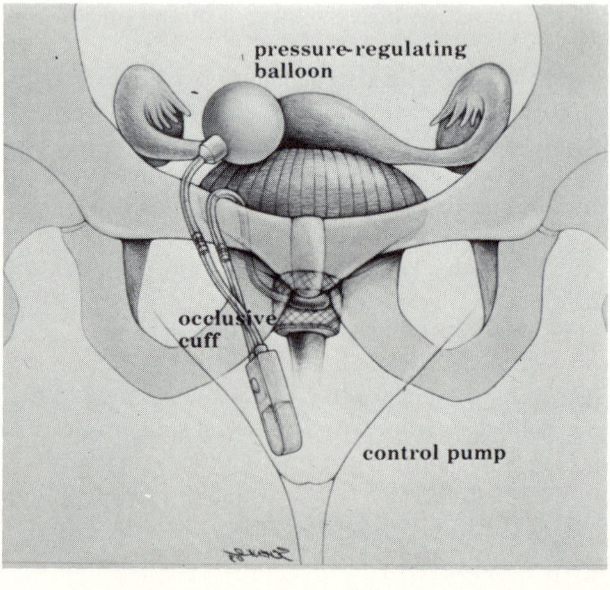

Figure 6. AS 800 artificial urinary sphincter in female patient with bladder neck cuff. *(Furlow WL: Artificial sphincter. In Stanton SL, Tanagho EA (eds): Surgery of Female Incontinence, 2nd ed. Berlin, Springer-Verlag, 1986, pp 155–173, with permission.)*

tissues at the 12 o'clock position on the urethra, the point at which dissection is most difficult and at which most urethral injuries occur.

If the urethra is injured, it may be possible to close the defect primarily with 4-0 or 5-0 absorbable suture. An alternative site on the urethra can then be selected for cuff placement. Unfortunately, some urethral injuries are not recognized and may result in early cuff erosion.

Once the urethral plane is established, the circumference is measured by using a calibrated (1 to 12 cm) measuring strap. The appropriately sized cuff, which for the bulbous urethra is almost always 4.5, 5.0, or 5.5 cm in length, is passed tab first under the urethra. The tab should be passed under the urethra toward the side where the pump is to be placed. The tubing is passed through an opening in the tab, and the cuff is snapped in place while gentle opposing traction is placed on the tab and tubing.

With use of a long curved forceps or a similar instrument, a tunnel is created in the subcutaneous tissues from the incision in the anterior abdominal wall down to the perineal incision. The cuff tubing is grasped and drawn into the upper incision through the subcutaneous tissues.

After the bulbous urethra is dissected and the quality of urethral tissue is assessed, the pressure of the balloon reservoir may be selected. We have used the 61- to 70-cm H_2O reservoir in most patients with uncomplicated bulbous urethral cuffs. In high-risk patients, the 51- to 60-cm H_2O reservoir is selected to preserve the integrity of the tissue.

A small incision (1 to 2 cm) is made in the rectus fascia, and the unfilled balloon is placed in a small pocket under the belly of the rectus muscle. The balloon tubing is passed through a separate puncture opening in the fascia, the balloon is filled with 22 ml (previously 18 ml) of isosmotic contrast medium, and the cuff is pressurized. Once the cuff is pressurized, the balloon is refilled to a maximum of 20 ml of fluid.

The AS 800 pump-control assembly is placed in a subcutaneous tunnel, most easily created with Hegar dilators in one side of the scrotum. The cuff tubing is attached to the appropriate control assembly tubing with a right-angle connector to prevent kinking. The balloon and the control assembly tubing are attached with a straight connector. Polypropylene (Prolene), 2-0 or 3-0, is used to tie the connectors in place.

Various techniques have been used to evaluate the cuff closing pressure and the degree of continence intraoperatively, but no perfect method exists. We have found that with urethral profilometry, an increase of 40 cm H_2O in urethral closing pressure when the cuff is closed usually predicts continence. A less scientific but useful method is to fill the bladder with fluid and apply limited external pressure to the suprapubic area. Continence can be predicted if no urine escapes the urethra. Generally, no drains are necessary. The catheter is left in place until the day after implantation. The patient leaves the operating room with the cuff pumped empty and the system deactivated (Fig. 7).

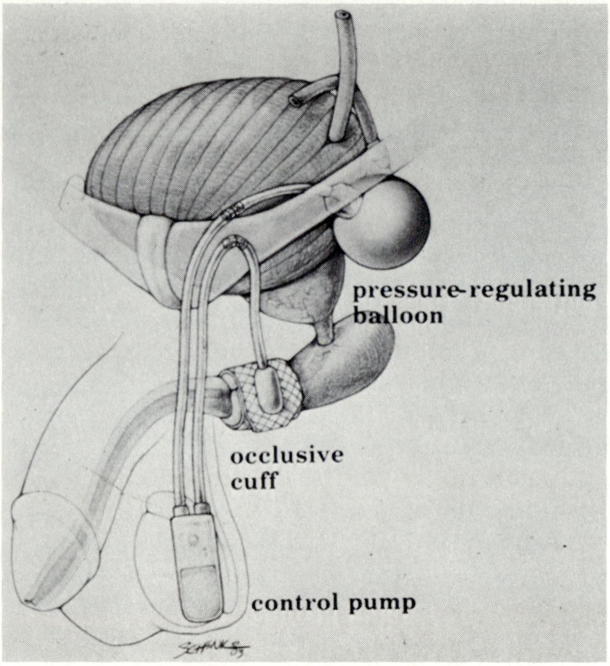

Figure 7. AS 800 artificial urinary sphincter with bulbous urethral cuff. (*Figures 7 through 12 from Barrett DM, Furlow WL, Goldwasser B: Artificial urinary sphincter. In Yalla SV, McGuire EJ, Blaivas JG, Elbadawi A (eds): Urodynamics and Neurourology: Principles and Practice. New York, Macmillan, 1988, with permission.)*

POSTOPERATIVE CARE AND ACTIVATION

The average hospital stay for a patient with bulbous urethral cuff placement is 3 to 4 days, and that for a patient with bladder neck placement is 2 to 3 days longer. Postoperative discomfort is moderate; some swelling and edema occur at the pump site in the scrotum or labia. For the first 24 to 48 hours, ice packs are placed in the region of the pump to help reduce postoperative edema. Except in unusual circumstances, the urethral catheter can be removed on the morning after implantation. Some patients report an immediate improvement in their urinary control, which can be explained on the basis of increased resistance due to swelling and edema at the cuff site. In almost all patients, this response is transient and incontinence is noticed again in a few days. Rarely, the patient is unable to urinate. In this event, intermittent catheterization with a small caliber urethral catheter is necessary until spontaneous voiding develops. Undoubtedly, prolonged intubation of the urethra or bladder neck through a recently implanted cuff enhances the risk of urethral cuff erosion.

Incontinence is expected to persist during the deactivation period, and some form of incontinence protection is worn until activation is undertaken. We discourage the use of clamps during this period and advise most patients to use diapers or condom drainage devices.

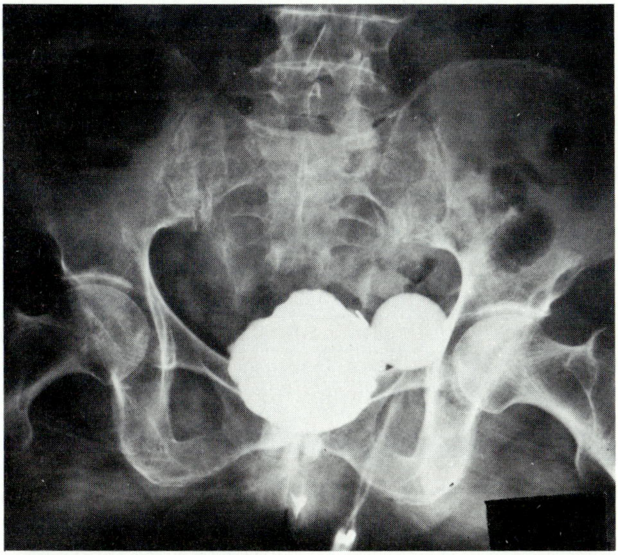

A

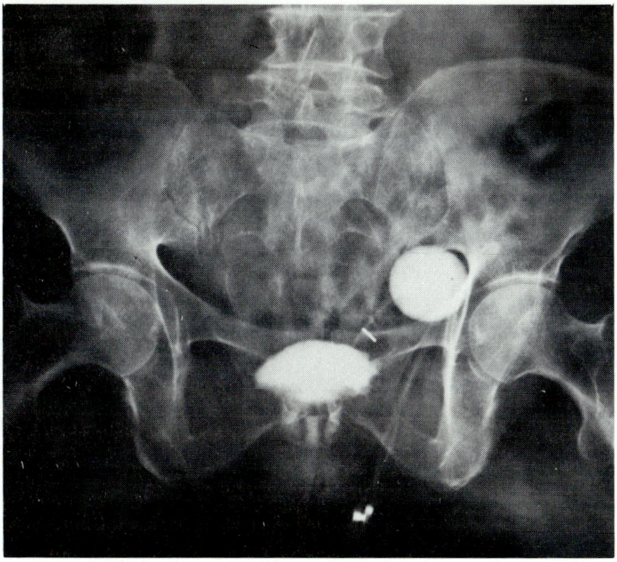

B

Figure 8. A. Cystogram of a female patient with AS 800 sphincter before voiding. **B.** Cystogram of the same patient after voiding.

Although ambulation is not limited after implantation, all patients are cautioned to avoid undue compression to their perineum and lower abdomen during the recovery period. Special emphasis is given to patients with bulbous urethral cuffs to avoid compression to the cuff area on the bulbous urethra. In our experience, patients are ready for activation in 6 to 8 weeks regardless of the location of the cuff site. Scrotal or labial tenderness generally subsides by that time, and the abdominal and perineal incisions are well healed. Activation is undertaken by compressing the pump firmly. The deactivation pin will "pop" into the activated configuration, allowing fluid to circulate through the control assembly The activation process can be monitored by obtaining deflation and inflation roentgenograms, which will confirm filling of the cuff after activation.

Instructing the patient about how the device functions generally begins before implantation. However, most patients require a direct demonstration of how to use the device after activation. Some patients are more nimble than others and learn to operate the sphincter pump easily (Fig. 8).

NOCTURNAL DEACTIVATION

Many patients are dry at night and do not require cuff compression for continence. We instruct these patients in nocturnal deactivation. This has the obvious benefit of reducing the risk of ischemia to the underlying urethra or bladder neck. Patients should be advised that after deflating the cuff, recompression requires 3 to 5 minutes, and that although bladder emptying was accomplished in less time, full continence can be expected only after the cuff is fully inflated. In patients with reduced flow rates, a second pumping may be required to empty the bladder adequately because cuff recompression will occur before voiding has been completed.

In patients who are unable to empty their bladders completely, intermittent self-catheterization is used.[24] Patients are advised to deflate the sphincter cuff before inserting the catheter into the bladder.

POSTOPERATIVE COMPLICATIONS

Hematoma

The most common minor complication of a sphincter operation is the formation of subcutaneous hematomas. Labial or scrotal hematomas cause the most problems because they may displace the pump into an unfavorable location for external manipulation. Although most hematomas resolve spontaneously, occasionally a large hematoma is drained to prevent discomfort and enhance healing.

Retention

Another minor problem that occasionally occurs is the inability to void completely after implantation. The initial assessment should include a check of the sphincter mechanism to confirm that the cuff is deactivated in the open position. Most patients, regardless of cuff location, begin to void after one or two in-and-out catheterizations with small caliber catheters (10 to 12 Fr). Patients who have had bladder neck cuff placement may do self-catheterization indefinitely, if necessary, without undue risk to the cuff and tissue. However, patients with bulbous urethral cuffs are at more risk for cuff-urethral injury from early repeated or prolonged catheterization.

Fortunately, the incidence of incomplete voiding in patients with bulbous urethral cuffs is rare; however, when it occurs we use a soft 10- or 12-Fr catheter for self-catheterization. The patient is asked to deactivate the cuff in the open position before insertion of the catheter; this technique ensures minimal external pressure on the urethra at the time of catheterization. The same technique is followed if emergency medical problems mandate the placement of an indwelling catheter. In the event of an elective need for prolonged bladder drainage, a suprapubic drainage system may be inserted with fluoroscopic monitoring to avoid the sphincter components.

Cuff Erosion

The most feared postoperative complications of sphincter operations are cuff erosion and infection. Although cuff erosion has become uncommon since delayed activation has been used, this problem still implies at least temporary failure. Erosion can occur at any time, but it is most common during the first 3 to 4 months after implantation. Cuff erosion has occurred before activation, and this complication usually implies an unrecognized surgical injury to the urethra or bladder neck.

Clinically, patients with cuff erosion may present with pain and swelling in the cuff or pump area, recurrent incontinence, and urosepsis. Urethrography or urethroscopy confirms erosion (Fig. 9). Surgical removal of the cuff is mandatory, and purulent drainage necessitates removal of the remaining sphincter components. An 18- or 20-Fr silicone Foley catheter is inserted and left in place for 3 to 4 weeks or until there is radiographic evidence of complete healing. Strictures are surprisingly rare after cuff erosion.

For "clean," uncomplicated erosion, we have had some success by removing only the cuff and temporarily occluding the tube leading to the pump with a stainless steel tubing plug. Generous irrigation of the surrounding area with antibiotic solutions and drainage may prevent subsequent infection around the device components. Several weeks later, after complete healing with no evidence of infection, a new cuff may be inserted. In the case of the urethra, an alternative location around the bulbar portion

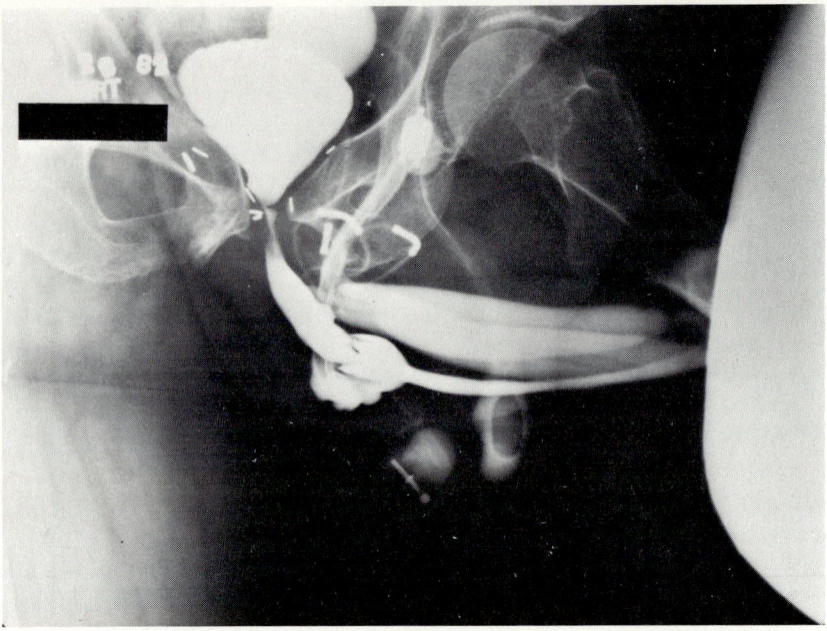

Figure 9. Urethrogram of patient with artificial urinary sphincter and penile prosthesis shows extravasation of contrast medium around sphincter cuff, a finding that is diagnostic of urethral cuff erosion.

is selected; for the bladder neck, the same site may be selected, but placement of the cuff cannot be guaranteed because of technical difficulty.

We have used two techniques to facilitate replacement of a bladder neck cuff:

1. The eroded opening in the bladder neck is closed with absorbable suture. The area is generously irrigated with antibiotic solution. A thin strap of silicone, approximately 2 cm wide, is passed around the bladder neck in the cuff bed and retained loosely. If infection is avoided, reoperation and cuff placement are facilitated by the plane maintained by the silicone strap.
2. The eroded bladder neck is closed and irrigated. The peritoneum is opened, and the omentum is tailored so that a tongue of this structure can be placed under and around the bladder neck. Redissection of the plane around the bladder neck is thus facilitated.

Infection

Purulent infection of the implanted sphincter may present as (1) an abscess and drainage from the incisions; (2) pain, swelling, and induration of the pump or cuff site; (3) fever; (4) pump erosion through the skin; or (5) cuff erosion. It is not always clear whether cuff erosion is the result of an underlying infection or is caused by pressure necrosis. Treatment generally requires removal of the sphincter. Although drainage of the infected pyogenic process around a sphincter component can be attempted with drains and antibiotic solutions, most devices must be removed for ultimate resolution of the infection. Reimplantation can be done later with the same inherent risks as those in patients with previous cuff erosion.

Mechanical Malfunction

The mechanical reliability of the AS 800 sphincter is a remarkable tribute to biomechanical engineering, and this device is relatively trouble free compared with all other sphincter models. Potential risks include tubing kinks, system leaks, and control pump malfunction.

From December 1982 to January 1986, we implanted 221 AS 800 sphincters. The mechanical reliability is depicted in Figure 10, but to date only six reoperations have been required: two for cuff leaks, two for tubing kinks, one for pump malfunction, and one for a connector leak. All patients had satisfactory repair. Although the exact longevity of this device cannot be predicted, the 5-year reliability rate will probably be more than 90 percent.

Recurrent or Persistent Incontinence

Recurrent urinary incontinence after successful reimplantation requires a systematic means of defining the problem. An "inflate-deflate" roentgenogram confirms the hydraulic function of the device. If the radiopaque fluid is not present in the system, a leak has occurred, but the exact location cannot be determined without surgical exploration.[25]

In our experience, the most common site for leakage is the lower surface of the cuff. The leaking point may be extremely small and not easily identifiable without removal of the cuff and close inspection. Because the cuff is the most difficult component to expose surgically, we recommend excluding leaks at the connector site and balloon stem before dissecting

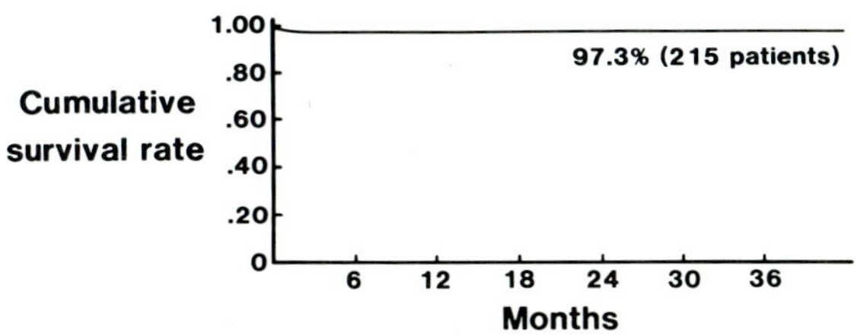

Figure 10. Mechanical reliability of 221 implanted AS 800 sphincters.

and removing the cuff. If fluid is present but the cuff fails to refill after pump compression, there may be a tubing kink or flow obstruction within the pump assembly. Again, surgical exploration is required to define the location of obstruction more adequately. If the roentgenogram confirms normal deflation and inflation of the sphincter cuff, a urethrogram followed by direct-vision urethroscopy will exclude cuff erosion.

A urethral pressure profile while the cuff is inflated and deflated allows for a determination of the closing pressure differential. However, quantitating the closing pressure may be misleading. A pressure differential of 40 cm H_2O is usually associated with enough closing pressure to afford satisfactory continence. Unfortunately, this is not an absolute rule because associated detrusor hyperreflexia and decreased detrusor compliance adversely influence differential pressure. If the differential pressure is low, an increase in the pressure of the balloon reservoir may enhance urinary control.

Of the 221 patients in our series, 14 underwent operations for an increase in balloon pressure to enhance the degree of continence. Five of these patients were unsatisfactorily wet after initial activation of the first device, and nine became insidiously incontinent some months after activation. This was presumably due to pressure atrophy of the tissue under the cuff, which ultimately results in reduced closing pressure. The recent recommended changes in the volume of the pressure-balloon reservoir described earlier are hoped to compensate for these changes and maintain adequate cuff compression.

Reduction of the cuff size is another option to be considered when compensating for recurrent or persistent incontinence in a patient with an otherwise normally functioning sphincter. The assumption is that because of erroneous measurement or underlying tissue atrophy, the closed cuff is unable to compress the underlying urethra or bladder neck adequately. Roentgenograms of this phenomenon are not helpful other than to confirm filling of the cuff. Differential closing pressure may be useful but, again, it may be misleading at times.

For persistent or recurrent incontinence in patients with bulbous urethral cuff placement, our policy is to increase the balloon pressure to the next highest pressure category, i.e., from 51 to 60 cm H_2O to 61 to 70 cm H_2O, if the initial cuff size is 5.5 cm or less. If the cuff size is more than 5.5 cm, we increase the balloon pressure, reexplore the cuff, and downgrade its size at least 0.5 cm.

Because the sizes of bladder neck cuffs are much more variable and dissection of the implanted cuff is more difficult, we are inclined to increase the balloon pressure initially. An intraoperative urethral closing pressure differential may be useful. If the closing pressure is not increased appreciably with the new balloon pressurized in the system, exploration and downsizing of the cuff are the next alternatives.

Despite optimal sphincter function and closing pressure, unacceptable incontinence occasionally persists. Results may be improved with pharmacologic agents, such as propantheline and oxybutynin, to decrease detrusor contractility or imipramine to enhance outlet resistance and decrease contractility.

SPECIAL CONSIDERATIONS

Inadequate detrusor compliance or hyperreflexia has historically excluded many patients from sphincter implantation. Recently, bladder augmentation techniques have increased the need for sphincter implantation (Fig. 11). Reports of combined augmentation cystoplasty and sphincter implantation emphasize the need for caution in this select group of patients for two reasons. First, although Light et al[26–28] mentioned use of the sphincter around bowel segments used as total bladder replacement, our experience with sphincter cuff around bowel has not been satisfactory. Second, the shape in which the cystoplasty is reconstructed has a bearing on the successful use of the artificial urinary sphincter. Tubular-shaped cystoplasties such as a conventional ileocecocystoplasty seem to be associated with high-pressure contractions produced by the bowel segment.[29] In association with the artificial urinary sphincter, these high-pressure contractions may overcome the obstruction produced by the sphincter cuff[30] or, alternatively, if they do

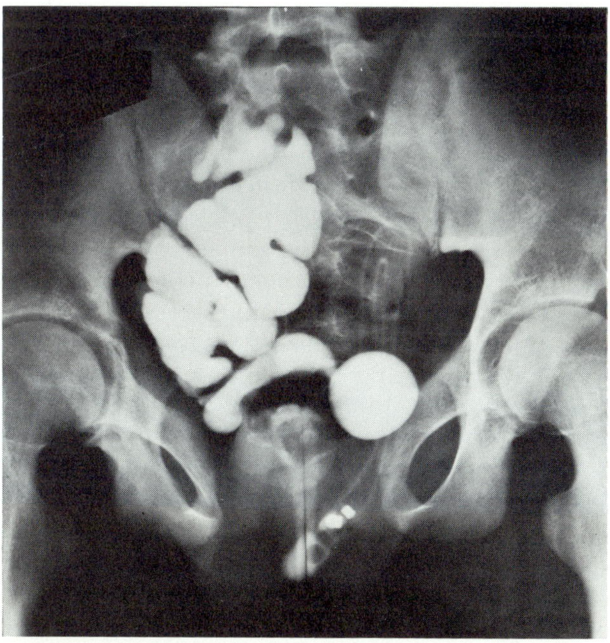

Figure 11. Cystogram shows cecocystoplasty and AS 800 artificial urinary sphincter with cuff open.

not, they may endanger the upper urinary tracts. Four technical considerations seem to be important in attempting to help prevent this problem:

1. Detubularizing the bowel segment used, thus interrupting the strong circular muscle layer of the bowel
2. Reconstructing the cystoplasty in a shape that will produce a large diameter
3. Providing a large capacity in which pressure produced by cystoplasty contraction will be dissipated
4. Placing the reconstructed bowel such that the peristaltic waves are directed away from the trigone

Goldwasser and Webster[29] described their experience with patients whose bladders were reconstructed according to these principles using the right colon. They found that although cystoplasty contractions still occur, they happen at a larger bladder capacity and they are low pressure. Advances in bladder reconstruction and in the artificial urinary sphincter will make their combined use more common in the future. One additional problem is infections associated with the use of bowel segments and the artificial urinary sphincter. Good bowel preparation, the use of prophylactic antibiotics, and copious irrigation during the operation of both the bowel segment and the area in which the cuff is placed may all help to reduce the incidence of infection around the device. Despite these measures, however, this problem still remains a deterrent for the use of the artificial urinary sphincter in combination with bowel segments.

RESULTS

What constitutes an optimal result in patients with an artificial urinary sphincter depends on the continence afforded by the device, safety to the tissues of the urinary tract, preservation of sexual function, and mechanical reliability of the device.

Although there are reports of upper tract decompensation related to sphincter implantation, in our experience this has been uncommon. Failure to empty adequately predisposes the patient to relative ureterovesical obstruction or reflux with resulting hydronephrosis and urosepsis. Regular indefinite follow-up of the patient to ensure upper tract stability and adequate emptying is mandatory, and most upper tract problems can thus be avoided.

We have not noted a significant change in erectile function in male patients or problems with intromission in female patients after implantation. Two women became pregnant and had delivery by cesarean section.

The percentage of successful implants in our series of 221 patients (203 male and 18 female) is shown in Figure 12. Of the male patients, 171 had

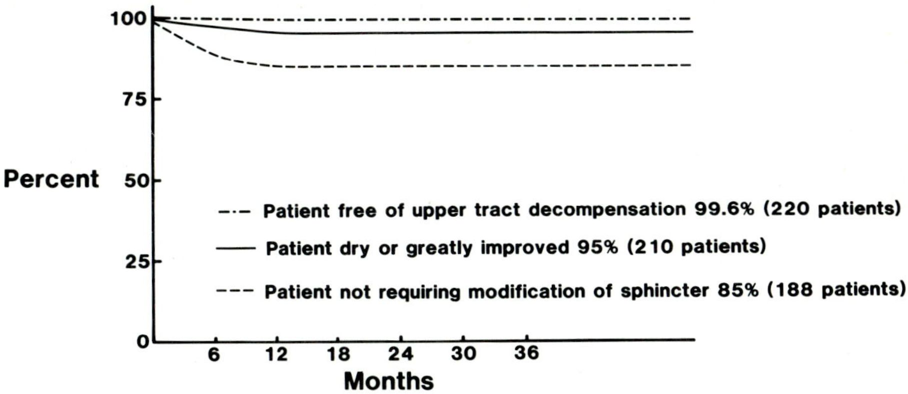

Figure 12. Percentage of successful implantations in 221 patients.

implantation at the bulbous urethra. Five devices were removed because of infection and three because of erosion (five were at the bulbous urethra and three at the bladder neck); four of these had successful reimplantation.

Seven patients with functioning sphincter devices were somewhat improved but unacceptably wet and had to wear multiple pads or diapers for protection. Thus, including the patients who had successful reoperation, the acceptably dry rate was 95 percent (210 patients).

FUTURE CONSIDERATIONS

Prosthetic implants for the management of urinary incontinence have evolved rapidly. This development is a tribute to biomedical engineering and the persistence of the clinician for constant improvement of the status quo. Our creativity with prosthetic materials and designs has many areas to pursue within the urinary tract. The future will undoubtedly provide exciting new advances not only for incontinence and impotency but also for replacements for the bladder, ureter, vas deferens, and urethra.

REFERENCES

1. Berry JL: A new procedure for correction of urinary incontinence: Preliminary report. J Urol 85:771, 1961
2. Kaufman JJ: A new operation for male incontinence. Surg Gynecol Obstet 131:295, 1970
3. Foley FEB: An artificial sphincter: A new device and operation for control of enuresis and urinary incontinence. J Urol 58:250, 1947

4. Scott FB, Bradley WE, Timm GW, Kothari D: Treatment of incontinence secondary to myelodysplasia by an implantable prosthetic urinary sphincter. South Med J 66:987, 1973
5. Scott FB, Bradley WE, Timm GW: Treatment of urinary incontinence by an implantable prosthetic urinary sphincter. J Urol 112:75, 1974
6. Rosen M: A simple artificial implantable sphincter. Br J Urol 48:675, 1976
7. Politano VA: Periurethral polytetrafluoroethylene injection for urinary incontinence. J Urol 127:439, 1982
8. Artificial Urinary Sphincter Investigational Study Group: American Medical Systems, Minnetonka, MN, 1980
9. Furlow WL: Implantation of a new semiautomatic artificial genitourinary sphincter: Experience with primary activation and deactivation in 47 patients. J Urol 126:741, 1981
10. Barrett DM, Furlow WL: Implantation of a new semi-automatic artificial genitourinary sphincter: Experience with patients utilizing a new concept of primary and secondary activation. Prog Clin Biol Res 78:375, 1981
11. Furlow WL, Barrett DM: The artificial urinary sphincter: Experience with the AS 800 pump-control assembly for single-stage primary deactivation and activation: A preliminary report. Mayo Clin Proc 60:255, 1985
12. Barrett DM, Furlow WL: The management of severe urinary incontinence in patients with myelodysplasia by implantation of the AS 791/792 urinary sphincter device. J Urol 128:484, 1982
13. Mitchell ME, Rink RC: Experience with the artificial urinary sphincter in children and young adults. J Pediatr Surg 18:700, 1983
14. Light JK, Scott FB: Management of urinary incontinence in women with the artificial urinary sphincter. J Urol 134:476, 1985
15. Donovan MG, Barrett DM, Furlow WL: Use of the artificial urinary sphincter in the management of severe incontinence in females. Surg Gynecol Obstet 161:17, 1985
16. Scott FB: The use of the artificial sphincter in the treatment of urinary incontinence in the female patient. Urol Clin North Am 12:305, 1985
17. Barrett DM, Furlow WL: Artificial urinary sphincter in the management of female incontinence. In Raz S (ed): Female Urology. Philadelphia, Saunders, 1983, pp 284–292
18. Barrett DM: Female incontinence and the artificial urinary sphincter. In Kaufman JJ (ed): Current Urologic Therapy, 2nd ed. Philadelphia, Saunders, 1986, pp 273–275
19. McGuire EJ, Wang C-C, Usitalo H, Savastano J: Modified pubovaginal sling in girls with myelodysplasia. J Urol 135:94, 1986
20. Barrett DM, Furlow WL: Radical prostatectomy incontinence and the AS791 artificial urinary sphincter. J Urol 129:528, 1983
21. Barrett DM, Furlow WL: Artificial urinary sphincter in children. In Kelalis PP, King LR, Belman AB (eds): Clinical Pediatric Urology, 2nd ed. Philadelphia, Saunders, 1985, pp 345–354
22. Barrett DM: Voiding dysfunction in children and the use of the artificial sphincter to correct sphincteric incontinence in the female child. Proc Symp Female Bladder Voiding Disturbances, Milan, Italy, December 17, 1983
23. AMS Sphincter 800 Urinary Prosthesis: New fluid-volume recommendation for the pressure-regulating balloon. Am Med Systems, Minnetonka, MN, 1986

24. Barrett DM, Furlow WL: Incontinence, intermittent self-catheterization and the artificial genitourinary sphincter. J Urol 132:268, 1984
25. Webster GD, Sihelnik SA: Troubleshooting the malfunctioning Scott artificial urinary sphincter. J Urol 131:269, 1984
26. Light JK, Engelmann UH: Reconstruction of the lower urinary tract: Observations on bowel dynamics and the artificial urinary sphincter. J Urol 133:594, 1985
27. Light JK: The artificial urinary sphincter in children: Experience with the AS 800 series and bowel reconstruction. Urol Clin North Am 12:103, 1985
28. Light JK, Scott FB: Total reconstruction of the lower urinary tract using bowel and the artificial urinary sphincter. J Urol 131:953, 1984
29. Goldwasser B, Webster GD: Augmentation and substitution enterocystoplasty. J Urol 135:215, 1986
30. Webster GD, Goldwasser B: Bladder reconstruction and continent urinary diversion. In King LR, Stone AR, Webster GD (eds): Replacement of the Urinary Bladder. Chicago, Year Book Medical Publishers, 1987, p 75

Current Management of Urethral Injuries

Norman E. Peterson

Traumatic injuries of the urethra constitute a maximum challenge to diagnostic and therapeutic resources. The opportunity for gratifying success with optimal management is balanced by the possibility for depressingly complicated sequelae in cases receiving inappropriate or untimely care. Anatomic distinctions account for the limitation to male patients of the majority of considerations regarding urethral trauma; female urethral injury commonly coexists with vaginal damage, and surgical correction will therefore incorporate urologic and gynecologic efforts.

The male urethra is anatomically classified into anterior and posterior segments. The anterior urethra is further subdivided into glanular, pendulous, and bulbar areas, and the posterior urethra is comprised of the membranous (sphincteric) and prostatic regions (Fig. 1). Trauma to either anterior or posterior urethra may result from external penetrating sources (bullet, impalement), or from internal, often iatrogenic, perforation from luminal instrumentation or foreign devices. Trauma to the pendulous anterior urethra may be self-inflicted or follow assault; damage to the bulbous urethra may result from assault, but is more common following straddle trauma to the perineum. Posterior urethral trauma is usually associated with pelvic fracture (crushing or deceleration-impact), with urethral fixation focusing shearing forces at the prostatomembranous junction.

Anterior urethral trauma often exists as an isolated injury, while posterior urethral damage more commonly occurs in a multi-injury setting.

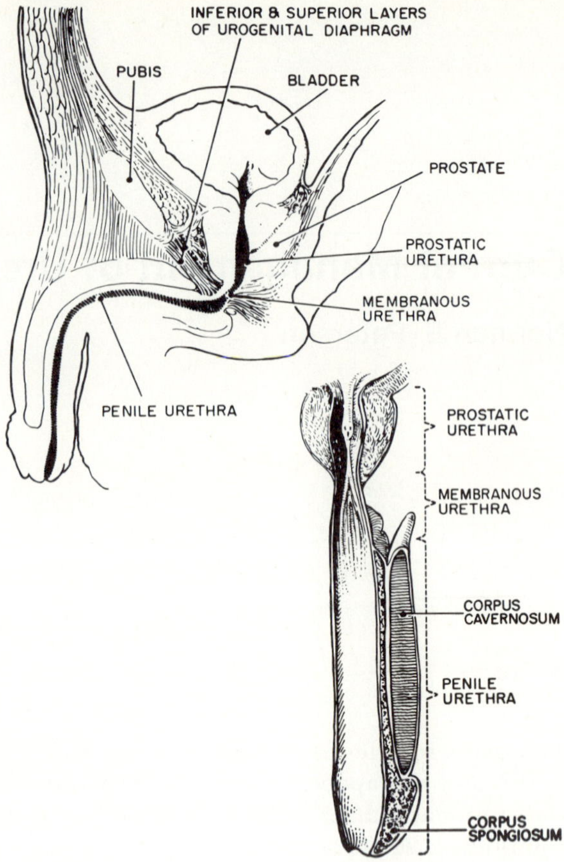

Figure 1. Anatomic divisions of the male urethra. *(Reprinted from Flock RH, Culp D (eds), Surgical Urology, 2nd ed, Chicago, Year Book Medical Pub, 1963, with permission.)*

ANTERIOR URETHRAL TRAUMA

Appraisal of severity of injury and appropriate management options are usually apparent at presentation. Nature of injury, anatomic site, delay between injury and presentation, and coexisting injury all impact upon therapeutic decisions. With gunshot wounds, missile caliber and velocity will identify the possibility for greater tissue destruction than apparent to inspection.

The history will commonly include penile or perineal trauma, with pain in the injured area. Voiding may initially be unimpaired, followed by progressive voiding dysfunction as tissues become suffused with blood or urine; tissue necrosis and septic complications may ensue. Urethral bleeding may range from none, to minimal, to excessive. Hematuria is initial, clearing with continued voiding. Periurethral or perineal edema and ecchymosis may wax and wane with voiding, and will reflect the site of injury according to fascial compartments (Fig. 2). It is repeatedly emphasized that a thorough understanding of penile–perineal fascial anatomy is mandatory for accurate diagnosis and appropriate management; in fact, intellectual precision is superfluous to the standard requirements for tissue drainage, urinary diversion, and antibacterial therapy, which in combination provide justifiable optimism for satisfactory results regardless of the site of injury. Briefly, one may consider Buck's fascia to ensleeve the penis, attaching distally at the corona and proximally at the triangular ligament; a defect in the urethra with Buck's fascia intact will therefore result in limitation of swelling and ecchymosis to the penis. Colle's fascia attaches posteriorly to the triangular ligament, where it fuses with the inferior fascial sheath of the urogenital diaphragm, and laterally to the fascia lata at the inguinal ligament, and also continues as Scarpa's fascia on the anterior abdominal wall. These attachments are responsible for the characteristic butterfly configuration of perineal ecchymosis (Fig. 3); they also account for the confinement within Colle's and Scarpa's compartments of extravasation from bulbomembranous, and most membranous, urethral injuries, and for the extension of extravasation from membranoprostatic ruptures into the pelvis, and possibly through the inguinal canals to more proximal sites. More simply, scrotal distortion by blood or urine will reflect a defect in Buck's fascia.

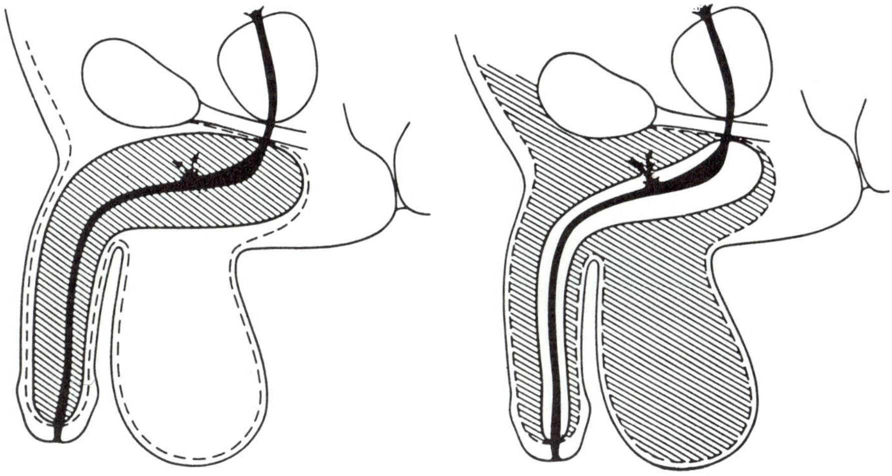

A B

Figure 2. Site of injury reflected by pattern of genital extravasation. **A.** Buck's fascia (*solid line*) intact, limiting deformity to penile shaft. **B.** Buck's fascial defect, permitting extravasation within the limits of Colles' fascia (*broken line*). *(Reprinted from Kiracofe L, Pfister R, Peterson N, J Urol 114:60, 1975, with permission.)*

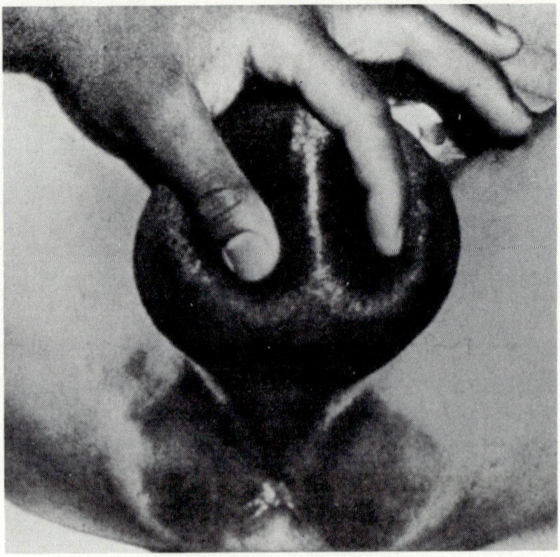

Figure 3. Scrotal and perineal hematoma, compatible with defect in Buck's fascia and confined by Colles' fascia.

More accurate appraisal of the site and degree of injury may be provided by voiding or retrograde urethrography, urethroscopy, or cavernosography. Voiding urethrography may be interdicted by the presence of extensive local extravasation or tissue necrosis. Urethroscopy is often limited by poor visibility and by the possibility for additional extravasation of irrigant delivered under hydrostatic pressure. Cavernosography has been indicted as potentially injurious, inducing scarring. These studies should therefore be obtained with deliberation and with an appreciation that initial management will likely be unchanged regardless of diagnostic verification beyond clinical impressions.

PENDULOUS URETHRAL INJURY

Penetrating wounds of the pendulous urethra will logically present with tissue damage reflecting the mode of injury, i.e., impalement, gunshot. Nonpenetrating injuries are most often straddle type, with assault also frequent. Tissue devitalization can occasionally be extensive. However, therapeutic results benefit from acknowledgment that tissue damage is frequently less profound than initially apparent, particularly if delay in presentation has permitted accumulation of hematoma, extravasation, and inflammation. Injudicious debridement may therefore be unnecessarily excessive. Management is more appropriately initiated conservatively, with the deliberate intention of further debridement as necessary following definitive tissue demarcation.

Penetrating wounds may routinely be considered as contaminated, as may nonpenetrating wounds that manifest tissue necrosis. Antibiotic administration is therefore elemental to management, including assurance of tissue levels before operative manipulation (2 hours intravenous; 6 hours intramuscular). Surgical efforts require sufficient exploration to expose possible coexisting injury, debridement of obviously devitalized tissue, and copious irrigation. With partial urethral injury (intact mucosal bridge), passage of a 14 Fr urethral catheter is permissible. Inability to catheterize, or contraindication to catheterization by tissue contamination, warrants perineal or suprapubic cystostomy. Tissue drainage, following evacuation of hematoma, is paramount. Edema or ecchymosis limited to the penile shaft (intact Buck's fascia) requires bilateral subcutaneous Penrose drains through generous transverse incisions in the proximal and distal penile skin. Buck's fascial defects (scrotal edema or extravasation confined by Colles' fascia) require an additional scrotal Penrose drain through proximal and dependent scrotal incisions. Anterior abdominal drainage is required only by obvious infection or necrosis. Tissue response to adequate drainage is characteristically prompt and dramatic, and drains may usually be removed after 48 to 72 hours.

Exploration will permit decisions regarding the permissibility of primary reconstruction and closure or the advisability of temporizing maneuvers intermediate to secondary urethroplasty. Obvious tissue contamination or indistinct margins of viability contraindicate primary repair. In addition, most distal urethral injuries are incomplete and therefore direct repair will be superfluous to anticipated spontaneous regeneration (stented or diverted).

Where primary repair is elected, debridement, irrigation, and preparation for tissue drainage is followed by generous mobilization of the urethra from the corpora in both directions, spatulation of the urethral remnants, and tension-free anastomosis with full thickness absorbable suture. Deliberate reapproximation of local spongiosium over the urethral anastomosis provides advantage. Indwelling 14 Fr Foley catheter (or cystostomy, according to judgment or preference) completes the procedure. Duration of catheterization is arbitrary; removal as early as 48 hours has been advocated, but there is no apparent advantage to early removal and no penalty with longer periods of drainage; catheterization for 5 to 7 days is standard.

Where primary anastomosis is considered inadvisable, acute management will require some form of urethral externalization and proximal urinary diversion. After conservative debridement, the urethral remnants are secured to local skin by fine absorbable suture. The marsupialized or missing segment is later addressed by any of several methods for urethral substitution.

Pendulous urethral injuries coexisting with significant penile skin loss are often characterized by a narrow circumferential remnant of skin at the corona, representing a tempting site for attachment of skin grafts. Chronic

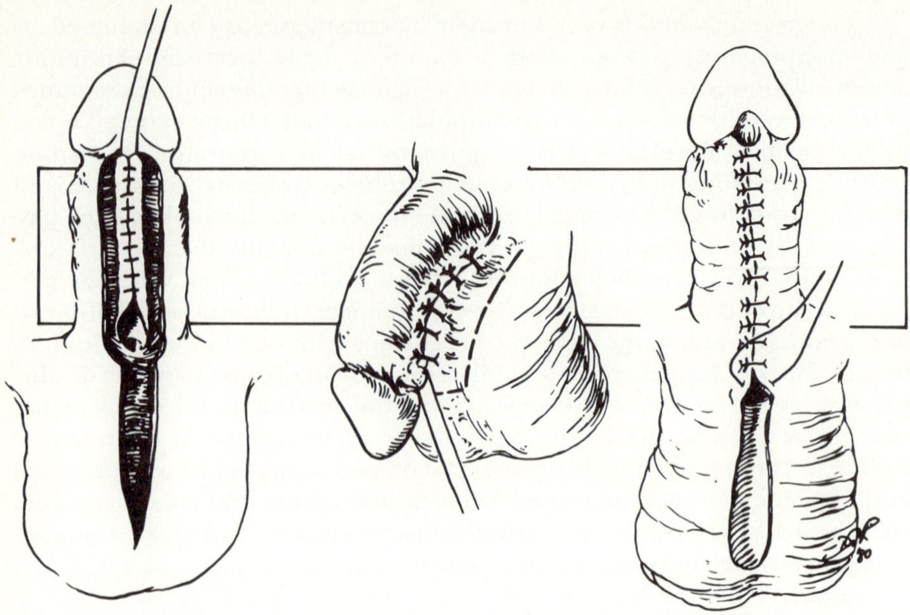

Figure 4. Scrotal burial method for covering penile cutaneous defect following completion of urethroplasty. For defects limited to the ventral penis, a midvertical scrotal incision is made and the corresponding margins of penile and scrotal skin are approximated. Alternately, transverse scrotal incisions will permit submersion of the involved area of the penis. Later cutaneous release incorporates individual closure of resulting penile and scrotal defects. *(Reprinted from Devine CJ, Devine PC: chap 22. In Stewart B: Operative Urology, Lower Urinary Tract, Pelvic Structures and Male Reproductive System, Baltimore, Williams & Wilkins, 1975, with permission.)*

edema of this collar remnant is virtually guaranteed and will become a cosmetic liability; excision during initial debridement is therefore advisable. Temporary burial of the denuded penis within the scrotum is a safe and expeditious maneuver for skin transfer (Fig. 4), but ultimate results following release are compromised by cosmetic imperfections, including the presence of hair. A free, split thickness graft from thigh, abdomen, or buttock is a second option; 0.015-inch thickness grafts are acknowledged as providing the most favorable combination of graft survival and cosmetic acceptability; thicker grafts contract less but are bulky and heal poorly. The presence of hair follicles and the absence of normal sensation compromise to varying degrees the results of all free skin grafts. The patient's own avulsed skin is surprisingly often available, but should never be employed in repair procedures; replantation survival is uncommon, and rates of infection are unacceptably high.

BULBAR URETHRAL INJURY

Most bulbar injuries result from straddle trauma; blunt trauma exceeds perineal impalement in incidence. The acute management of bulbar urethral trauma differs little from that described for the pendulous urethra. Assessment for genital and rectal injury is mandatory, after which decisions focus upon requirements for surgical drainage and eligibility for immediate reanastomosis.

A patient presenting with minor perineal bruising, who also denies having attempted voiding, may be exempted from surgical drainage; immediate urethrography will appraise the presence and degree of urethral damage. Equivocal manifestations may be managed by 7 to 10 days of urethral catheterization (14 to 16 Fr adult; 8 Fr child). More severe injuries will require operative intervention for initiation of perineal drainage, and inspection for extent of urethral devitalization or evidence of contamination (penetrating injuries). Simple debridement and closure of bulbar defects is a common temptation owing to the compliance and capacity of the bulbous urethra; however, unappreciated tissue ischemia will guarantee marked stricturing. Liberal debridement with circumferential spatulated reanastamosis is often advisable, including careful approximation of local spongiosum. Stenting urethral drainage for 7 to 14 days is usually adequate.

Where damage exceeds the limits for excision and reanastomosis, or where contamination is present or suspect, debridement should be followed by exteriorization to the adjacent scrotoperineal skin, with proximal urinary diversion by cystostomy. Following a judgmental interval for stabilization of tissue conditions, secondary urethroplasty may be undertaken.

ENDOURETHRAL RUPTURE

Perforation of the urethra during instrumentation by endoscope, sound, lithotriptor, biopsy instrument, urethrotome, mandarin catheter, or filiform and follower may occur despite all appropriate precautions. Identification seldom requires radiographic verification. During manipulation of the instrument, a characteristic sensation is transmitted to the examiner which signals an extraurethral position. In addition manipulation is impeded, and endoscopic visibility is either obscured, or shaggy nonurothelial tissue is identified. Bleeding may be sufficient to obstruct visibility without being externally manifested. Employment of irrigant may produce a discrepancy between influx and egress, and penoscrotal or pelvic extravasation may be reflected by local tissue cooling or obvious accumulation.

Management requires immediate discontinuance and catheter drainage. Not uncommonly urethral access to the bladder may be accomplished by coudé catheter, mandarin catheter, or filiforms and followers. Otherwise perineal urethrostomy (for pendulous defects) or suprapubic cystostomy will be necessary. Surgical drainage of fluid accumulation is rarely necessary and dilutional syndromes or hypervolemic complications following absorption are infrequent. Local conditions will usually stabilize within 7 days, sufficient to allow repetition of the original transurethral procedure.

URETHROPLASTY AND STRICTURE REPAIR

Reconstitution of anterior urethral integrity will involve plastic reconstruction of exteriorized defects or methods for reducing or eliminating urethral stricturing subsequent to operative maneuvers. (Unacceptable results after dilation or urethrotomy will occasionally require exteriorization preparatory to urethroplasty.) The surgical procedure selected will be influenced by site and length of defect and tissue conditions. It has also been advocated that surgical selection should await operative exposure for definitive delineation of length and thickness of the scarring process, since extension into adjacent unstrictured urethral and periurethral (spongiosal) tissues, inconspicuous to endoscopic and radiographic analysis, may require more extensive correction than otherwise anticipated.[1]

Operative remedies may be categorized as anastomotic (excision and reapproximation), substitution (applications of extraneous tissue), and regenerative (from intact urothelium in the area of involvement). *Anastomotic* techniques are suitable only for short segments which will permit tension-free approximation. *Substitution* techniques may employ pedicled (vascularized) local tissue or free (unsupported) tissue from more remote sites; application of either as patch or tube graft is possible. Lengthy segments are eligible for substitution, although failure and complication rates increase directly with the length of substitution. *Regenerative* maneuvers include re-epithelialization following endoscopic incision of stricture or spontaneous tubularization from an intact remnant of urethral mucosa (buried strip). Longer strictures, multiple strictures, anterior urethral strictures, and those involving older patients have been variously described as less amenable to regenerative methods. Management of the majority of urethral strictures is best initiated by visual internal urethrotomy, owing to a high rate of success and low order of complications, expense, and inconvenience. Unacceptable results of urethrotomy, or patient noncompliance, will warrant formal urethroplasty. Excision-reanastomosis for short segments (Figs. 5 and 6), or buried strip techniques for longer segments are the next most dependable options, followed by pedicled, then free graft applications. Ultimate success of any method is greatly dependent upon the absence of local tissue inflammation and ischemia, and upon the availability of intact corpus spongiosum to provide vascularized coverage. Extension of the fibrotic process into the spongiosum generally reduces expectations for favorable results.

Patients managed initially by pendulous urethral exteriorization (mar-

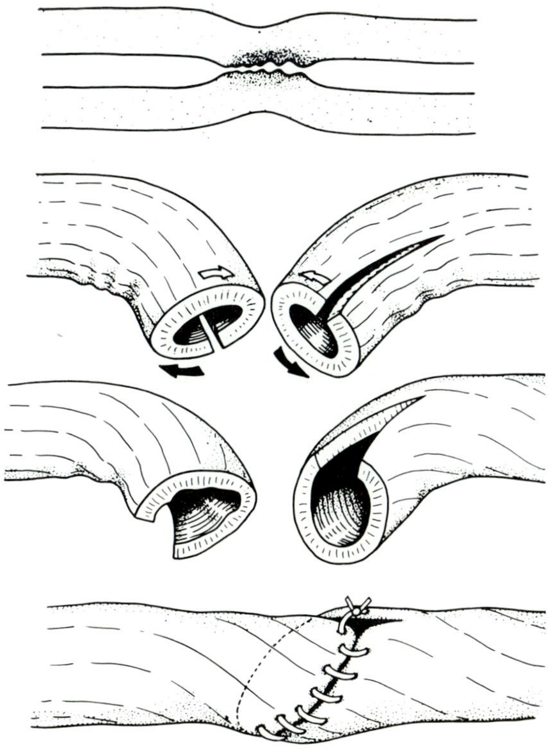

Figure 5. Excision of scarred urethra, with end-to-end anastomosis. Important features include generous urethral mobilization, adequate excision, spatulation well into normal urethra, and elliptical anastomosis. *(Reprinted from Blandy J (ed): Urology, vol II, London, Blackwell Scientific, 1976, with permission.)*

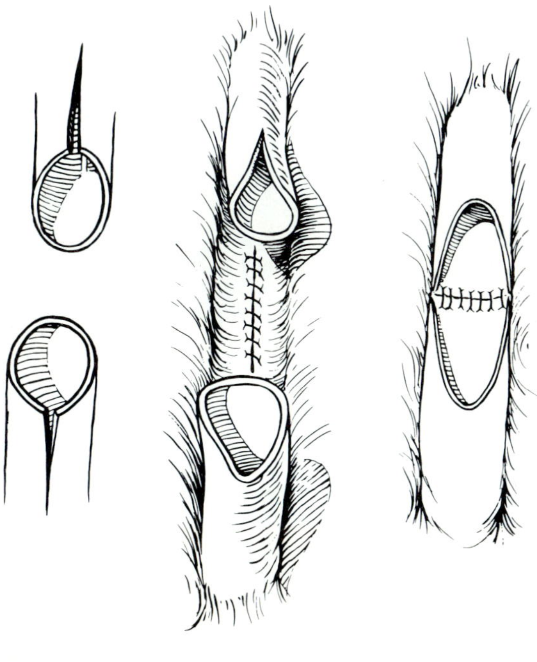

Figure 6. Technique for pendulous urethral remnants of inadequate length to permit tension-free repair. After debridement, dissection, and spatulation, the dorsal segments of the urethral remnants are connected. The remaining defect may then be closed with a pedicled or free patch graft, or managed as a buried skin strip (with proximal urinary diversion) for spontaneous regeneration. *(Reprinted from Devine CJ, Devine PC: chap 22. In Stewart B: Opertive Urology, Lower Urinary Tract, Pelvic Structures and Male Reproductive System, Baltimore, Williams & Wilkins, 1975, with permission.)*

supialization) are readily correctable by any of several methods designed to reconstruct an epithelialized tube of even caliber. Available methods include incorporation of adjacent penile skin (two-stage Johanson procedure),[2] patch or tube graft application of pedicled, full-thickness skin from the prepuce or penile shaft,[3,4] or free, defatted, full thickness skin from more remote sites (prepuce, inner or upper arm, lateral chest wall) (Figs. 7 through 12).[5] Scrotal skin is compromised by the presence of hair follicles, unsightly thickness, and vulnerability to eczematoid reactions upon exposure to urine. Where grafting from the penis leaves a cutaneous defect, closure may involve rotation of available preputial (Nesbit or Byers) or scrotal skin flaps, temporary burial in the scrotum (Cecil), or free skin grafting.

Similar methods are available for urethral strictures unresponsive to internal urethrotomy. Simple meatal strictures require only generous ventral meatotomy; coaption and restenosis must be prevented by temporary daily dilation or suture separation. Dense strictures of the fossa navicularis

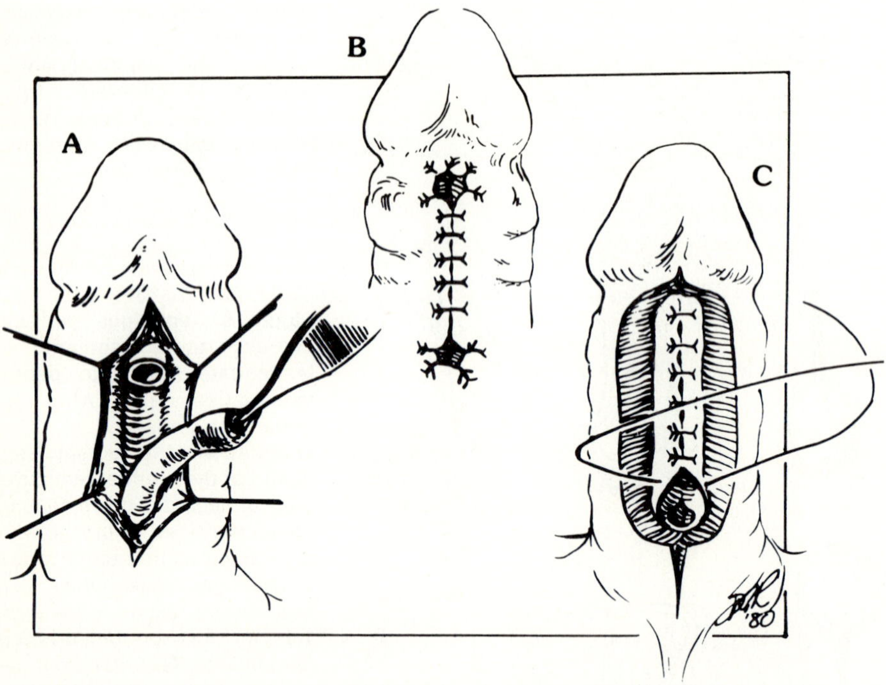

Figure 7. Optional method for acute management of pendulous urethral injury (Steward). After debridement (**A**), the proximal and distal remnants are secured to the skin (**B**). Delayed urethroplasty (**C**) follows tissue stabilization. *(Reprinted from Devine CJ, Devine PC: Chapter 22. In Stewart B: Operative Urology, Lower Urinary Tract, Pelvic Structures and Male Reproductive System, Baltimore, Williams & Wilkins, 1975, with permission.)*

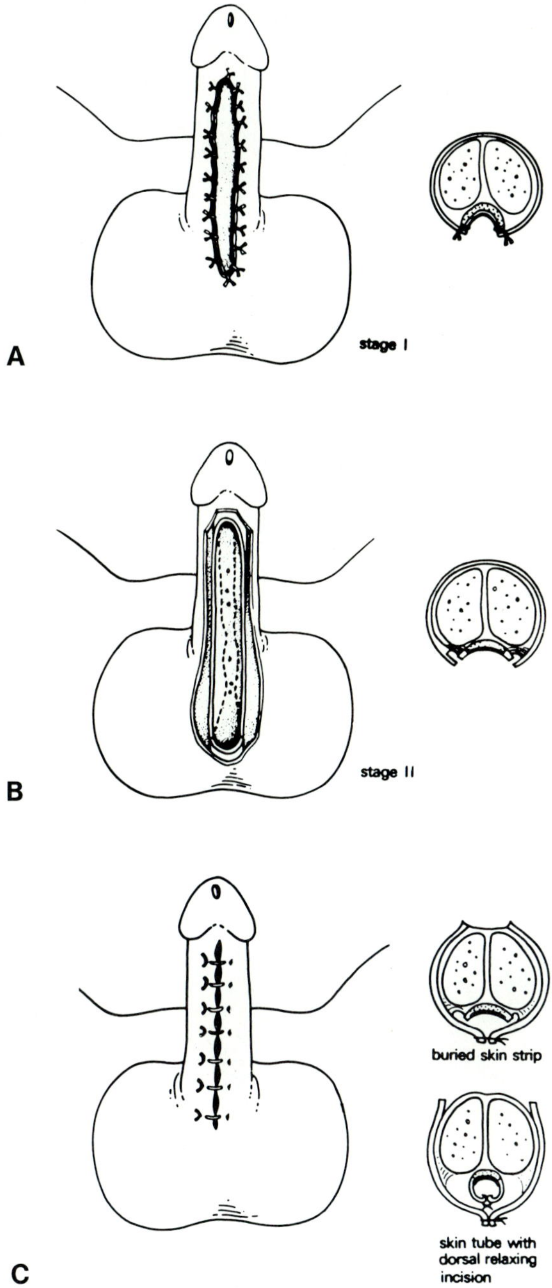

Figure 8. Anterior urethroplasty (Swinney). **A.** (Stage 1) incision of strictured urethra into uninvolved tissue at either end and circumferential anastomosis to local skin. **B.** Stage 2 involves circumferential incision to form a skin strip, which may then be buried for spontaneous tubularization (Denis-Browne), or converted into a closed tube. **C.** Skin is closed. Dorsal relaxation incision is optional and judgmental. (*Reprinted from Blandy J. (ed): Urology. vol II, London, Blackwell Scientific, 1976, with permission.)*

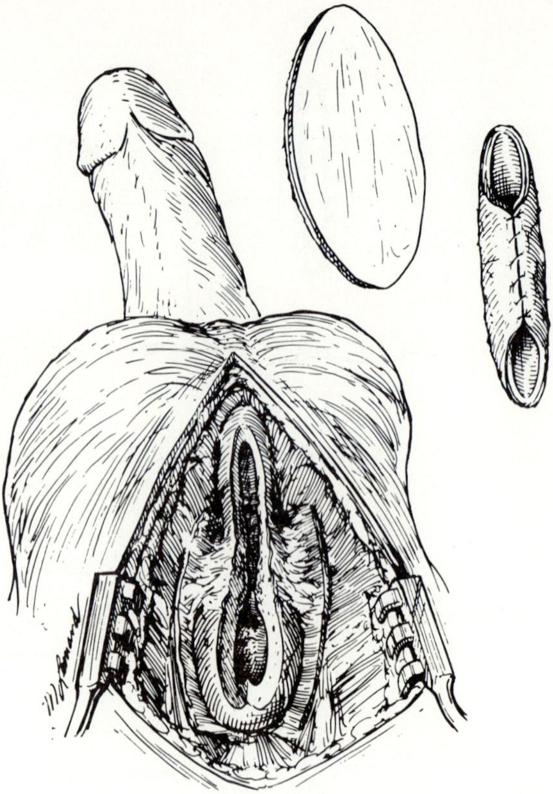

Figure 9. Full thickness patch and tube graft applications to pendulous and bulbar urethral strictures, after generous resection of scar, and spatulated exposure of 2 cm of normal proximal and distal urethra. *(Reprinted from Webster G, Koefoot R, Sihelnik S: Urethroplasty management in 100 cases of urethral stricture: A rationale for procedure selection. J Urol 134:894, 1985, with permission.)*

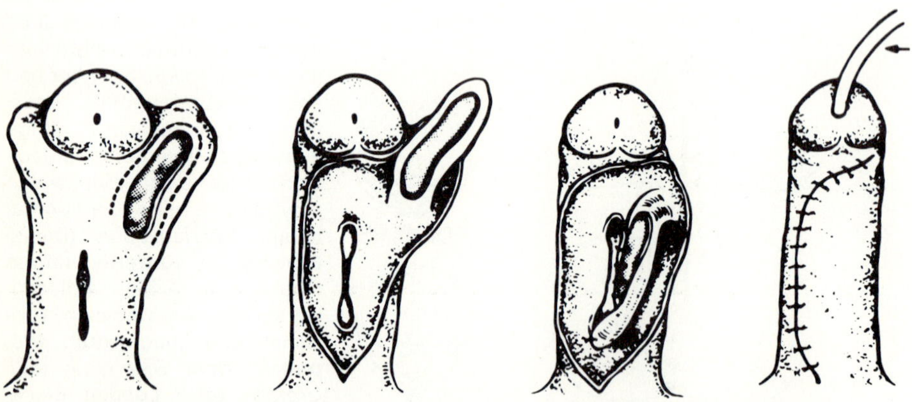

Figure 10. Pedicled skin inlay procedure for one-stage repair of pendulous urethral stricture (available from prepuce, penis, scrotum). After preparation of scarred urethra, a cutaneous area of appropriate shape and dimensions is selected and dissected, retaining continuity at the pivoting margin. Anastomosis to urethra with epithelial surface toward the urethral lumen. *(Reprinted from Turner-Warwick RT: Chapter 49. In Glenn (ed): Urologic Surgery, 2nd ed, New York, Harper & Row, 1975, with permission.)*

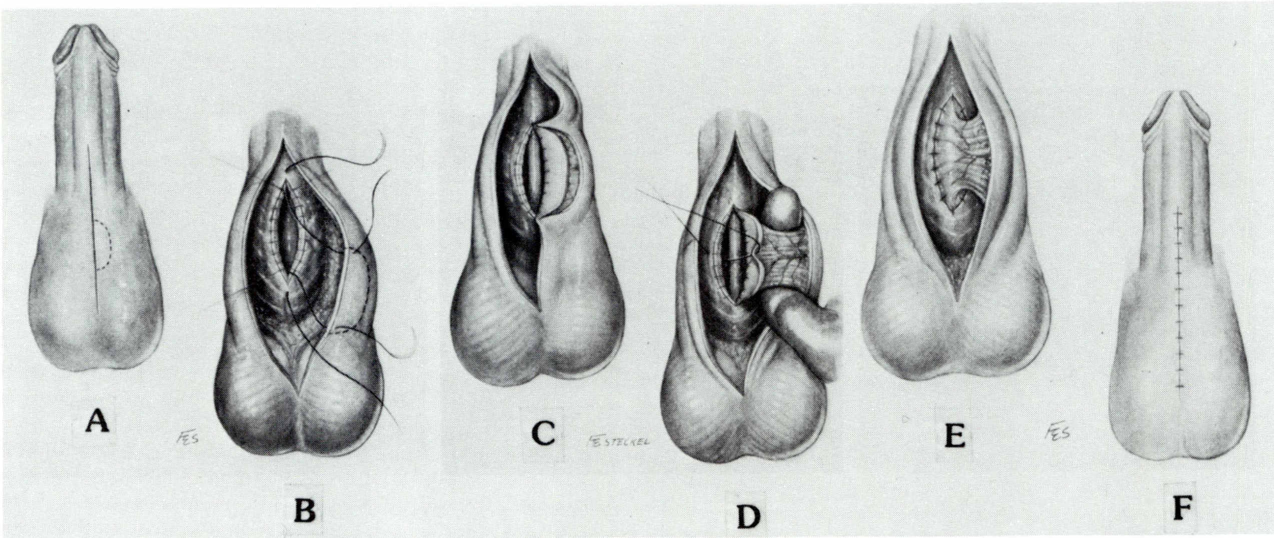

Figure 11. Technique for pedicled cutaneous urethroplasty for pendulous urethral stricture. **A.** Selection of site and dimensions of proposed graft for transposition (adjacent to skin incision over stricture). **B.** Initiation of anastomosis to apices of urethrotomy. **C,D.** Incision and dissection of the lateral aspect of the graft, with preservation of the subcutaneous pedicle. **E.** Completion of anastomosis (epithelial surface toward urethral lumen). **F.** Skin closure. *(Reprinted from Blandy J: Chapter 24. In Libertino JA, Zinman L (eds): Reconstructive Urologic Surgery, Baltimore, Williams & Wilkins, 1977, with permission.)*

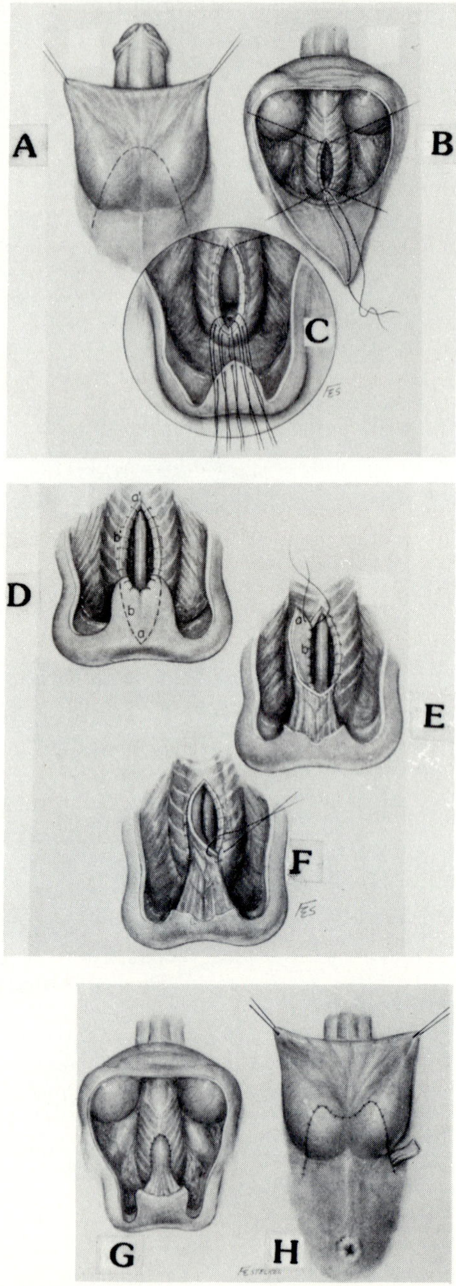

Figure 12. Modification for provision of postdepilation graft to bulbous urethral strictures. **A.** U-shaped scrotal skin incision. **B.** Development of scrotal flap; urethral exposure and urethrotomy. **C.** Suture approximation of apex of scrotal flap to proximal urethrotomy. **D.** Outline of patch graft of appropriate dimensions. **E,F.** Dissection of patch, maintaining subcutaneous attachments, and application to urethrotomy (epithelial surface to lumen). **G.** Graft completed. **H.** Cutaneous closure. *(Reprinted from Blandy J: Chapter 24. In Libertino JA, Zinman L (eds): Reconstructive Urologic Surgery, Baltimore, Williams&Wilkins,1977,with permission.)*

may require more formal meatoplasty. Surgical correction of pendulous and penoscrotal stricturing may be managed by simple excision and anastomosis for strictures less than 2 cm in length, by free or pedicled patch or tube graft substitution for longer strictures, or by two-stage marsupialization techniques for circumstances requiring stabilization of inflammation or infection. It is routinely recommended that incision or excision be carried 1 to 2 cm into apparently normal urethra at either end, that normal urethra be mobilized 2 to 4 cm (for anastomosis), that repairs be constructed over a 24 Fr stent (to be replaced by a 14 to 16 Fr drainage catheter for 7 to 14 days), and that available local spongiosum be included in all repairs.

In addition to the applicability of these methods to bulbourethral strictures, two-stage methods involving rotation of scrotoperineal skin flaps represent additional options for strictures extending proximally into the membranous urethra (Fig. 13). These procedures carry the disadvantages of

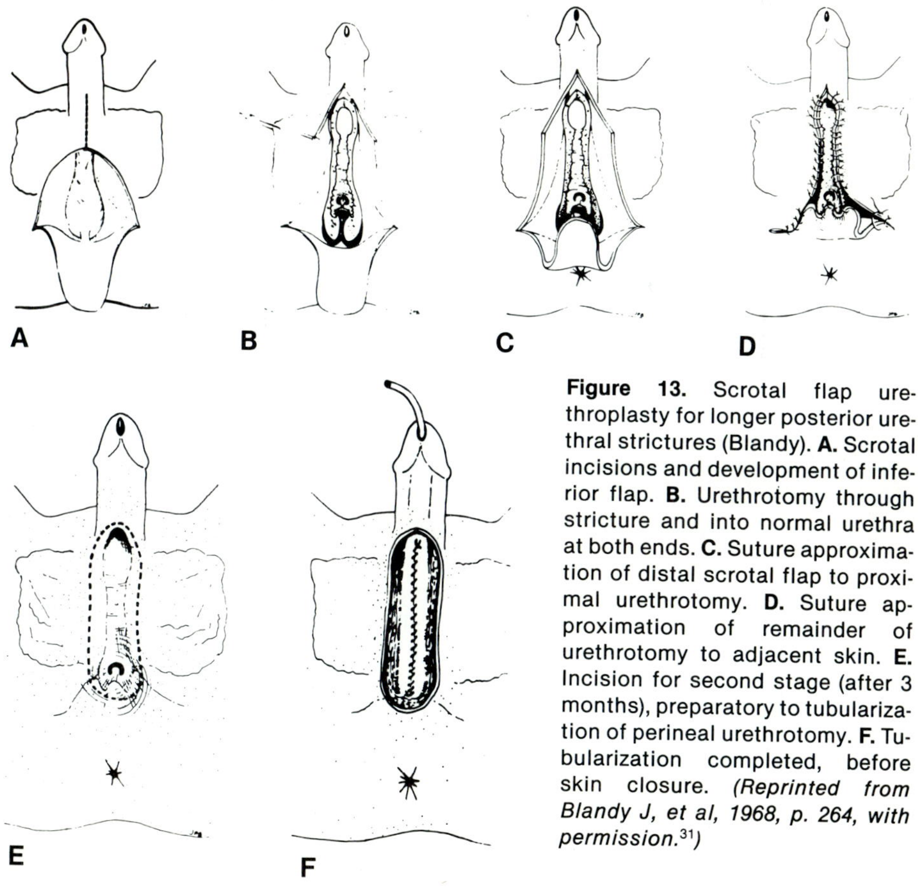

Figure 13. Scrotal flap urethroplasty for longer posterior urethral strictures (Blandy). **A.** Scrotal incisions and development of inferior flap. **B.** Urethrotomy through stricture and into normal urethra at both ends. **C.** Suture approximation of distal scrotal flap to proximal urethrotomy. **D.** Suture approximation of remainder of urethrotomy to adjacent skin. **E.** Incision for second stage (after 3 months), preparatory to tubularization of perineal urethrotomy. **F.** Tubularization completed, before skin closure. *(Reprinted from Blandy J, et al, 1968, p. 264, with permission.[31])*

technical difficulty, limited exposure, and the frequent need for special instruments, but two-stage repairs are mandatory for tissue conditions requiring drainage and subsidence of inflammation.

In general, free patch grafts on the pendulous urethra are discouraged owing to the availability of shaft or preputial skin for pedicled grafting. Similarly, unpedicled tube grafts are less desirable owing to their unreliability in comparison with pedicled and patch procedures. Comparative success rates have been estimated at 95 percent (bulbourethral anastomosis), 86 percent (free patch graft), 70 percent (scrotal inlay), and 60 to 70 percent (internal urethrotomy). Overall stricture recurrence has been estimated at 20 percent, of which the majority is amenable to internal urethrotomy.

PENILE AMPUTATION

Partial penile amputation may become unavoidable when irrevocable soft tissue damage or loss accompanies genital trauma. Alternately, deliberate penile amputation is occasionally encountered, requiring judgments regarding candidacy for replantation. Contraindications to replantation, or failed replantation, incorporate the necessity for plastic revision of the penile remnant.

Avoidance of unnecessarily excessive debridement will be permitted by limiting initial efforts to removal of only grossly nonviable tissue, allowing sufficient time for additional tissue demarcation during urinary diversion, antibiotic administration, and local tissue hygiene. Although tissue trauma may interfere with interpretation, marginal tissue viability may also be reflected by tissue fluorescence after intravenous injection of fluorescein, employing either a Wood's lamp (35 mg/kg) or dermofluorometer (1.5 mg/kg).[6]

Surgical objectives include debridement proximally into viable tissue sufficient to permit tension-free closure (with 1-cm overlap of dorsal skin and 1 cm of additional urethra), individual closure of the corporal tunics and skin, and meatoplasty designed to discourage subsequent stenosis (Fig. 14).[7]

Cases elected for replantation ideally incorporate microscopic anastomosis of vessels and nerve.[8] Success is uncommon after intervals exceeding 18 hours and loss of the skin of the amputated segment is frequent after a 2-hour delay. The amputated segment should be immersed in iced Ringer's lactate with heparin (1500 units/150 cc) and antibiotic. The urethra, fascial compartments, and skin are reconnected, the urethra is anastomosed elliptically over an indwelling catheter, the distal skin is amputated if more than 2 hours have elapsed, and a bulky dressing is applied for immobilization. Cystostomy diversion has been advocated. Administration of broad-spectrum antibiotics and antiplatelet therapy (aspirin, indomethacin) is mandatory. Development of distal gangrene mandates amputation. (Before microvascular techniques, sporadic success of penile replantation was re-

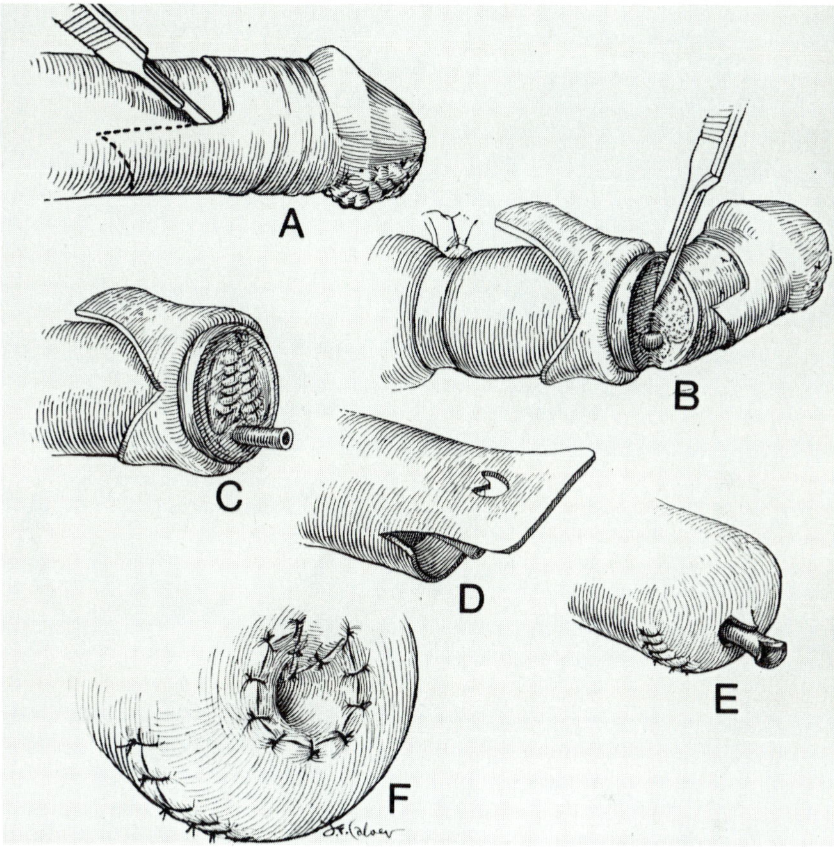

Figure 14. Partial penectomy. **A.** After demarcation and debridement, incisions to permit dorsal skin flap to exceed ventral flap by 1 to 1½ inches. **B,C.** Amputation through viable tissue, with at least 1 inch of additional urethra; closure of corpora. **D,E.** Fashioned buttonhole of dorsal skin flap to accommodate urethra **F.** Followed by skin closure and plastic meatoplasty. *(Reprinted from Peters P (ed): Complications of Urologic Surgery, p 413, Philadelphia, Saunders, 1976, with permission.)*

ported despite omission of efforts to revascularize. These cases exclusively involved distal amputations.[9])

PROXIMAL URETHRAL AVULSION

The fixation of the membranous urethra within the pelvic diaphragm is responsible for the concentration of shearing traumatic forces at the prostatomembranous junction as the prostate is forcefully displaced because of its puboprostatic attachments (Fig. 15). Anatomic differences exempt female

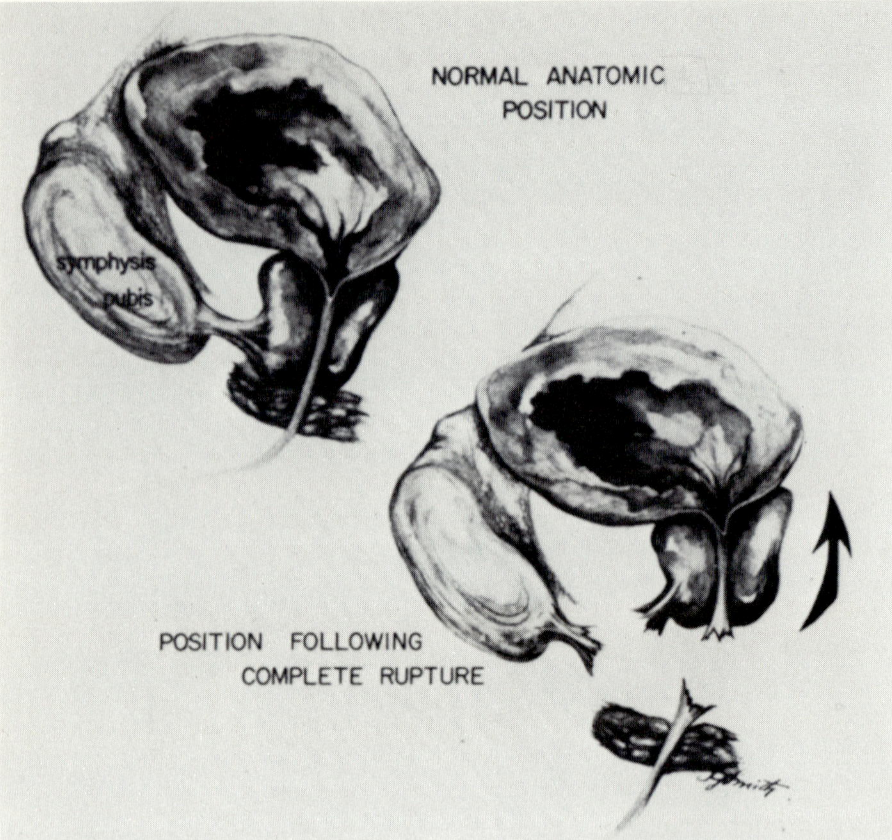

Figure 15. Anatomic explanation for traumatic membranoprostatic avulsion. Prostatic fixation by the pelvic diaphragm and puboprostatic ligaments focus shearing forces at the site of least resistance. Intact puboprostatic ligaments may carry prostate away from the pelvic diaphragm with displaced bony fragments. *(Reprinted from Morehouse DD, et al, 1969, p 482, with permission.[21])*

patients from significant traumatic urethral insult; when injury is encountered, it is characteristically located at the vesicourethral junction, often occurs in association with other severe (often life-threatening) injuries, and frequently coexists with vaginal damage resulting in urethrovaginal communication, requiring efforts directed toward prevention or correction of urovaginal fistula. More proximal urethral trauma has also been described in preadolescent males, attributed to immature prostatic volume, but this distinction is subtle and of little consequence to sequelae and management.

Any combination of the potential complications of proximal urethral avulsion may place the patient in jeopardy of a protracted convalescence, even despite the advantages of contemporary management over methods previously available; a lifetime of suffering commonly resulted from the need for multiple operative revisions, e.g., chronic infection, calculous formation, vulnerability to sepsis, and irrevocable incontinence and impotence. Remedies were often imperfect and frequently suspect of compounding the patient's misery. Emotional and psychogenic reactions were understandable. Therapeutic advances have dramatically improved prognosis but timely, precise, and comprehensive management remains essential to the achievement of satisfactory results.

Associated Injuries

Injuries commonly associated with prostatomembranous avulsion include pelvic fracture, distal ureteral damage, vesical laceration, pelvic hemorrhage, and anorectal injury. Responsibility for diagnosis and management will incorporate urologic consultation.

Prostatomembranous avulsion usually occurs in the setting of deceleration injuries or crushing pelvic trauma, and *pelvic fracture* most often initiates diagnostic inquiry. (The prevalence of pelvic fracture is statistically supported, accounting for 3 percent of all fractures and 0.1 percent of all hospitalizations, and represents the third most common injury sustained in motor vehicle fatalities.) A compilation of published reports totalling 6000 cases of pelvic fracture yields an incidence of "urologic" injury (usually designated as urethral) of 12 percent, with a range of 5 to 25 percent.[10] Complications of pelvic fracture are documented in 43 to 74 percent and high risk injuries are frequent, including a reported mortality of 30 percent. A mortality of 42 percent is associated with hemodynamic instability accompanying pelvic fracture versus only 3.4 percent with hemodynamic stability. Although open pelvic fractures account for only 5 to 20 percent of the total, they are associated with a 50 percent mortality as opposed to a 10 percent mortality with closed fractures. Extraperitoneal pelvic bleeding has been incriminated as the cause of death in 60 percent of related mortalities, and Malgaigne fractures (unstable pelvic ring) are reported as responsible for the majority of cases manifesting fatal pelvic hemorrhage.[11-14] Attempts to correlate the likelihood of urethral damage with type and degree of pelvic fracture (bilateral, symphyseal, Malgaigne) are both unreliable and irrelevant to the requirement for diagnostic urethrography in patients sustaining pelvic trauma. Physical manifestations of proximal urethral injury include blood at the urethral meatus, prostatic displacement, perineal ecchymosis, inability to void, and inability to catheterize (Fig. 16). These signs are not unequivocal, are helpful only if present and appreciated, and serve only to endorse the requirement for urethrography in a patient usually already demonstrating indications for that study.

Distal ureteral injuries are uncommon, but should be suspected in the presence of fractures of the posterior pelvic ring. Diagnosis depends upon clinical suspicion, since injury may go undetected by routine screening maneuvers. Excretory (or retrograde) urography during the first 36 hours will

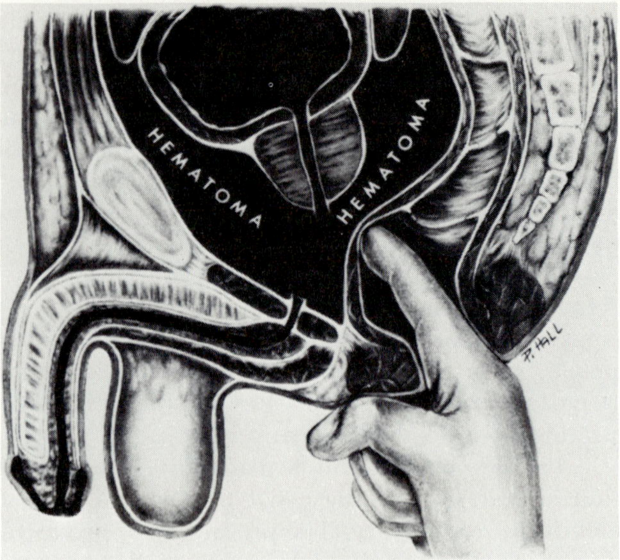

Figure 16. Rectal examination of total proximal urethral avulsion may disclose proximal displacement of prostate and retropubic hematoma. *(Reprinted from Bellinger WF, Rutherford RB, Zuidema GD (eds) Management of Trauma, 2nd ed, p 474, Philadelphia, Saunders, 1973, with permission.)*

commonly demonstrate contrast extravasation. After this period, obstructing edema at the injury site will limit excretory extravasation and produce proximal dilatation; therefore, retrograde ureterography is more dependable and recommended. Management of ureteral injury may involve temporary stenting catheterization (operative or endoscopic) or formal ureteroneocystostomy.

Comprehensive reviews have identified an incidence of coexisting bladder and urethral injury of 5 to 16 percent. (*Bladder injury* is sustained in 5 to 25 percent of pelvic fractures; conversely, 70 percent of patients with bladder injury will have sustained pelvic fracture.) Mortality associated with bladder injury has been variously reported as 21 to 30 percent, with higher figures accompanying intraperitoneal rupture; causes of death are invariably due to associated injury, including hemorrhage, sepsis, and anorectal trauma. Diagnosis is provided by retrograde urethrocystography, or contrast instillation after passage of a catheter. (Bladder injury is demonstrated by excretory urography in only 15 percent of cases.[15]) Another indicator of intraperitoneal urine leakage in cases with delayed diagnosis is an exaggeration of the serum urea: creatinine ratio, often approaching 30:1 (n = 10:1).[16] Mode of injury may involve intraperitoneal blowout rupture of a distended bladder (20 percent) or extraperitoneal laceration of the bladder base by bony spicule (80 percent). Intraperitoneal injuries will require operative repair to prevent interference with coaption by bowel or omentum and to inspect for possible injury to bowel or mesentery. Extraperitoneal bladder injures are amenable to prompt spontaneous resolution with temporary (5 to 7 days) urethral catheter drainage.

Local hemorrhage accompanying pelvic fracture is most commonly of venous origin and consequently subject to spontaneous tamponade. Operative exposure will therefore not only fail to disclose controllable sources of bleeding, but will also risk initiating fresh hemorrhage or sustaining established bleeding. Despite this feature, the hemorrhagic complications of pelvic fracture already described testify to the possibility of pelvic arterial injury, usually involving distal hypogastric (pudendal, obturator) branches and therefore not readily accessible to operative exposure and control. Verification requires hypogastric arteriography, with incorporation of selective therapeutic embolization. (Conscientious effort is also required to prevent an attitude of complacency with apparently routine pelvic hemorrhage from interfering with a thorough appraisal for less apparent sources of bleeding. An example is provided by femur fracture in elderly patients, in whom destabilizing volumes of blood may be lost into the thigh.)

A paramount consideration when confronted by severe pelvic fracture (particularly crushing trauma, in which urethral injury is virtually guaranteed) is the requirement for thorough investigation for coexisting *anorectal laceration.* Associated mortality figures as high as 60 percent have been attributed mainly to septic complications;[17,18] although these figures may have improved considerably with contemporary diagnotic and therapeutic management, the undiminished significance of anorectal injury is reflected in reported hospitalization requirements exceeding 50 days in more than 50 percent of patients and exceeding 100 days in another 31 percent.[19] Diagnosis relies upon clinical suspicion. Blood on the examining rectal finger is significant and diagnostic confirmation relies upon rectosigmoidoscopy or contrast enema. (Contiguous bladder injury may permit disclosure by excretory or retrograde cystography.) Injuries are often compounded through the perineum, in which event direct digital inspection is mandatory. Irrigation maneuvers demonstrating continuity between colon and perineum are also diagnostically helpful. Management includes proximal colostomy, thorough irrigation, presacral drainage, and appropriate antibiotic coverage.

Complications

Although a number of deleterious consequences of prostatomembranous avulsion are possible, attention has classically focused upon stricturing, impotence, and incontinence, and upon efforts to reduce their incidence and to attenuate their influence once they develop.

Stricture. It may be anticipated that some degree of urethral stricturing will follow every instance of prostatomembranous avulsion. Factors have been suggested as increasing or decreasing the magnitude of scarring, but connections are inconclusive. Among those most commonly cited are distraction of the prostate from the triangular ligament by displaced bony fragments, fibrous organization of pelvic hematoma, iatrogenic contamination of the pelvic hematoma, and premature operative intervention before subsidence of tissue inflammation.

Obviously distracted pelvic fractures will require orthopedic reduction.

Opinion regarding the significance of the pelvic hematoma is divided. One view holds that large pelvic hematomas resist prompt spontaneous resolution, thus obstructing urethral restoration; another view considers urethral coaption to be unlikely in the presence of any hematoma, regardless of size; still another claims prompt spontaneous resolution of all pelvic hematomas, thereby representing no obstacle to urethral reconstitution, and permitting omission of pelvic evacuation with its potential sequelae of renewed hemorrhage, iatrogenic impotence, and introduction of contamination. Contamination of the hematoma is an acknowledged source of exaggerated scarring and omission of avoidable manipulation is therefore advisable. Suboptimal tissue conditions are often difficult to evaluate and may therefore be considered as an unalterable aspect of the operative process. Known contamination or infection can be appropriately managed by irrigation, drainage, antibiotics, and allowing sufficient intervals for resolution, with no guarantee that optimum conditions for operative success will have become established. A particular example is represented by attempted primary suture reapproximation at presentation, when tissue edema, hemorrhage, and poor exposure may collaborate to defeat the most careful and skillful efforts.

The magnitude of ultimate post-traumatic urethral stricturing varies unpredictably. Moreover, important distinctions pertain to anatomic (apparent) and functional (symptomatic) strictures; uroflowmetry is largely unaffected until urethral dimensions have become compromised to a caliber of 10 Fr. Management will be selected not only according to symptomatic manifestations and functional disorder, but also by a lack of improvement with more conservative efforts; for example, urethroplasty may become necessary only after intolerance to, or failure of, periodic urethral dilation or internal urethrotomy. Numerous reviews have attempted to correlate management selected at presentation with the extent of subsequent urethral stricturing. Favorable results as high as 57 percent have been claimed by proponents of primary suture anastomosis, whereas others have criticized this form of management as impractical owing to initial tissue damage, hemorrhage, contamination, and poor exposure. At least one investigator has attributed exaggerated stricturing to this method for these reasons.[20]

The alternative method of initial diverting cystostomy followed by urethroplasty after 3 to 6 months to allow tissue stabilization became immediately popular upon its introduction not only because of its proposed advantages of eliminating both iatrogenic impotency and exogenous contamination of the pelvic hematoma, but also because it provided an acceptable temporizing interval permitting optimal preparation of the patient or referral for qualified operative care.[21] Further endorsements followed the recognition that subsequent stricturing, although virtually assured, was characteristically limited and easily managed operatively.

The major competing therapeutic option involves primary catheter splinting for variable periods, allowing urethral coaption and maintenance of the urethral lumen during normalization of local tissue conditions. Subsequent operative requirements will vary according to the results observed. Collective experience has identified a final rate of stricturing of 36 to 70 percent and a requirement for urethroplasty of 25 to 64 percent. Arguments supporting stenting catheterization include (1) the possibility for stricture-free results, thereby eliminating need for further intervention; (2) attenuation of urethral scarring, amenable to more conservative remedies; (3) expediency provided by accessibility during emergency laparotomy for other reasons; and (4) avoidance of extensive scarring and complex stricturing occasionally observed in patients managed by primary cystostomy.[10]

Impotence. Rates of impotence as high as 80 percent have been reported following pelvic trauma, but correlations are often questionable, including descriptions of impotence coexisting with injuries unlikely to damage the neuroerectile apparatus, i.e., incomplete proximal urethral avulsion, isolated bulbar urethral injury, pelvic fracture without urethral damage, pelvic trauma without fracture, recovery of potency after incongruous intervals and after exhaustion of litigation and compensation benefits, and with psychotherapy. A more accurate correlation is suggested from reviews of patients managed by primary cystostomy only, thereby eliminating iatrogenic contributions; such reports claim impotency rates of only 3 to 10 percent.[22] If one can presume these injuries to be accurately diagnosed as total prostatomembranous avulsions, the reported figures then infer that iatrogenic factors are largely responsible for any additional impotence developing after alternate methods of management.

Incontinence. Correlations of urinary incontinence with pelvic fracture and proximal urethral avulsion range from 0 to 33 percent.[10] Credibility of these figures is again questioned. The integrity of the internal sphincter (vesical outlet) is rarely affected and the external sphincter is likewise protected by its incorporation within the pelvic diaphragm. The urethra is avulsed immediately above the fixed external sphincter complex. Although the membranous urethral mucosa may be included in the avulsion process, thereby explaining membranous urethral stricturing, integrity of the muscular sphincteric apparatus should remain unaffected. Injudicious or indelicate retropubic instrumentation, particularly primary suturing attempts or traction sutures from the prostate through the perineum (Vest), has been indicted as contributory.

Operative Options

Final results are variable and unpredictable regardless of initial management. Available remedies may be selected according to the perceived magnitude of stricturing and personal preference.

Narrow, compliant strictures often respond to simple periodic urethral dilation, which represents an attractive option for patients who refuse surgery or are poor operative candidates. Periodic dilation is generally acceptable only if well tolerated and infrequently required. Application to pediatric patients is contraindicated.

Visual internal urethrotomy has supplanted blind (Otis) internal urethrotomy as a conservative method for managing urethral stricturing not requiring formal urethroplasty. Outpatient facilities and local anesthesia are generally permissible. Adjuncts to urethrotomy have included intralesional steroid injection, long-term catheterization, exaggerated incision, and multiple incisions, but these methods have produced uneven results. Their inclusion is judgmental.

Proximal urethroplasty is a technically challenging procedure, with operative exposure constituting the major limiting obstacle. Perineal access has permitted straightforward excision-reanastomosis (Figs. 17 and 18), ure-

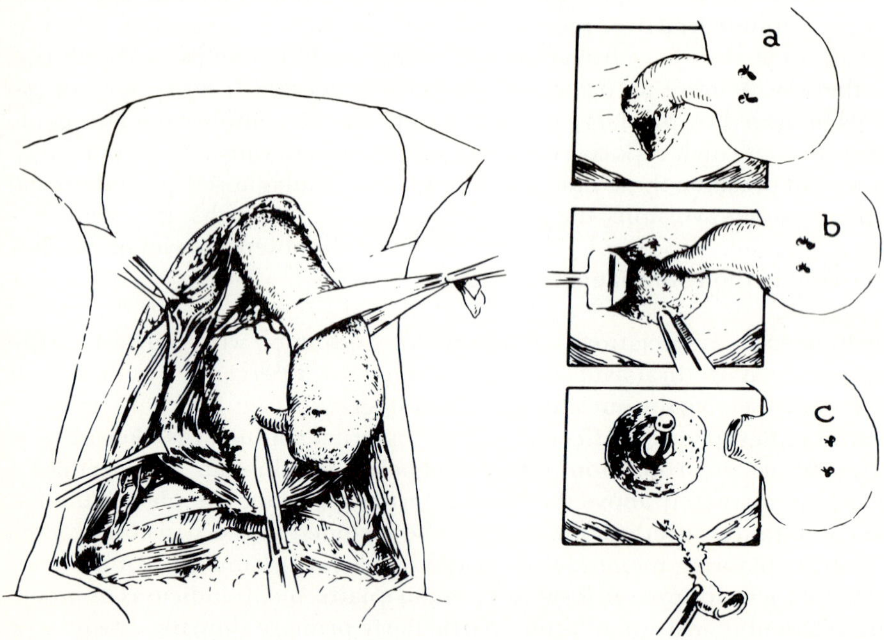

A B

Figure 17. A. Surgical correction of bulbomembranous urethral stricture. (*Left*) exposure of the bulb and proximal dissection of strictured urethra. **B.** (a) vertical midline incision of urogenital diaphragm, posterior to scarred membranous urethra; (b) preparation for excision of scarred remnant; (c) adequacy of excision reflected in antegrade passage of urethral sound. Preparation for suture anastomosis. *(Reprinted from Pierce JM Jr: Posterior urethral stricture repair. J Urol 121:741, 1979, with permission.)*

thral invagination (Solovov) techniques (for narrowly limited indications)[23] (Fig. 19), and a variety of other methods which incorporate the rotation of scrotal and perineal skin into the strictured site for enlargement of the lumen at the expense of sphincteric integrity (Fig. 20).[24-31] Enthusiasm for these methods has been attenuated by a significant learning curve, poor exposure, a need for special instruments, the requirement for multistaged procedures and operative revisions, and the development of more facile and dependable methods.

Transpubic exposure through an osteal window has improved retropubic access for segmental urethral resection and reapproximation or bypass of the strictured segment (Figs. 21 and 22). Exposure may be tedious and prolonged because of pelvic displacement, bony callous, and fibrotic reaction. Moreover, tissue compliance may be severely compromised. Combining transpubic and perineal approaches may provide a crucial advantage and also permits more precise localization of the strictured segment.[32] The bony defect created is innocuous to ambulation. Incorporation of adjunctive pedicled omentum for the purpose of eliminating dead space and

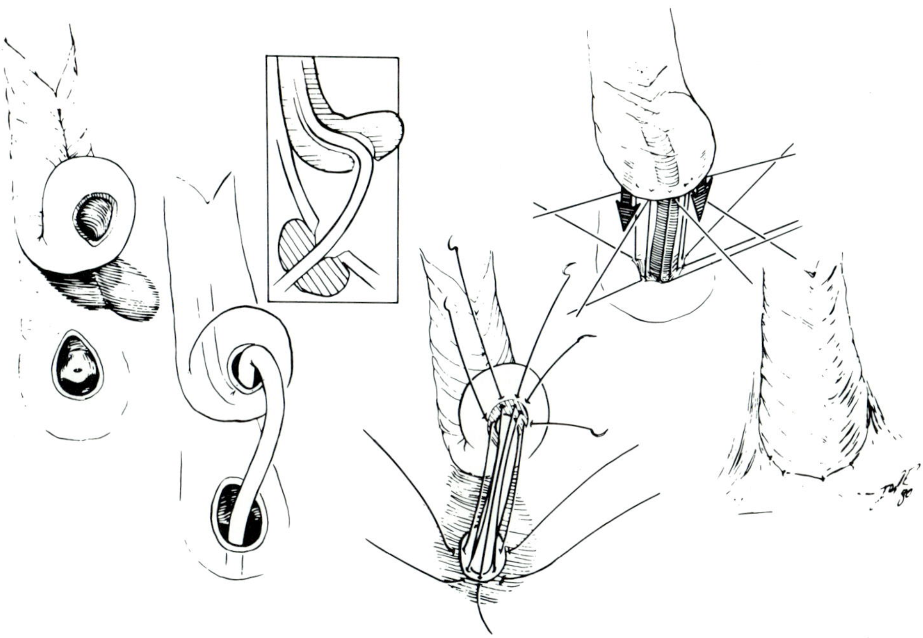

Figure 18. Alternate method for membranous urethral strictures (Turner-Warwick). After perineal dissection, excision, mobilization, and spatulation, urethral anastomosis is performed with a 2-cm overlap. (This procedure is claimed to permit the bridging of longer defects.) *(Reprinted from Devine CJ, Devine PC: Chapter 22. In Stewart B (ed): Operative Urology, Lower Urinary Tract, Pelvic Structures and Male Reproductive System, Baltimore, Williams & Wilkins, 1975, with permission.)*

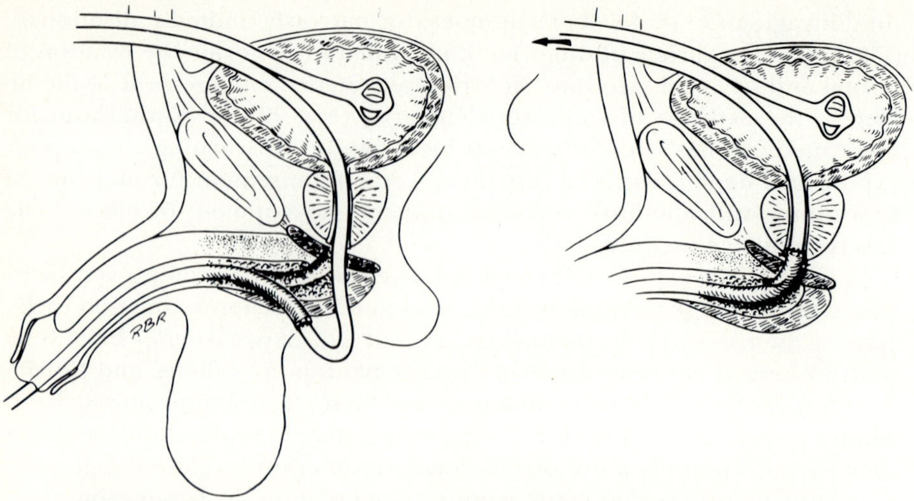

Figure 19. Perineal or perineal-suprapubic urethral intussusception method (Solovov–Badenoch) for proximal urethral strictures. After exposure, dissection, and excision of the strictured segment, the proximal end of the mobilized distal urethra is secured to an indwelling catheter passed antegrade (*left*), which is then employed to draw the distal urethra into the proximal segment, where it may be transfixed (*right*). *(Reprinted from Devine CJ, Devine PC: Chapter 22. In Stewart B (ed): Operative Urology, Lower Urinary Tract, Pelvic Structures and Male Reproductive System, Baltimore, Williams & Wilkins, 1975, with permission.)*

offering vascularized support to anastomotic suture lines provides additional advantage to selected cases (Fig. 23).[33]

Emergency Management

Management upon emergency arrival will be supervised by emergency or surgical personnel, with attention directed to priorities adjusted to clinical stability and nature and extent of injuries. Airway assurance, control of active hemorrhage, and vascular access and institution of volume repletion precede additional diagnostic efforts. The latter are initiated by priority appraisal of central neurologic injury which would demand expeditious computerized scanning or arteriographic assessment. Similar importance is applied to thoracic injuries which jeopardize cardiac or pulmonary function, including pericardiocentesis, thoracentesis, and thoracostomy.

Diagnostic peritoneal lavage has justifiably assumed prominence in the appraisal of the trauma victim. An overall accuracy of 97 percent has been extracted from a collective review of over 10,000 cases, contrasting with a false-negative rate of 20 percent with simple paracentesis. A minor complication rate of only 0.5 percent has been observed, composed almost entirely of perforations of hollow organs. Technique involves infraumbilical punc-

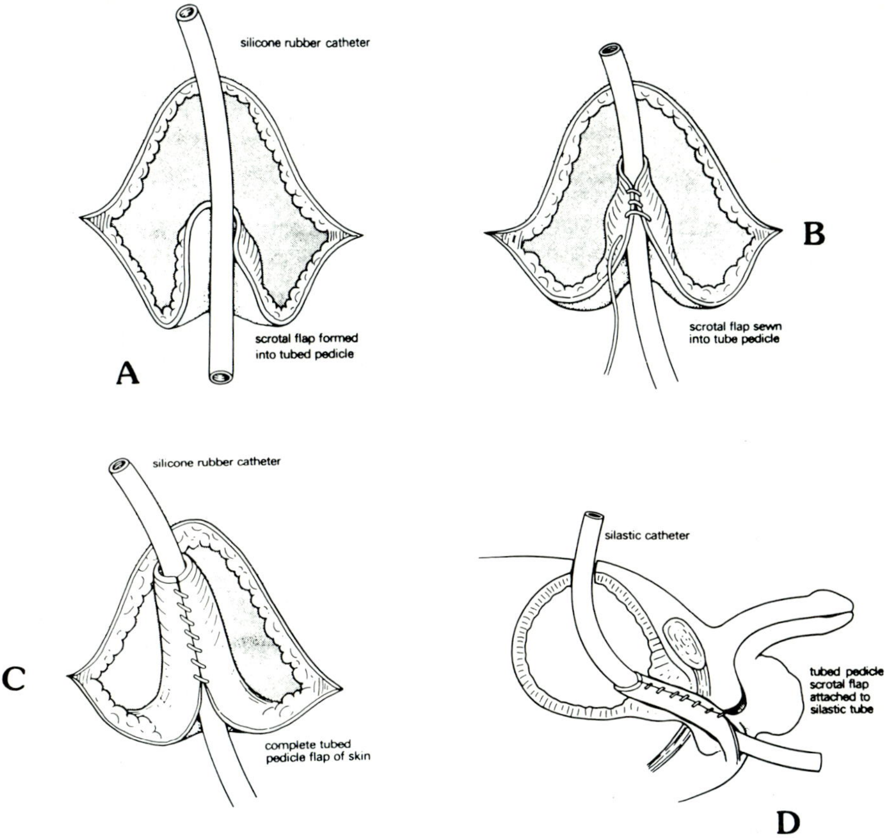

Figure 20. Scrotal pedicle urethroplasty. After preparation of inferior flap, tubularization is fashioned over a catheter with previously depilated skin toward the lumen. **A–C.** Catheter and neo-tube are then drawn into the bladder and transfixed to bladder outlet or suprapubic skin **D.** Second stage urethroplasty follows an arbitrary interval. *(Reprinted from Blandy J (ed): Urology, vol II, chap 39, London, Blackwell Scientific, 1976, with permission.)*

ture after stomach and bladder decompression, initial aspiration, instillation of 1 L (adult) or 15 cc/kg (pediatric) of irrigant, and drainage. Evidence of intraperitoneal injury is reflected by (1) 10 to 20 cc gross blood at paracentesis, (2) return of lavage fluid through chest or bladder drainage tubes, (3) grossly bloody lavage, (4) 50,000 to 100,000 RBC/mm^3, (5) 500 WBC/HPF, (6) amylase content exceeding serum level, or (7) bacteria or food fibers on Gram stain.

Hemodynamically stable patients with equivocal peritoneal lavage and suspicion of trauma to duodenum, pancreas, or diaphragm are candidates for ultrasonagraphy, computerized scanning, or radiocontrast studies.

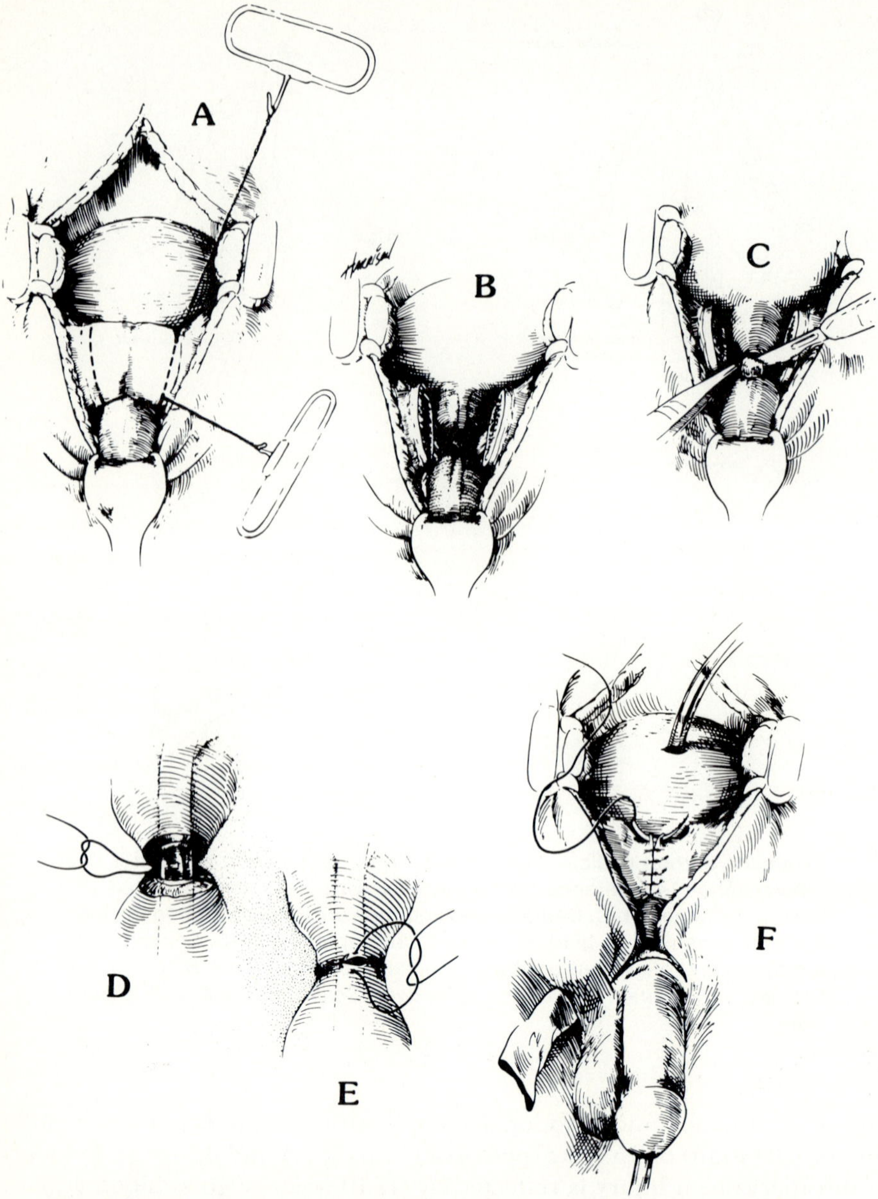

Figure 21. Transpubic urethroplasty. **A.** Removal of symphysis (Gigli saw, rongeur, chisel, mechanical burr). **B.** Operative exposure. **C.** Dissection and excision of scarred segment. **D,E.** Reanastomosis over stenting catheter. **F.** Wound closure, including reapproximation of symphseal periosteum (optional). *(Reprinted from Allen TD: The transpubic approach for strictures of the membranous urethra. J Urol 114:67, 1975, with permission.)*

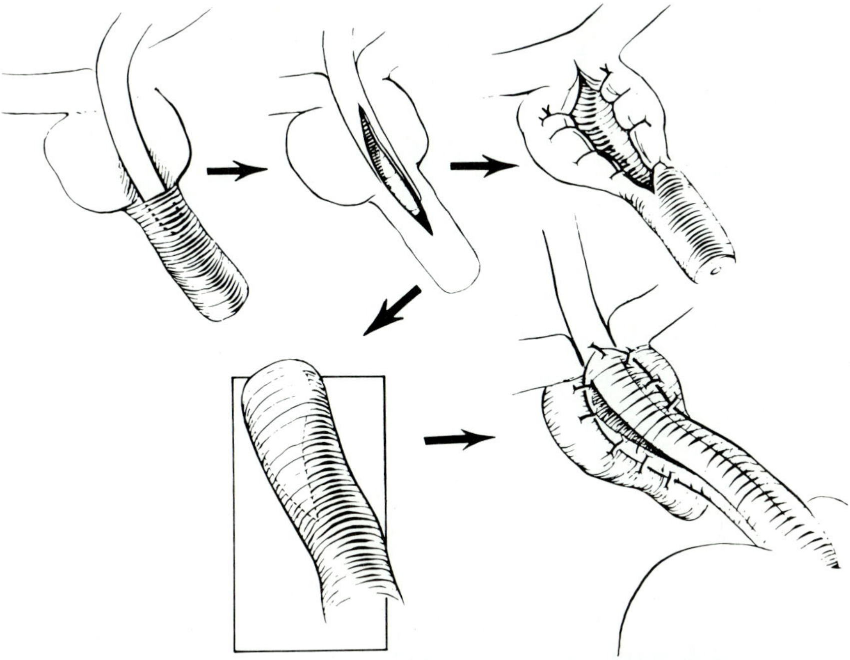

Figure 22. Membranous urethral stricture correction, with transpubic exposure. After exposure and dissection, the distal urethra is mobilized extensively to permit tension-free anastomosis and spatulated. The strictured distal prostatic urethral lumen is disregarded in favor of creating an anterior prostatic urethral defect (Waterhouse), to which the spatulated urethra is anastomosed. *(Reprinted from Devine CJ, Devine PC: Chapter 22. In Stewart B (ed): Operative Urology, Lower Urinary Tract, Pelvic Structures and Male Reproductive System, Baltimore, Williams & Wilkins, 1975, with permission.)*

Hemodynamically unstable patients with pelvic trauma and negative diagnostic lavage become suspect for extraordinary pelvic hemorrhage, involving distal hypogastric arterial vessels, or proximal iliac or hypogastric veins. Such patients are best managed by urgent selective arteriography with incorporation of methodology for therapeutic embolization. An added advantage is the opportunity for elective study of carotid, celiac, and renal vessels. Apparent pelvic hemorrhage undemonstrated by angiography, or continued pelvic bleeding after embolic maneuvers have been implemented, indicate a possible venous disruption; venous catheterization will identify the source. Since embolic control is unlikely with venous injuries, proximal occlusion by balloon catheter will provide local control preparatory to operative repair.

Application of military antishock trousers (MAST) as a means of achieving external tamponade during clinical stabilization and vascular re-

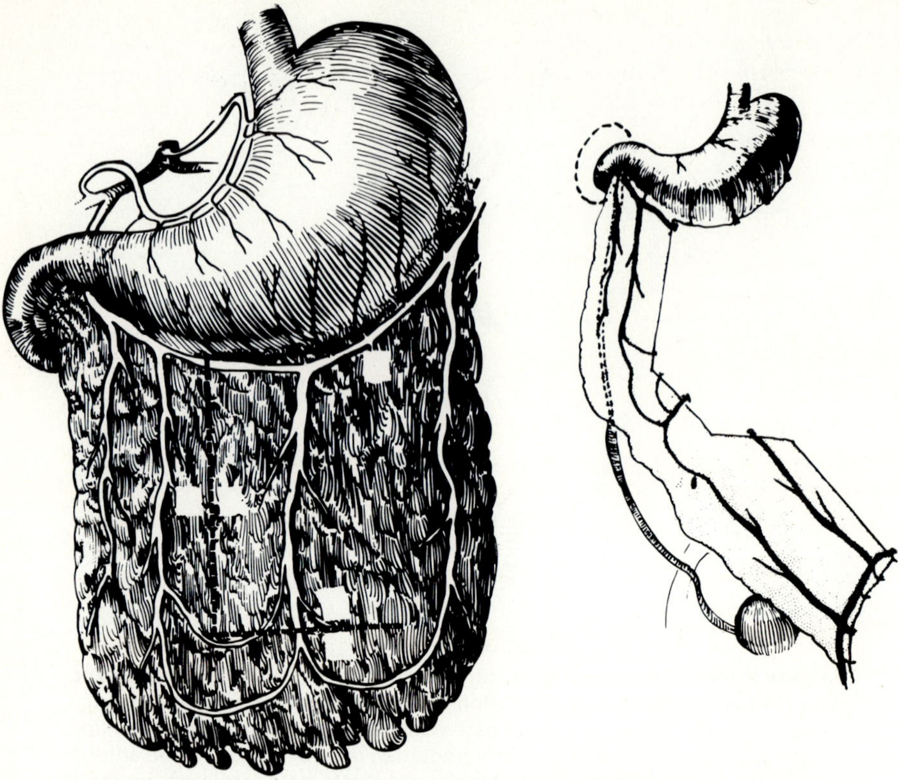

Figure 23. Example of incisions permitting development of vascularized pedicle of adequate length to accommodate support for membranous urethral procedure. *(Reprinted from Malloy T, Wein A, Carpiniello V: Transpubic urethroplasty for prostatomembranous urethral disruption. J Urol 124:360, 1980, with permission.)*

pletion has undergone reappraisal following initial unconditional enthusiasm for their employment. Despite several reservations, there is broad agreement that MAST trousers remain of particular value to patients with intraperitoneal or pelvic trauma with hemorrhage, and to those requiring transport or other delay between injury and intervention. Advantage with pelvic fractures pertains to orthopedic stabilization as well as vascular tamponade; more accurately, diversion of blood volume to head and chest.

UROLOGIC EVALUATION

Urologic evaluation of the patient with traumatic hematuria has classically included both excretory urography and retrograde urethrocystography. While comprehensive uroradiography is often advisable, selective urologic appraisal is permissible in many circumstances. A personal experience with 250 blunt urologic injuries, and a review of 2250 cases from the literature has identifed a coexistence of significant upper and lower urinary tract injury in less than 1 percent of involved patients.[34] In addition, the majority of combination injuries is characterized by a nominal significance of the lesser injury; moreover, where both injuries are severe the overall trauma sustained is frequently incompatible with survival. These observations endorse the acceptable limitation of uroradiographic evaluation to the obvious site of major injury in selected patients.

Lower urinary tract evaluation following trauma assumes responsibility for the bony pelvis, anorectum and distal ureters, as well as the urethra and bladder; evaluation for the former injuries will relate to clinical suspicion and will rely upon additional studies according to judgment. Proximal urethral injury is classified in degree as complete (total avulsion) or incomplete (partial integrity) and in location as to supramembranous, membranous, inframembranous, or combined. Although correlations have been suggested between site of injury and prognosis, validity is unestablished. It is conceded that urethral damage without total avulsion will be readily reconstituted without compromise over a stenting catheter or during cystostomy diversion. Despite occasional exceptions, incomplete urethral interuption will be identified by urethrographic coexistence of local urethral extravasation and bladder opacification (Fig. 24); total urethral avulsion will prevent contrast medium from entering the bladder. Techniques of urethrography include employment of a Brodny clamp specific for the pur-

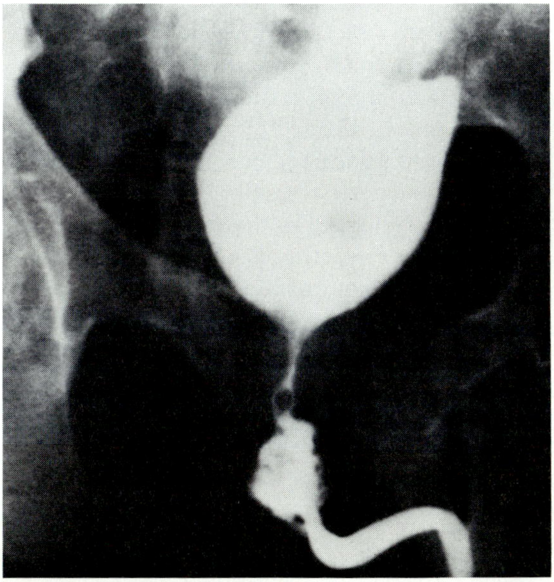

Figure 24. Retrograde urethrogram. Local extravasation coexisting with bladder opacification reflects incomplete urethral damage (absence of total avulsion).

pose, inflation of a balloon catheter within the pendulous urethra (appropriate to the size of the patient), placement of a small feeding tube into the pediatric pendulous urethra with sealing of the meatus by a drop of collodian, or (preferred) simple retrograde syringe injection through the urethral meatus. Fifteen to 30 cc of water-soluble contrast medium is injected, exposures are immediate, and sufficient re-exposures are obtained until information is considered diagnostic. Oblique positioning is advisable when permissible. Since bladder opacification is of diagnostic interest, urethrography should precede other procedures employing contrast agents (excretory urography).

Cystography may be obtained by continued retrograde filling until the bladder is distended or until residual urine is opacified, or, in the event of an uninjured urethra, through a catheter passed into the bladder. Exposures during distention and after decompression are adequate. Inspection for rectal opacification is important and may be modified by staining of the contrast medium with indigo carmine or methylene blue and observance for discoloration of rectal contents or an inserted sponge. An opacified bladder apparently lifted out of the pelvis ("pie in the sky"), or laterally compressed ("teardrop"), reflects the presence of significant pelvic bleeding.

Preferred Management

Therapeutic options are often limited by the priority status of severe coexisting injury or by an unstable clinical status. Where options are unrestricted, stenting catheter realignment has been locally endorsed because of several potential advantages. A virtual assurance of stricturing in patients managed by initial diverting cystostomy is commonly addressed by transpubic urethroplasty, frequently modified by additional perineal dissection, and occasionally by transperitoneal access for preparation of a buttressing omental pedicle; moreover, a small percentage of patients so managed will develop extensive, complicated strictures, deviating markedly from the small, limited stricture usually seen, and profoundly exaggerating the operative challenge. The possibility for stricture-free results by catheter alignment is acknowledged and subsequent stricturing in the remainder is often manageable by conservative (nonoperative) methods, including urethrotomy and dilation. Indeed, retrospective reviews have suggested that many patients undergoing urethroplasty may well have responded to more conservative management.[35] Other surveys have favorably compared the results of parallel groups of patients managed by these competing methods.[36]

The requirement for emergency post-trauma laparotomy for coexisting injury provides access which affords the opportunity to appraise pelvic damage and exploit the advantages of stenting without additional definitive surgery. An appreciation of the likely correlation between retropubic manipulation and iatrogenic complications (impotence, infection) emphasize the admonition to limit activities to atraumatic catheter introduction, with deliberate avoidance of attempting prostatic repositioning or evacuation of the retropubic hematoma.

Method

Diagnosis of posterior urethral injury will stipulate partial or complete transection. Partial injuries will respond promptly to either cystostomy diversion or to urethral stenting. Retrograde catheterization should be attempted only by experienced personnel (urology) with atraumatic technique and limited attempts. Anticipated laparotomy for other purposes will permit diverting cystostomy and the possibility of traumatic catheterization can therefore be avoided altogether. Following either method, reconstitution is usually complete by 10 days and may be verified by urethrography (antegrade voiding, after contrast instillation through the cystostomy, or retrograde through a pediatric feeding tube passed parallel to the stenting catheter to the site of injury). Absence of extravasation signals permission to discontinue drainage. Subsequent complications will be reflected by voiding dysfunction or urinary infection, but are uncommon.

Management of complete proximal urethral avulsion is incorporated into overall management in the presence of priority-associated injuries. Once permissible, initial management is contingent upon the apparent status of pelvic hemorrhage. Patients whose overall condition dictates avoidance of pelvic exploration because of operative or anesthetic instability or unestablished pelvic tamponade are best managed by simple cystostomy. Reintervention exclusively for bridging catheterization after a few days will permit clinical stabilization and subsidence of pelvic hemorrhage.

The technique for bridging catheterization stresses a deliberate and rigid attention to avoiding prostatic manipulation and therefore employment of interlocking sounds, or retropubic attachments of bidirectional catheters, is discouraged. The index finger is passed across the opened bladder into the prostatic urethra. A Van Buren sound is passed retrograde into the urethral bulb where gentle manipulation during further advancement will be identified by the probing finger, which then guides it into the bladder. The open end of a Robinson catheter is inserted over the sound, which is withdrawn antegrade to the meatus. A Foley catheter (20 to 24 Fr) is attached by suture to the Robinson catheter, which draws the Foley retrograde into the bladder. The Robinson is discarded, and a No. 1 Prolene suture is affixed to the Foley tip, then brought through the wound and secured. Balloon distention may be limited to 5 cc. Bladder spasms (rare) are correctable by balloon deflation, permissible because of the anchoring suture. (This process may be simplified by substituting for the Van Buren sound by a Foley catheter on a mandarin, although experience has taught that mandarins are often too flexible to permit adequate manipulation.) The wound is closed routinely. Neither Vest sutures nor catheter traction is required or advisable. The catheter is secured to the abdomen to discourage bulbar urethral erosion. Meatal cleansing and application of neosporin ointment twice daily is recommended; antibiotic suppression is advisable.

The catheter-anchoring suture serves the dual purpose of preventing accidental catheter extrusion and of providing a means for catheter replacement.

After a selected interval dependent upon clinical status and initial local conditions, restoration of urethral integrity may be tested. Retrograde urethrography employing a pediatric feeding tube passed alongside the indwelling urethral catheter may be employed. A second maneuver involves removal of the stenting catheter, with access maintained by the anchoring suture, and contrast introduction by syringe at the meatus. A third method involves contrast cystography through the catheter, followed by voiding urethrography after removal of the stenting catheter.

Coaption is usually complete by 14 days of stented catheter drainage. Presence of extravasation requires continuation for a selected period, followed by re-examination. Once continuity is verified, catheterization is discontinued. Initial urethrography will improve because of subsidence of local mucosal edema, but observation for stricture compromise is indicated. Experience has identified a significant advantage to daily self-catheterization for maintenance of prostatomembranous urethral caliber during maturation of the healing process. The recommended technique involves lubricated clean self-catheterization by 18 to 20 Fr Robinson or Foley catheter on arising, before voiding, with return of urine considered the end point (to insure adequate insertion). The catheter is then cleaned with soap and water and stored in clean water until the following day. Rigid compliance is mandatory; haphazard efforts are typically reflected by prompt restricturing manifested by voiding dysfunction, urinary infection, or identification at scheduled urethrography and will require visual urethrotomy and reinitiation of the self-catheterization routine. Duration of this program is arbitrary, but weaning is usually permissible within 1 to 3 months. Follow-up thereafter is judgmental, but late recurrences have not been encountered in compliant patients.

The particular morbidity and operative challenges associated with prostatomembranous urethral obliteration resulting from primary cystostomy or from failed operative repairs are acknowledged. As noted, such conditions are commonly addressed by transpubic methods and may require the inclusion of perineal and intra-abdominal modifications. These methods are stressful to the patient and may tax the competence of surgeons who are called upon only infrequently to employ them. A simplified remedy to this dilemma has produced gratifying and competitive results.[37]

The bladder is exposed routinely, and a probing index finger is passed into the prostatic urethra to the site of obstruction. A Van Buren sound (14 to 18 Fr) is passed retrograde into the urethral bulb, where gentle manipulation during further advancement will be transmitted to the probing finger (despite even extensive fibrotic obliteration identified by double contrast urethrography or double endoscopy) (Fig. 25).[38] The probing finger then guides the sound into the bladder during modestly forceful advancement. Once access is established, transurethral resection may be employed to remove excessive local scarring. Less extensive scarring may require only Otis or visual urethrotomy. Following reconstitution, with or without modification, indwelling urethral catheterization is maintained for approximately 1 week, after which the protocol is identical as for catheter removal following alignment. Local restricturing is more likely in this setting and therefore diligent compliance with daily self-catheterization is especially critical. Visual urethrotomy at intervals may be temporarily required, but is usually tolerated as an outpatient under local anesthesia. The ultimate achievement of normal voiding without resorting to transpubic procedures has constituted a gratifying endorsement of this maneuver.

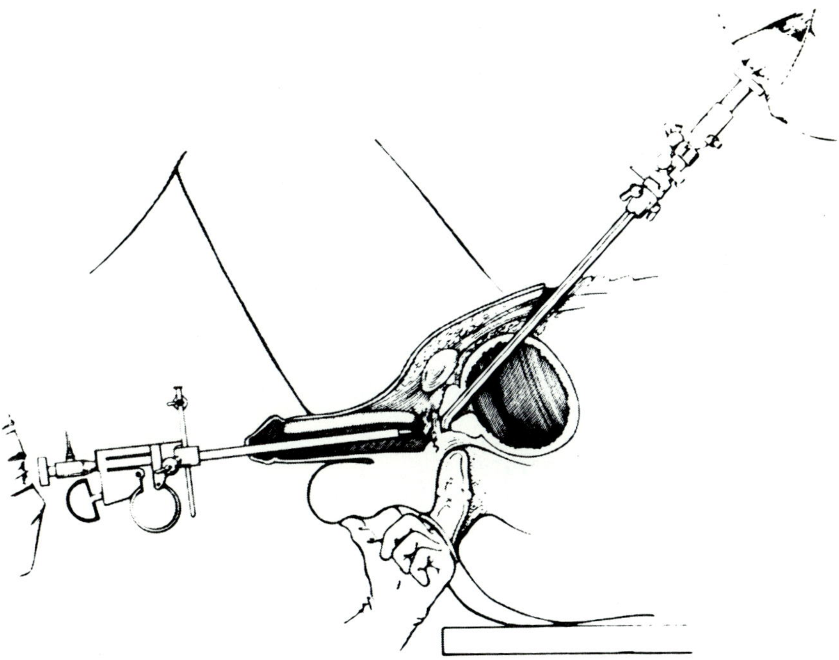

Figure 25. Bidirectional endoscopy for delineation of limits of stricture or for visual transection of stricture by urethrotome ("cutting toward the light"). *(Reprinted from Gonzalez R, Chiou R, Hekmat K, Fraley E: Endoscopic re-establishment of urethral continuity after traumatic disruption of the membranous urethra. J Urol 130:786, 1983, with permission.)*

REFERENCES

1. Turner-Warwick RT: Management of urethral strictures. Contemp Surg 16:52, 1980
2. Johanson B: Reconstruction of the male urethra in strictures. Acta Chir Scand 106 (suppl 176):483, 1953
3. Quartey JKM: One-stage penile/preputial cutaneous island urethroplasty for urethral stricture. J Urol 129:284, 1983
4. Webster GD, Robertson CN: The vascularized skin island urethroplasty. J Urol 133:31, 1985
5. Devine PC, Fallon B, Devine CJ Jr: Free full thickness skin graft urethroplasty. J Urol 116:444, 1976
6. Walker RD, Graham B: Measurement of blood flow in hypospadias flaps with subvisual doses of fluorescein. J Urol 136:266, 1986
7. Engelman ER, Polito G, Perley J, et al: Traumatic amputation of the penis. J Urol 112:774, 1974
8. Heymann AD, Bell-Thompson J, Rathod DM, Heller LE: Successful reimplantation of the penis using microvascular techniques. J Urol 118:879, 1977
9. Peterson NE: Penile amputation. Urologists' Letter Club, September 1976
10. Peterson NE: Traumatic posterior urethral avulsion. Monogr Urol 7:61, 1986
11. Margolies MN, Ring EJ, Waltman AC, et al: Arteriography in the management of hemorrhage from pelvic fractures. N Engl J Med 287:317, 1972
12. Ring EJ, Waltman AC, Athanasoulis C, et al: Angiography in pelvic trauma. Surg Gynec Obstet 139:375, 1974
13. Weems WL: Management of genitourinary injuries in patients with pelvic fractures. Ann Surg 189:717, 1979
14. Mucha P Jr: Recognizing and avoiding complications with pelvic fractures. Infect Surg p 53, January 1985
15. Brosman SA: Trauma of the bladder. Surg Gynec Obstet 143:605, 1976
16. Sullivan MJ, Lackner H, Banowsky LHW: Intraperitoneal extravasation of urine. JAMA 221:491, 1978
17. Wanebo HJ, Hunt TK, Mathewson C Jr: Rectal injuries. J Trauma 9:712, 1969
18. Raffa J, Christenson NM: Compound fractures of the pelvis. Am J Surg 132:282, 1976
19. Shrock TR, Christenson N: Management of perforating injuries of the colon. Surg Gynec Obstet 135:65, 1972
20. Turner-Warwick RT: A personal view of the management of traumatic posterior urethral strictures. Urol Clin North Am 4:111, 1977
21. Morehouse DD, MacKinnon KJ: Urological injuries associated with pelvic fractures. J Trauma 9:479, 1969
22. Morehouse DD, Belitsky P, MacKinnon KJ: Rupture of posterior urethra. J Urol 107:255, 1972
23. Solovov PD: Fracture of pelvis with injury of bladder and urethra. Vestn Khir 37:36, 1935
24. Turner-Warwick R: The repair of urethral strictures in the region of the membranous urethra. J Urol 100:303, 1968
25. Gil-Vernet JM: Un traitement des stenoses traumatiques et inflammatories del l'urethre posterieure. J Urol Nephrol 72:97, 1966

26. Swinney J: Urethroplasty. Br J Urol 29:293, 1957
27. Wilke TF, Cowan RJ, Balfour J: Urethroplasties for strictures. Br J Urol 32:16, 1960
28. Cowan RJ, Sullivan LD: Experience with perineal urethroplasty for stricture. Plast Reconstr Surg 41:137, 1968
29. Turner-Warwick RT: A technique for posterior urethroplasty. J Urol 83:416, 1960
30. Leadbetter GW Jr: A simplified urethroplasty for strictures of the posterior urethra. J Urol 83:54, 1960
31. Blandy JP, Singh M. Tresidder GC: Urethroplasty by scrotal flap for long urethral strictures. Br J Urol 40:261, 1968
32. Waterhouse K, Abrahams JI, Gruber H, et al: The transpubic approach to the lower urinary tract. J Urol 109:486, 1973
33. Turner-Warwick RT, Wynne EJC, Handly-Ashken M: The use of the omental pedicle graft and reconstruction of the urinary tract. Br J Surg 54:849, 1967
34. Peterson NE, Schulze K: Selective uro-radiography for trauma. J Urol 137:449, 1987
35. Chilton CP, Shah PJR, Fowler CG, et al: The impact of optical urethrotomy on the management of urethral strictures. Br J Urol 55:705, 1983
36. Ruutu M, Alfthan O, Standertsjold-Nordenstam CG: Treatment of urethral strictures by urethroplasty or direct vision urethrotomy. Scand J Urol Nephrol 17:1, 1983
37. Peterson NE: Perforation-reconstitution of posterior urethral obliteration. J Urol 137:507, 1987
38. Glass RE, Flynn JT, King JB, Blandy JP: Urethral injury and fractured pelvis. Br J Urol 50:578, 1978

The Role of Pyridoxine in Stone Prevention of Hyperoxaluric Patients

G. Alan Rose

INTRODUCTION

General

Vitamin B_6 has been used in the treatment of calcium oxalate urolithiasis for quite a few years. When the author reviewed the rationale for this 6 years ago,[1] he could find little to commend it. Since then, however, there have been important developments which have made it important to reconsider this matter. First, with improved methods for measurement of urinary oxalate, it has become evident that hyperoxaluria is much more common than used to be supposed. Second, it has become clear that hyperoxaluria is much more important than hypercalciuria as a risk factor for calcium oxalate urolithiasis.[2] Third, it is clear that certain types of hyperoxaluria do respond to vitamin B_6 therapy.[3] This chapter is therefore an attempt to indicate the role of B_6 therapy for treating calcium oxalate urolithiasis.

Measurement of Urinary Oxalate

Any departments devoted to treatment of calcium oxalate urolithiasis need to be able to measure urinary oxalate precisely in view of its critical role as a risk factor. Furthermore, they need to be able to measure it with the frequency that calcium is currently measured. Unfortunately, there are few laboratories that can meet these requirements. Although many methods have been developed, most of them are tedious and not easily susceptible to automation. Many result in spontaneous conversion of ascorbate to oxalate, a nonenzymatic reaction discovered in 1933,[4] forgotten and rediscovered in 1983.[5,6] This is not the place to review methodology. Suffice it to say that the author uses an "autoanalyzer" method based on immobilized oxalate oxidase which operates at some 25 samples per hour and is unaffected by ascorbate.[7] The normal range by this method is 0.06 to 0.42 mmol/24 hr.

Measurement of Plasma Oxalate

Methods for this assay are much less available than for urinary oxalate. This is because the normal plasma oxalate is as low as approximately 2 μmol/L and the ratio of ascorbate to oxalate is much higher than in urine. Consequently more care is required to prevent interference by ascorbate. Fortunately, however, in ordinary urolithiasis studies, it is not necessary to measure plasma oxalate except in the case of hyperoxaluria complicated by oxalosis. The increasing availability of renal transplantation then makes the plasma oxalate an important consideration. Practical, reliable methods for measuring plasma oxalate are now becoming available. The method in use by the author[8] again depends upon immobilized oxalate oxidase and a continuous flow automatic analysis system. The normal range by this method is 1.3 to 3.1 μmol/L.

Figure 1 shows how the plasma oxalate rises in chronic renal failure. The plasma oxalate:creatinine ratio remains constant whether primary hy-

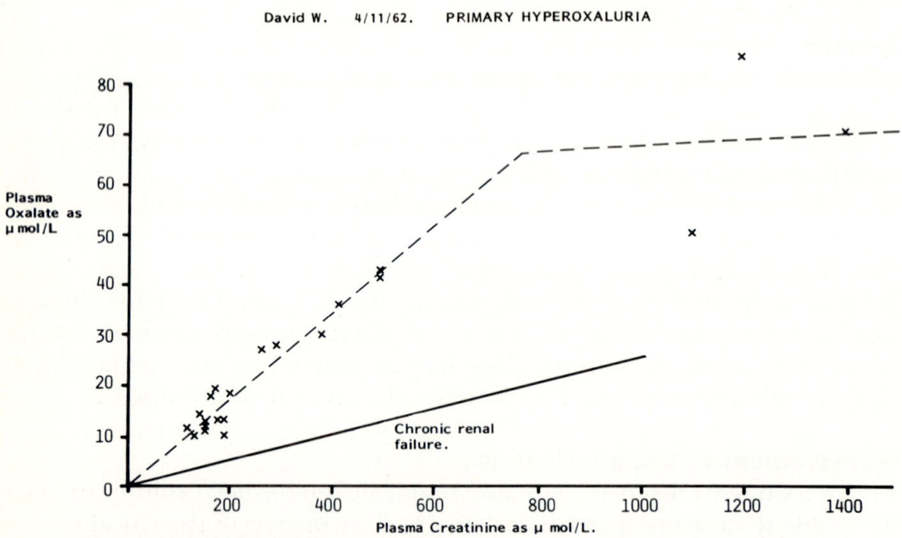

Figure 1. Plasma oxalate values in chronic renal failure alone (*solid line*) and accompanied by primary hyperoxaluria (*x and broken line*). The solid line is the regression line from many points.[8] Note that plasma oxalate is proportional to creatinine at plasma oxalate levels below 50 μmol/L. By noting the relationship of plasma oxalate to creatinine, one can recognize those patients with renal failure who also have primary hyperoxaluria.

peroxaluria is present or not. However, the ratio is much higher if primary hyperoxaluria is present. Oxalosis occurs when levels of plasma oxalate reach about 60 μmol/L and Figure 1 shows that this occurs in primary hyperoxaluria with a plasma creatinine of only 700 μmol/L (7.9 mg/100 ml), whereas without primary hyperoxaluria it requires a plasma creatinine as high as 2200 μmol/L (25 mg/100 ml).

Vitamin B_6 Physiology

The term vitamin B_6 refers to a group of chemically related compounds. These are pyridoxine, pyridoxal, pyridoxamine, and their corresponding phosphates. The chemical structures of these are shown in Figure 2. The active form seems to be pyridoxal phosphate which is generated from the other forms in the liver and transported bound to plasma albumin to the various tissues, where it acts as a coenzyme in a whole variety of enzyme systems which include transminases, decarboxylases, transmethylations, and transulfurations. It is also involved in the formation of nicotinic acid from tryptophane so that vitamin B_6 deficiency results in increased urinary xanthurenic acid after an oral tryptophane load.[9] At the clinical level, vitamin B_6 deficiency can cause sideroblastic anemia,[10] dermatitis, peripheral neuropathy, and convulsions.[11] It can also cause hyperoxaluria in cats,[12] rats,[13] and in man.[14] The precise cause of this is not known, but it may be due to reduced transamination of glyoxylate to glycine which results in increased diversion of glyoxylate to glycollate and oxalate (Fig. 3).

A number of metabolic abnormalities characterized by raised daily requirement for vitamin B_6 have been identified. A curious feature is that in each case only one of the end organs requiring the vitamin is affected giving frequent convulsions,[15] or sideroblastic anemia,[16] or mental retardation caused by accumulation of homocystine,[17] cystathionine,[18] or xanthurenic acid. In each of these disorders, it seems that it must be the enzyme system

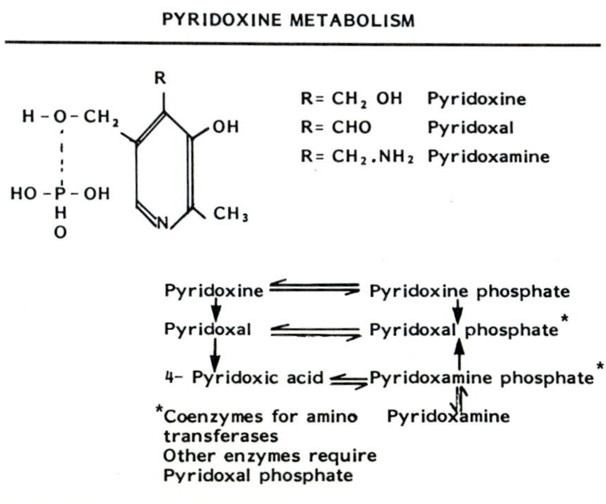

Figure 2. Structural formula of the various forms of vitamin B_6. The metabolic pathway of pyridoxine to the active metabolites pyridoxal-5-phosphate and pyridoxamine phosphate, and to the main excretory product pyridoxic acid.

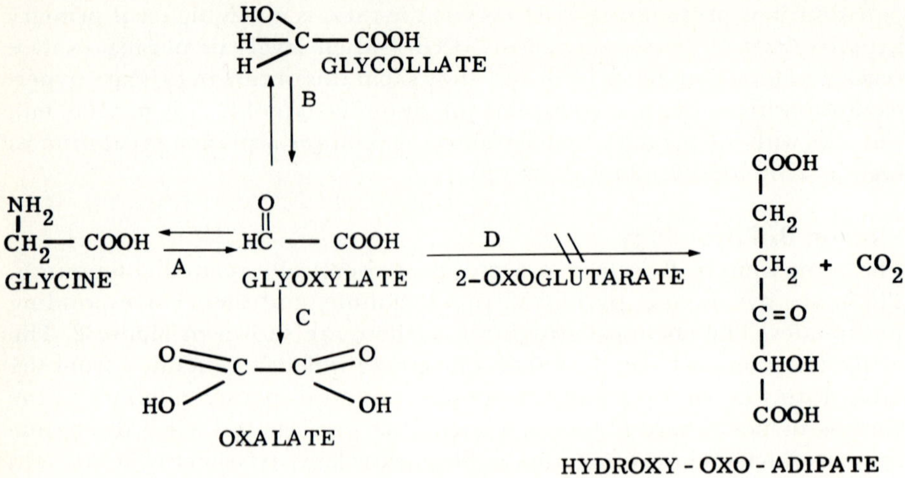

TYPE 1 PRIMARY HYPEROXALURIA

Figure 3. Metabolic production of oxalate from glycine. **A.** Reversible oxidative deamination of glycine; the reamination is thought to be dependent upon pyridoxal phosphate as coenzyme. **C.** One-way only reaction. **D.** Site of the supposed enzyme block in type I primary hyperoxaluria, leading to excess production of glycollate and oxalate. *(Reproduced from Rose GA, 1982, with permission.[58])*

that is abnormal and not the vitamin B_6 itself, since in each case only one system is affected and in none of them has hyperoxaluria been reported. The only exception to this rule is that certain cases of B_6-dependent sideroblastic anemias have been found to respond to intramuscular pyridoxal phosphate.[19] These are important points when considering the possible cause of mild metabolic hyperoxaluria and primary hyperoxaluria.

The normal daily requirement of vitamin B_6 is 20 to 30 μg/g protein in the diet giving an adult need of about 2 mg/day. The vitamin is water soluble and found in wheat, corn, meat, fish, milk, eggs, and vegetables and a daily intake of 10 mg is not uncommon in developed countries where deficiency is unusual.

Toxicity with vitamin B_6 was not recognized until 1983 when seven cases were described who had taken up to 6 g/day[20] with onset of sensory neuropathy. More cases have since been described[21] and it seems advisable not to exceed 1 g/day for adults and proportionally less according to body weight in children.[22]

Increased requirements for vitamin B_6 may be induced by treatment with isonicotinic acid hydrazide [INAH],[23] or D-penicillamine[24] and certain other drugs.

Pyridoxine is excreted mainly as pyridoxic acid and measurement of this product in urine provides a convenient way of checking on compliance of pyridoxine therapy.

Types of Hyperoxaluria

Types of hyperoxaluria are itemized in Table 1 but a few words of explanation are required. Of the inherited types, the variety with raised urinary glycollate is more common. Type II has been recognized in only a handful of cases throughout the world, mainly from a single family. In part this may reflect difficulties in analyzing urine for glycerate, but even allowing for this it probably is an extremely rare condition which can be ignored in the remainder of this chapter.

The acquired hyperoxalurias can conveniently be divided into those with raised urinary glycollate and those without, since the finding of raised urinary glycollate indicates a metabolic abnormality affecting the pathway of oxalate formation via glyoxylate and rules out simple excessive oxalate ingestion or absorption as a cause of hyperoxaluria. Hence once hyperoxaluria is recognized, it becomes important to measure urinary glycollate as the next step. Again, however, very few laboratories can perform this measurement at the present time. The author's laboratory uses a method based on glycollate oxidase[28] and the normal range is 0.05 to 0.33 mmol/24 hr. In hyperoxaluria induced by methoxyflurane[26] and aspergillosis,[27] there is no report in the literature of whether the hyperoxaluria is accompanied by raised urinary glycollate but it is assumed for the time being that this is not the case.

Ethylene glycol has been used in the form of antifreeze as a cheap

TABLE 1. THE TYPES OF HYPEROXALURIA

Inherited
- Type I—Primary hyperoxaluria (with raised urinary glycollate)
- Type II—Primary hyperoxaluria (with raised urinary glycerate)

Acquired
- With raised urinary glycollate:
  - Ethylene glycol and diethylene glycol poisoning
  - Excess glycine absorption during transurethral resection of prostate[25]
  - Mild metabolic hyperoxaluria
    - Without renal tubular acidosis
    - With renal tubular acidosis[3]
  - Vitamin B_6 deficiency
- Without raised urinary glycollate
  - Intestinal (steatorrhea, jejunal bypass)
  - Excess dietary oxalate
  - Methoxylurane anesthesia[26]
  - Aspergillosis[27]
  - ?Idiopathic hypercalciuria

intoxicant and is well known as a cause of hyperoxaluria. Diethylene glycol is also used as antifreeze and was recently found to have been added to certain European wines. This too leads to hyperoxaluria[29] and raised the question as to whether this could have led to urolithiasis in regular wine drinkers. The final item in Table 1 is of very great importance. There is increasing evidence in recent literature that idiopathic hypercalciuria may be accompanied by raised urinary oxalate. It is thought that overabsorption of dietary calcium causes reduced intestinal binding of oxalate by calcium and hence overabsorption of dietary oxalate. This leads to either hyperoxaluria[30–32] or simply a rise in the mean urinary oxalate even though many of the values remain within the normal range.[3,33] It seems that small variations in urinary oxalate even within the normal range can be an important risk factor for calcium oxalate urolithiasis. More work is needed on these small deviations from the normal. If it is confirmed, however, the implication would be that more stress should be placed on restricting oxalate rich foods in the treatment of idiopathic hyperoxaluria.

Mild metabolic hyperoxaluria (accompanied by raised urinary glycollate) is a condition which has been recognized in very few centers as yet. This is because in order to recognize it, one must be able to measure urinary oxalate with considerable precision and also be able to measure it in all cases of calcium oxalate urolithiasis and to measure urinary glycollate as well. It has, however, been recognized in London, England[3,34] and in Canada.[35] It may respond to vitamin B_6 and hence is of great interest in the present context and will therefore be considered in detail below.

TYPE I PRIMARY HYPEROXALURIA

General

This condition is defined as an inborn error of metabolism transmitted by a rare autosomal recessive gene in which there is increased metabolic production of glycollate and oxalate. This is thought to be due to lack of a carboligase enzyme which normally converts glycollate to hydroxy-oxo-adipate (Fig. 3). It should be stressed, however, that the evidence that this is the enzyme block is based upon a single study of only five cases.[36] One would expect that the disease would be present from birth and affect males and females in equal proportions, but both of these propositions may be incorrect.

The author's experience of primary hyperoxaluria is based upon a personal series of 50 cases. Some have been under the care of other physicians but in all cases the urine and plasma oxalate and glycollate measurements have been repeatedly performed in the author's laboratory and there has been close liaison between the clinicians and the laboratory. There were six examples of multiple cases in sibships each of which contained two cases. There were no examples of cases in more than one generation per family.

All this is in accordance with transmission by a recessive gene. Of these 50 cases, 38 were male and 12 female giving a ratio of 3.17:1 and a similar bias was reported in the smaller series of 17 cases from Scandinavia.[37] At least two possible explanations come to mind. First, we may be looking at a mixture of genetic abnormalities. Second, the disease may be expressed more severely in males than in females. A possible reason for this is suggested by the work of Nath and colleagues in India[38] who found that testosterone increased the formation of oxalate in rats' livers.

Natural History

Primary hyperoxaluria goes through several distinct phases although the time span of the phases is extremely variable. Death may occur after only a few months of life but, on the other hand, the first symptoms may be delayed for 10 or 15 years, and death of the untreated patient may be delayed into the 20s or 30s. Phase one of the disease is an asymptomatic hyperoxaluria with normal renal function. Urinary oxalate is raised to 1 to 5 mmol/24 hr and plasma oxalate is raised in proportion but not to a level that can cause oxalosis. Phase two is characterized by recurrent stone formation, the stones usually being made of almost pure calcium oxalate, and stone episodes which eventually cause severe renal glomerular damage. The plasma oxalate rises steeply and when calcium oxalate deposition in tissues begins to occur this leads into phase three of accelerated renal failure. The oxalosis causes further renal glomerular impairment and hence even worse oxalosis and this vicious circle ends in death unless reversed by medical intervention. Urinary oxalate concentration remains high throughout and it is usually possible to demonstrate calcium oxalate crystals in warm fresh urine. These are often the monohydrate of the "dumbbell" variety (Fig. 4) but may be the dihydrate "envelope" type (Fig. 5).

Response to Pyridoxine

One of the most remarkable features of primary hyperoxaluria is the response to pyridoxine. Although tried with little success previously by others, 1970 saw the first impressive report of successful therapy by pyridoxine.[39] Since then there have been numerous similar reports. They agree that some cases respond and some do not, but the proportion of responders has varied from paper to paper, probably because of the small numbers of cases in each paper. The experience at St. Peter's Hospitals (London, England) to date is summarized in Figure 6. Thirty-four patients have been given long-term trials with high dose pyridoxine (up to 800 mg/70 kg body weight). Of these patients 26 were male and 8 female; 29.4 percent of the total number gave an unequivocably good result with fall in urinary oxalate and glycollate to normal for as long as the vitamin was given. The response rate was slightly different in the two sexes being 26.9 percent for males and 37.5 percent for females but this might not be statistically significant. No significant response was found in 41.2 percent with values for males and females

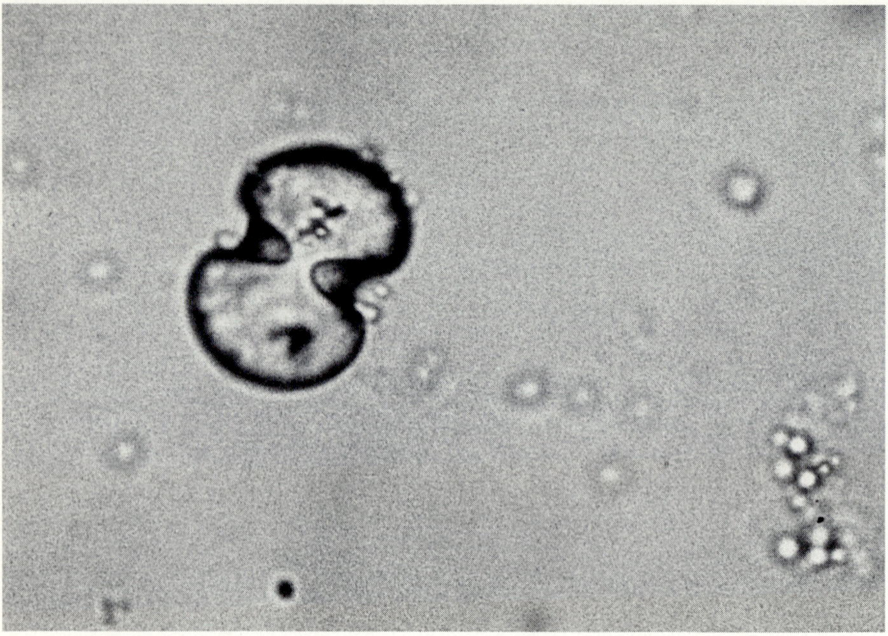

Figure 4. "Dumbbell" calcium oxalate monohydrate crystal in urine and characteristic of hyperoxaluria.

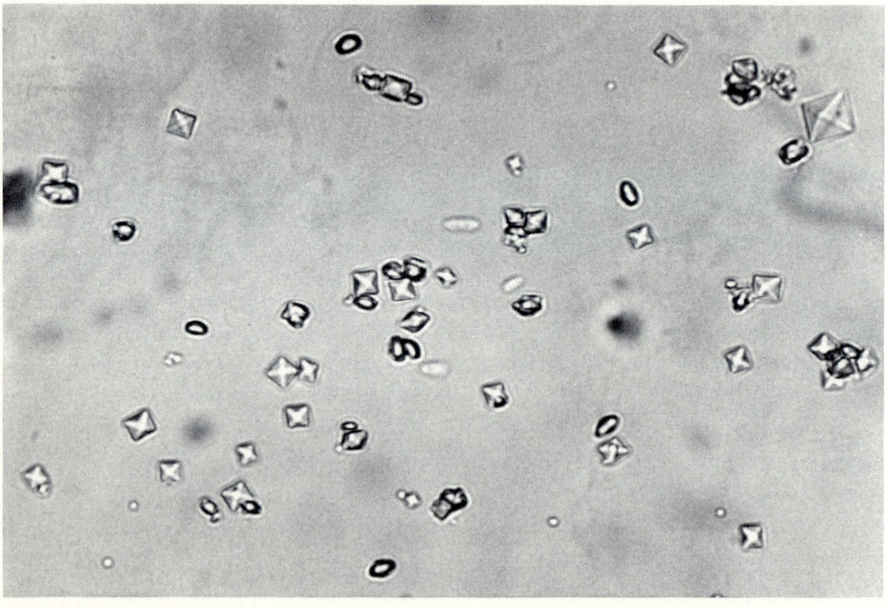

Figure 5. Multiple "envelope" calcium oxalate dihydrate crystals in urine and characteristic of hypercalciuria.

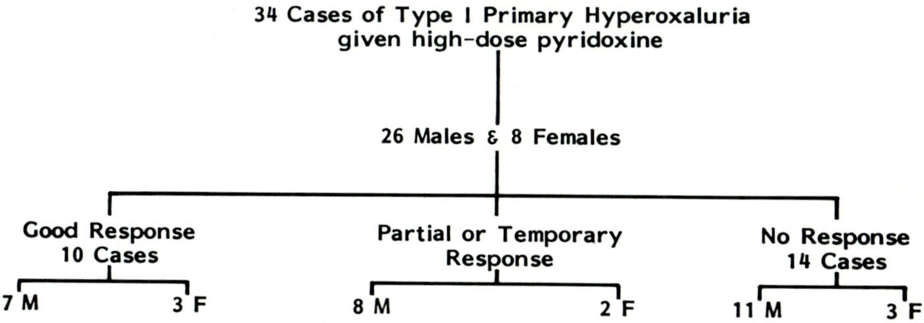

Figure 6. Response of patients with primary hyperoxaluria to high dose pyridoxine. Note that response is not always clearly positive or negative, but there are various in-between types of response.

being 42.3 and 37.5 percent respectively. In addition there was a third group comprising 29.4 percent of the total in whom the response was either partial with a fall in urinary oxalate, but not to normal, or temporary when a fall to normal urinary oxalate was followed by relapse. This group comprised 30.8 percent of the males and 25 percent of the females. There were four sibships in whom two sibs were treated. In sibship R (two brothers), both responded well; in sibships V and C (brother and sister in each case), all were unresponsive; in sibship S (two sisters), one responded completely and the other partially.

Reversal of Renal Failure with Pyridoxine

Robert C was born of unrelated parents on September 10, 1955. In April 1958, he developed hematuria and later passed two small stones. In September 1958, he suddenly became anuric and 12 stones were removed from the penis. He was then found to have bilateral renal calcification; 24-hour urinary calcium was 1.5 to 1.8 mmol (60 to 70 mg) and oxalate was 57 μmol (5.1 mg). With an ammonium chloride test, the minimum urinary pH was 5.6 and he was thought to have an incomplete form of renal tubular acidosis and treated with sodium bicarbonate 4 g/day. The main diagnosis was recognized in July 1964 when the urinary oxalate was found to be 0.52 mmol/24 hr which was thought to be three times normal for his age. In June 1967, in an attempt to prevent further nephrocalcinosis, treatment was started with magnesium hydroxide suspension 16 ml/24 hr. It was thought that this treatment was beneficial and 3 years later the case history up to that time was reported.[40] In July 1975, he was found to be hypertensive with a diastolic blood pressure of 120 mm Hg and guanethidine was given. In June 1976, the plasma urate was 503 μmol/L (8.5 mg/100 ml) and treatment with allopurinol was started. By this time, the plasma creatinine which had been rising very slowly began to rise increasingly fast and he was admitted to University College Hospital, London to determine the reason for this. The renogram showed symmetric excretion with no evidence of urinary tract obstruction. Renal biopsy showed many calcium oxalate crystals and it was concluded that the nephrocalcinosis was the cause of the rapidly progressing renal failure. He was therefore transfered to these hospitals to consider hemodialysis treatment. On admission here, he was a healthy looking young man of 70.5 kg, blood pressure was 120/80. His plasma results were as follows (mmol/L except where otherwise stated): urea, 23; creatinine, 0.67; sodium, 141; potassium, 4.6; bicarbonate, 26; calcium, 2.58; phosphate, 1.6; urate, 0.35; magnesium, 1.2; alkaline phosphatase, 10 KAU; SGPT, 24 IU/L; SGOT, 9.2 IU/L. Twenty-four-hour urine contained (mmol/L) creatinine, 14.6; sodium, 177; potassium, 65; calcium, 1.4; phosphate, 26; urate, 3.1; oxalate, 1.88; magnesium, 6.5; and protein, 0.1 g. Hemoglobin was 8.9 g/100 ml; MCV, 90 cm; MCHC, 32.5 percent. Midstream urine showed 50 WBC per mm^3, a trace of protein but no bacteria, and sterile on culture.

As he had never been treated with pyridoxine, it was decided to add this to the other drugs before starting regular hemodialysis. The results of this are shown in Figures 7 and 8. After a few days, the urinary oxalate fell and reached almost normal limits after 1 month of therapy and did not rise again. Soon after the fall in urinary oxalate took place, the plasma creatinine stopped rising and in fact began to fall and soon became stationary at about 0.3 mmol/L. Hemodialysis has therefore proved unnecessary to date and long-term follow-up on pyridoxine continues. The reason for the improved renal function is thought to be that a fall in plasma oxalate presumably matched the fall in urinary oxalate so that some of the oxalosis could

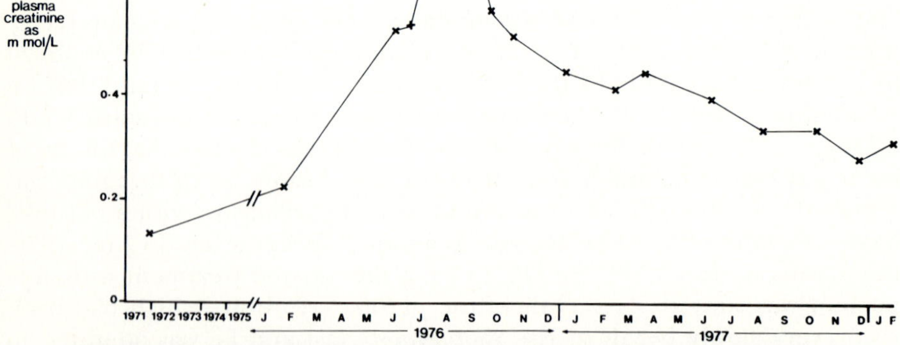

Figure 7. Rise and fall in plasma calcium of a patient with primary hyperoxaluria before and during pyridoxine therapy. Ten years later the plasma creatinine remains at 0.3 mmol/L. (Same patient as Figure 8.)

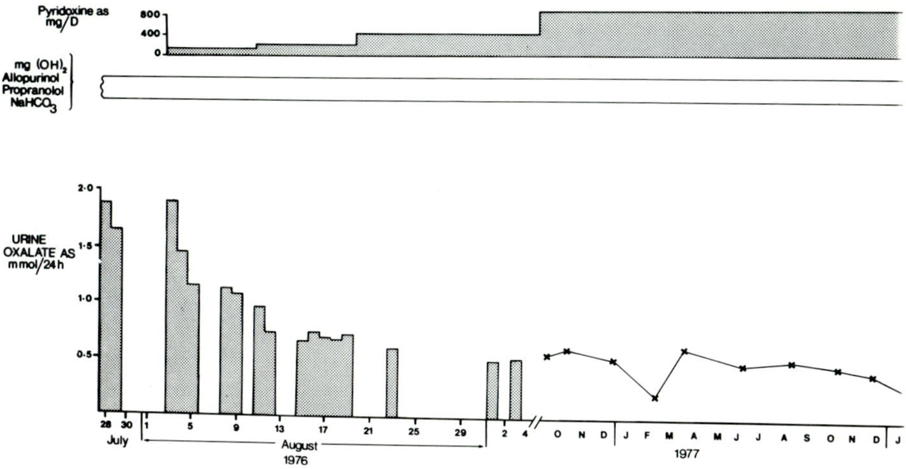

Figure 8. Decline in urinary oxalate of a patient with primary hyperoxaluria when given pyridoxine. Note how urinary oxalate persisted at just above the normal value for about 16 months after which it dropped to and remained well within the normal range. During these 16 months tissue calcium oxalate was perhaps dissolving away. (Same patient as Figure 7.)

dissolve away leading to improved renal glomerular function. This theory is supported by the observation in Figure 7 that urinary oxalate remained very slightly elevated during the first 16 months of treatment. Since that time urinary oxalate has remained well within normal limits and plasma creatinine has remained at 300 μmol/L (about 3.0 mg/100 ml).

Temporary Response to Pyridoxine

Andrew P was born July 26, 1971. At 9 years of age, he was investigated on account of abdominal pains and stones found in both kidneys. Blood urea was 7.3 mmol/L and plasma creatinine was 96 μmol/L. He was found to have hyperoxaluria and was given a low oxalate diet to which he kept. Pyridoxine treatment began in October 1980, the dose being 150 mg/day, but was doubled on November 7, 1980. The response to pyridoxine is shown in Figure 9. It is clear that there was a substantial fall in urinary oxalate and glycollate which lasted approximately 6 months, but the trend reversed and nothing we were able to do has since yielded any further improvement. He was admitted to St. Peter's Hospitals for further studies and received first a 7-day course of vitamin B_1 300 mg t.d. and then a course of daily injections of pyridoxamine phosphate 250 mg IM for a week, but this led to no improvement. He is therefore now treated by other means reserved for those who fail to respond to pyridoxine. Not only did he fail to improve but during the first few days in hospital the urinary oxalate and glycollate actually doubled without change in urinary creatinine or pyridoxic acid, and this reversed when he went home.

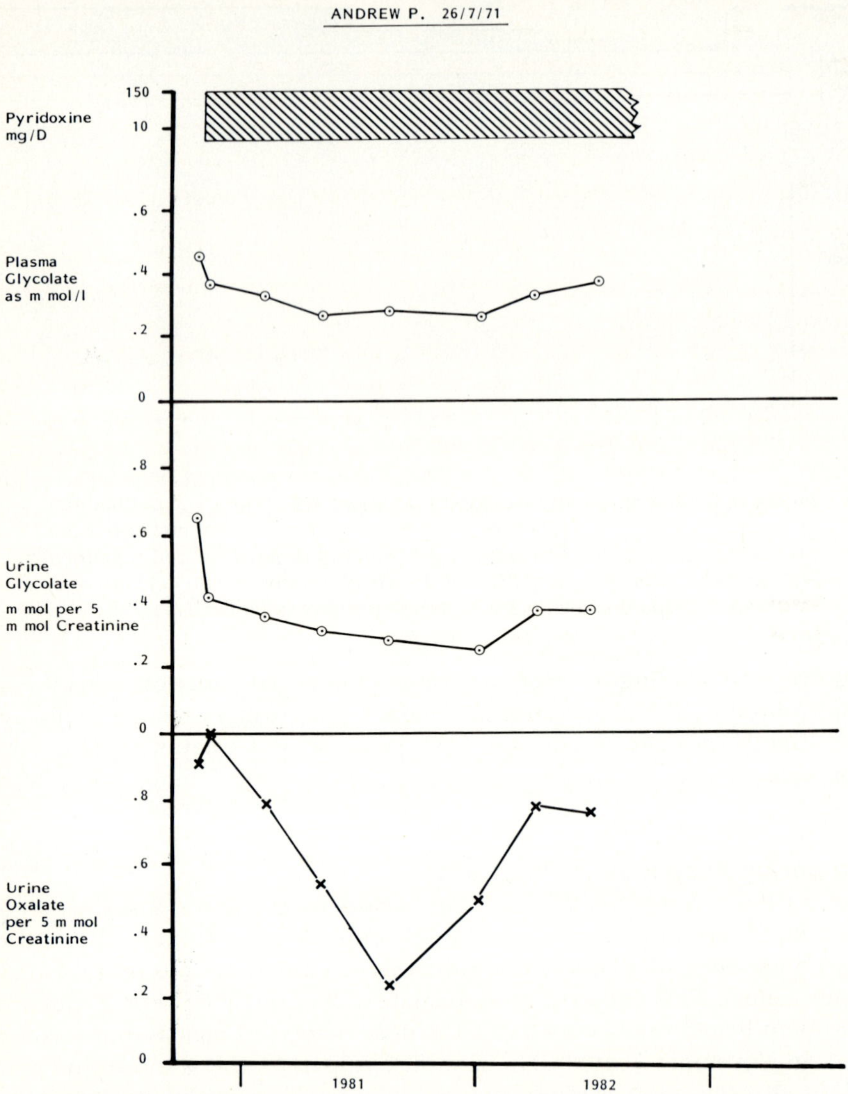

Figure 9. Example of patient with primary hyperoxaluria showing temporary response to pyridoxine. *(Reproduced from Kasidas GP, Rose GA, 1984 with permission.[3])*

Why this should have occurred is not clear but an environmental factor seems possible, although what this could be is unknown.

Delayed Response to Pyridoxine

The boy now to be mentioned, Scott C, is remarkable for several reasons. First, he was not hyperoxaluric at 1 week of age but clearly was so a month later. Second, treatment was initiated at the age of 2 months and still continues, he now being 7 years of age. Third, full response was delayed for about 8 months but once achieved he never relapsed. Fourth, an attempt was made to diagnose the disease or its absence in utero. Details have been published elsewhere[41] but are summarized here for convenience. An older brother had died at 6 months of age from hyperoxaluria and oxalosis.[42] When Scott's fetal age was 15 to 16 weeks, amniocentesis was performed and the fluid oxalate found to be detectable and therefore raised according to our criteria at that time. A urine sample at the age of 7 days was found to have normal oxalate and glycollate concentrations relative to creatinine. A further sample at age 6 weeks was clearly hyperoxaluric. In disbelief, both samples were reassayed with the same results. Subsequent biochemical course is shown in Figure 10. It is clear that full response to pyridoxine was delayed for about 8 months but fortunately the treatment was not abandoned. The child thrived, now 7 years of age at the time of writing, and the urinary oxalate and glycollate which are checked every few months have remained normal. He suffered one small stone which was removed in 1984 and which was made before response was complete but there have been no other stone events. It is difficult to know why the disease was not present at birth, but one possible hypothesis is that although the enzyme abnormally is present at birth there is an environmental factor which is required to produce the full biochemical expression.

Renal Transplantation in Primary Hyperoxaluria

The onset of chronic renal failure in primary hyperoxaluria raises the question of renal transplantation. What is the risk of oxalosis rapidly developing in the newly transplanted kidney? In 1975, a report from the American College of Surgeons/National Institute of Health Renal Transplant Registry concluded that "oxalosis is a form of chronic renal failure that is unsuitable for treatment by transplantation."[43] In the last 10 years, however, this conclusion has been proved to be incorrect. First, it is stressed that transplantation should not be performed until the patient has had a 6-month trial of high dose pyridoxine, i.e., 800 mg/day for a 70-kg man, or equivalent dose in a child. Response is best followed by oxalate:creatinine ratio in the urine but if there is no urine the same ratio may be used in plasma (Fig. 1). A complete response means that renal transplantation can then proceed without increased risk to the donor kidney. An example of this successful method of treatment was published five years ago[44] when previous attempts at transplantation were also reviewed.

Second, even should the patient not respond to pyridoxine, renal transplantation can still be entertained provided that the plasma oxalate can be maintained sufficiently low to prevent any (further) oxalosis. One precaution is to try and undertake transplantation early in chronic renal failure. Present experience makes us think that the critical level of plasma oxalate is 16 times the upper limit of normal (about 50 μmol/L) and this requires a plasma creatinine of only about 600 μmol/L (6.8 mg/100 ml) in a patient with primary hyperoxaluria. If this level has been exceeded and ox-

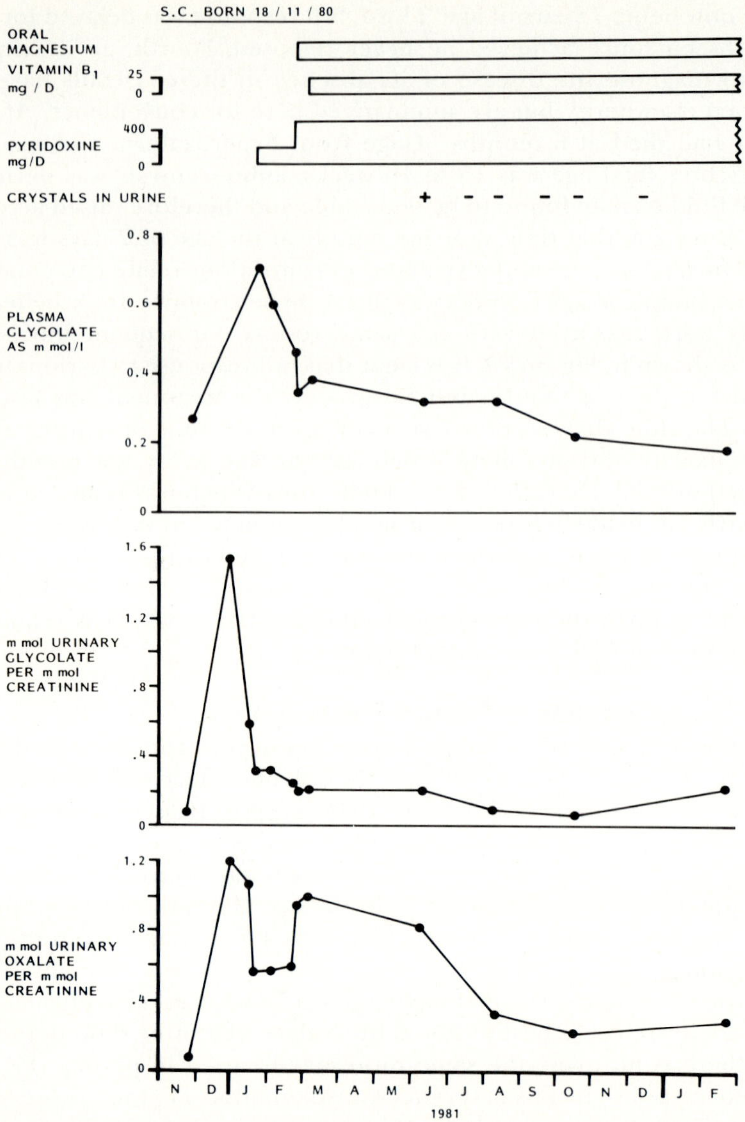

Figure 10. Example of patient with primary hyperoxaluria showing delayed response to pyridoxine which, however, was permanent once established. Note also that he did not show primary hyperoxaluria soon after birth. *(Reproduced from Rose GA, 1979, with permission.[1])*

alosis has occurred, then vigorous hemodialysis may reduce the plasma creatinine to a safe level. The plasma oxalate and creatinine levels must be held down to safe levels during any periods of nonfunction or reduced function of the donor kidney. Very vigorous hemodialysis is then required. Given these circumstances, renal transplantation can be successful and a number of such cases have recently been described[45] and the author has personal experience of several other cases treated along these lines. The following is an example. David W was born November 4, 1962 with horseshoe kidney. In 1968, a live related donor renal transplant failed as a result of oxalosis and he went back on hemodialysis and was given pyridoxine 500 mg/day. The first plasma oxalate and creatinine values were 71 and 1400 μmol/L respectively and these confirmed hyperoxaluria resistant to pyridoxine, and with the former being high enough to cause oxalosis. On November 4, 1984, he received a cadaver renal transplant (Mr. Rudge at Guy's Hospital, London) which functioned immediately. He was also given IV pyridoxine 600 mg/day, phosphate and magnesium, and 10 mg b.i.d. of bendrofluazide. The serial values of plasma oxalate and creatinine are shown in Figure 11 and reveal that they moved together very closely once the oxalate level had fallen below 79 μmol/L. In May 1985, a 24-hour urine collection contained 1.6 mmol/L oxalate, 0.59 mmol/L glycollate, and 287 mg pyridoxic acid (confirming the intake of pyridoxine). He therefore has type I primary hyperoxaluria unresponsive to pyridoxine despite which the second renal transplant was successful and is still functioning well after over 1 year.

It is worth noting at this point that the excess oxalate is probably produced in the liver and that it might be better to consider liver transplantation before oxalosis and renal failure begins, than to undertake renal transplantation after oxalosis has occurred.

It is important in transplanting the patient with oxalosis for the surgeon to remember that oxalosis in blood vessel walls can be a hazard leading to ruptured vessel walls.

Alternative Treatment When Pyridoxine Fails

Even when cases of primary hyperoxaluria fail to respond to pyridoxine, there is a lot that can be done to reduce the incidence of urolithiasis and onset of renal failure and oxalosis. First, raising urinary volume by water drinking and restricting dietary oxalate intake reduces the oxalate concentration in the urine. Water therapy is not as easy as it sounds and the patients should be given written instructions on how much water to drink, how to spread it through the day (and night), how to anticipate high risk situations such as dehydration caused by travel, hot occupations, and sporting activities, and how the color of urine is a good indication of concentration. The instructions might also list the oxalate-rich foods to avoid and this must include nuts, chocolate, and iced tea.

Second, it has been claimed that oral magnesium and inorganic phosphate therapy will reduce the tendency of calcium oxalate to precipitate in urine and improve the prognosis.[40,46] It is easy to understand how raising urinary magnesium is beneficial since it has been shown that this does reduce calcium oxalate precipitation when dilute whole urine is evaporated to high but physiologic concentration.[47] The way in which inorganic phos-

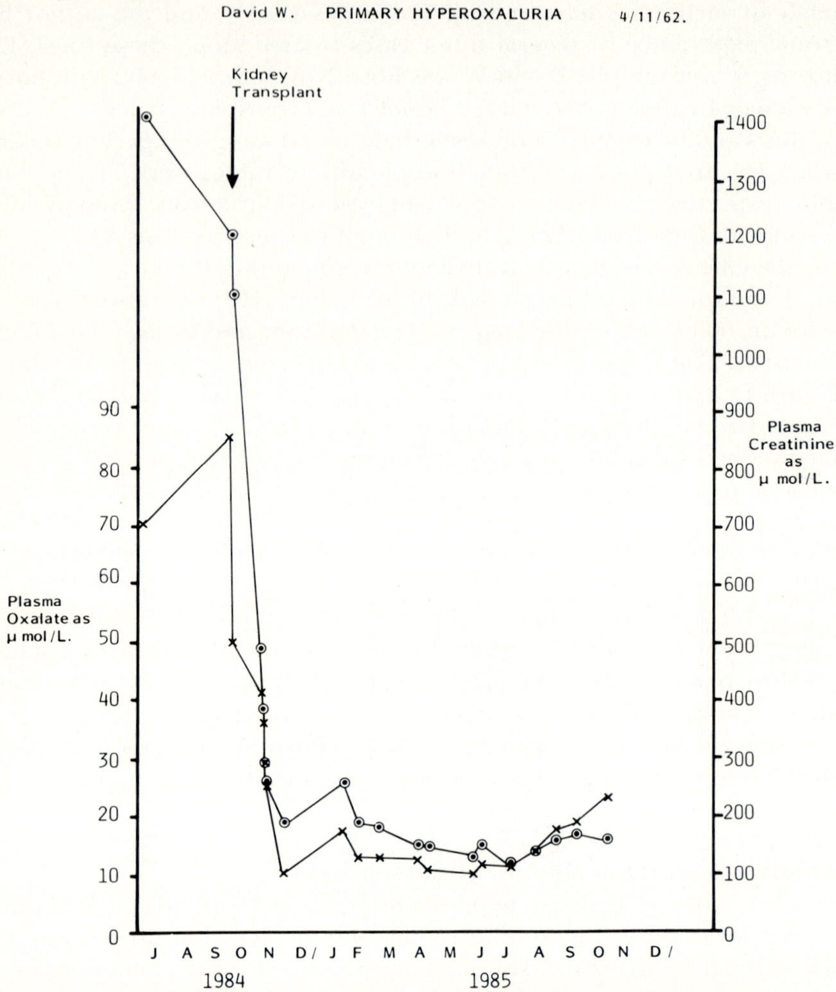

Figure 11. Serial plasma oxalate and creatinine levels in a patient with primary hyperoxaluria nonresponsive to pyridoxine, who received a cadaver kidney transplant in November 1984. Circles = creatinine, crosses = oxalate.

phate helps is not clear because the metabolic changes that result are rather complex, with a fall in urinary calcium, and rises in urinary phosphate, pyrophosphate, pH, and citrate. Both milk of magnesia and neutral phosphate are bowel laxatives and the dose of either may have to be small at first but then raised to the limits of tolerance. When renal glomerular impairment is present or threatening, magnesia is a safer therapy than phosphate (sodium and potassium loads) and the latter also carries the risk of aggravating hypertension. For these reasons, the author favors magnesia.

The following case illustrates the beneficial effects of "alternative therapy." Alan R was born December 19, 1968. In 1979, he had painless hematuria and in 1980 stones were removed from the left kidney. In November 1980, a stone was removed from the right ureter. In November 1981, he passed another stone and in 1982 was found to have a cluster of stones in the lower pole of the right kidney. When first seen in the St. Peter's Hospital Metabolic Stone Clinic, in May 1980, plasma findings were all normal (Na, 140; K, 3.8; urea, 4.1; creatinine, 0.08; calcium, 2.29; phosphate, 1.32; urate, 0.44; and Mg, 0.77 mmol/L; alkaline phosphatase, 640 IU/L). A 24-hour urine volume was 1200 ml and it contained 0.3 mmol calcium, 9.4 mmol creatinine, 1.23 mmol oxalate, 3.1 mmol glycollate, and 4.0 mmol magnesium. A random fresh sample of urine contained numerous rectangular and aggregated crystals and also many dumbbell and hourglass crystals characteristic of hyperoxaluria. He was started on pyridoxine 20 mg/day but as there was no fall in urinary oxalate, the dose was raised progressively to 800 mg/day by the end of June 1982. Despite continuing this dose until December 1985, there has been no definite evidence of response. In August 1982, he was started on milk of magnesia and was gradually able to raise the dose to 10 ml, two or three times a day. Urinary volume rose progressively over a year or two to about 4 liters per 24 hours. In August 1984, a stone was removed from the left kidney percutaneously (Mr. J.E.A. Wickham) and this proved to be almost pure calcium oxalate monohydrate. There has been no evidence of stone growth since 1982 and he now has a possible small calculus in the right kidney, but no others. Plasma urea and creatinine levels remain well in the normal range.

Conclusions

Type I primary hyperoxaluria is not a homogenous condition. It can be subdivided into those that respond to pyridoxine and those who do not. This division is not as sharp as previously thought, however, since there are delayed responses, partial responses, and some who respond for a limited period and then relapse. The condition is more common in males than females. It may be that certain environmental factors affect the severity of the expression of the disease. Pyridoxine in high dose is the treatment of choice and can return an individual to clinical normality and reverse chronic renal failure caused by oxalosis, and greatly improve the risk of oxalosis in a renal transplant. Even when there is no response to pyridoxine, treatment by water, low oxalate diet, and milk of magnesia can greatly improve the prognosis.

MILD METABOLIC HYPEROXALURIA WITH RECURRENT UROLITHIASIS

Introduction

In 1972, we introduced a new enzyme method for urinary oxalate[48] that was highly reproducible and generated reliable results within the normal range. Following this it was possible to measure urinary oxalate in all patients with calcium oxalate urolithiasis when it seemed that there was a special need to do so, i.e., when the cause of the stones could not be found by the usual other investigations. In 1983 we developed an automated method for urinary oxalate and since that time have been able to make the measurements in virtually unlimited numbers. Currently the hospital routine biochemistry laboratory measures urinary oxalate more frequently than urinary calcium. As a result, hyperoxaluria is being observed more frequently and a number of cases of severe recurrent urolithiasis with mild metabolic hyperoxaluria have been uncovered. This condition is characterized by:

1. Urinary oxalate usually 0.6 to 0.8 mmol/24 hr although higher values sometimes occur
2. Normal dietary oxalate
3. Raised urinary glycollate, thereby excluding excessive dietary intake or absorption as the cause of hyperoxaluria
4. A preponderance of males
5. Varying response to pyridoxine. Some have responded to low dose (10 to 20 mg/day), some have responded to low dose but then needed higher doses, some have responded only to high dose but then relapsed
6. Age of onset has varied between childhood and the sixth decade of life
7. Each case so far has been sporadic and without family history
8. One group of patients has had cellulose phosphate therapy for many years and the condition seems related to this treatment. These patients will not be considered in detail here
9. Most of the patients have not received cellulose phosphate but have often shown other medical conditions, i.e., primary hyperparathyroidism, medullary sponge kidney, idiopathic hypercalciuria, and renal tubular acidosis (RTA). The patients with RTA have been discussed previously[3] and will not be considered further here. Examples of the remaining cases will now be considered and some brief clinical details are given in Table 2

Complete Response to Short Course of High Dose Pyridoxine Without Relapse on Stopping

These cases have been described elsewhere[34] and the complete clinical details will not be repeated here. Both of these cases were given high doses of pyridoxine because it was not then appreciated that they might respond to lower doses. The effects of the pyridoxine on urinary oxalate and glycollate are reproduced in Figure 12. Both of these cases suffered from recurrent calcium oxalate urolithiasis. In the case of David M (born October 6, 1939), no cause had been detected until he was found to have metabolic hyperoxaluria at St. Peter's Hospitals in 1977. On 400 mg/day of pyridoxine, urinary oxalate and glycollate rapidly fell to normal and remained there for over 2 years after stopping pyridoxine. Stone formation ceased and he then stopped attending but is presumed to have remained well. Nicola Y (born August 17, 1955) was investigated at St. Peter's Hospitals for renal tubular acidosis but found to have metabolic hyperoxaluria as well. With only 10 mg/day of pyridoxine, urinary oxalate and glycollate fell to normal, but before this was appreciated the dose was raised to 100 mg/day. On stopping the treatment, urinary oxalate and glycollate remained normal for 8 years until the time of writing (1985).

Response to Low Dose Pyridoxine But With Rising Requirement

The clinical history and investigations on Arthur D, born November 14, 1957, have been reported in detail before[3] but are summarized here for convenience. In 1976, he reported right loin pain of 6 years' duration and was found to have stones in the right kidney. One stone was removed from the right ureter and was said to have been "mainly oxalate." In 1981, eight stones were removed from both ureters but he passed nine more stones later that year. He was then referred to St. Peter's Hospitals and more stones were visualized in both kidneys. Plasma and urinary biochemical findings were all normal, including urinary oxalate. Five stones from earlier episodes were analyzed and found to be 90 to 97 percent calcium oxalate. Stone formation was attributed to previous high dietary calcium and a period of immobilization following industrial injury and he was advised to increase fluid intake.

The urinary oxalate and glycollate values and response to pyridoxine are shown in Figure 13. This is remarkable for several reasons. First the urinary oxalate was normal at first but presumably he had suffered from hyperoxaluria previously because all the earlier stones analyzed proved to be virtually pure calcium oxalate. Second, he responded at first to quite a low dose (20 mg/day) of pyridoxine but quickly relapsed when this was stopped. Hence there seems little doubt that the pyridoxine was the effective agent in reducing urinary oxalate and glycollate. Third, the requirement for pyridoxine has been rising. Thus, it has not been possible during 1985 to keep the urinary oxalate normal, even though the urinary pyridoxic acid levels have constantly indicated that he has taken all the vitamins prescribed.

Primary Hyperparathyroidism With Hyperoxaluria and Good Response to Low Dose Pyridoxine

This patient will be described in more detail elsewhere (in preparation) but brief clinical information can be given here. Raja J, born March 14, 1933, came to the United Kingdom, from Sri Lanka in 1961. He had passed over ten stones between 1959 and 1984. Radiology then revealed multiple calculi in the left kidney and renal pelvis. Plasma calcium was persistently raised at 2.52 to 2.59 mmol/L but urinary oxalate was also raised at 0.58 mmol/24 hr with raised glycollate.

TABLE 2. BRIEF CLINICAL DATA ON 14 PATIENTS WITH MILD METABOLIC HYPEROXALURIA WITH RECURRENT UROLITHIASIS

Patient	Sex	Age at Diagnosis of Hyperoxaluria	Other Clinical Data
Sidney E	M	62	Idiopathic hypercalciuria
Brent P	M	43	Idiopathic hypercalciuria
Terrence M	M	52	Idiopathic hypercalciuria
Sheila G	F	38	Idiopathic hypercalciuria
Simon M	M	18	Medullary sponge, kidney, and hypercalciuria
Anthony M	M	34	Idiopathic hypercalciuria
Raja J	M	51	Primary hyperparathyroidism
Julie J	F	12	No metabolic abnormality
Bryn D	M	10	Nephrocalcinosis, vesicoureteric reflux
David M	M	37	See ref. 35
Geoffrey S	M	34	See ref. 3
Arthur D	M	25	See ref. 3
Nicola Y	F	22	See ref. 35
Sape S	M	57	Brain surgery "spinal fluid bypass"

His biochemical response to pyridoxine is shown in Figure 14. He was first given 20 mg/day of pyridoxine and the urinary oxalate and glycollate fell to normal. On May 2, 1985, he had a neck exploration (Mr. J.P. Williams) and two parathyroid adenomas weighing 110 and 180 mg respectively were removed. The plasma calcium then fell to normal and remained there. Pyridoxine was stopped on June 6, 1985 and after an interval of 3 months the

Treatment	Response to B_6	Mean (mmol) or Range of Pretreatment Urinary Oxalate	Mean (mmol) or Range of Pretreatment Urinary Glycollate
Cellulose phosphate for 4 years	None so far to 40 mg/day	0.54	0.40
Cellulose phosphate for 16 years	No response to 200 mg/day	0.56	0.60
Cellulose phosphate for 4 years	No response to 100 mg/day	0.51	0.38
Cellulose phosphate for 6 years	Good response to 10 mg/day after stopping cellulose phosphate	0.39–0.63	—
Magnesia and bendrofluazide	Short response to 800 mg/day followed by relapse	0.62	0.75
	? Good response to 20 mg/day	0.55	0.62
2 Parathyroid adenomas removed	Good response to 20 mg/day	0.53	0.47
	Good response to 20 mg/day. Returned to USA, no follow-up	0.83	0.6 per 10 mmol creat
	Good response to 20 mg/day but ? requirement rising	2.88	3.5 per 10 mmol creat
	Good initial response, no further follow-up	0.81	0.79
Hypotensive drugs	Remained normo-oxaluric on 10 mg/day for 3½ years so far	0.65	0.45
	Good initial response, requirement rose steadily to 400 mg/day	0.37–1.77	0.93
	Off B_6 since January 1980 and urinary oxalate remained normal	0.66	0.82
Bendrofluazide	Partial response to 50 mg/day	0.65	0.67

hyperoxaluria returned. Pyridoxine (same dose) was restarted in November 1985.

This patient had two entirely separate causes for urolithiasis, namely primary hyperparathyroidism and hyperoxaluria. It is interesting to note that before availability of the automated method, urinary oxalate would probably not have been measured because the diagnosis of primary hyper-

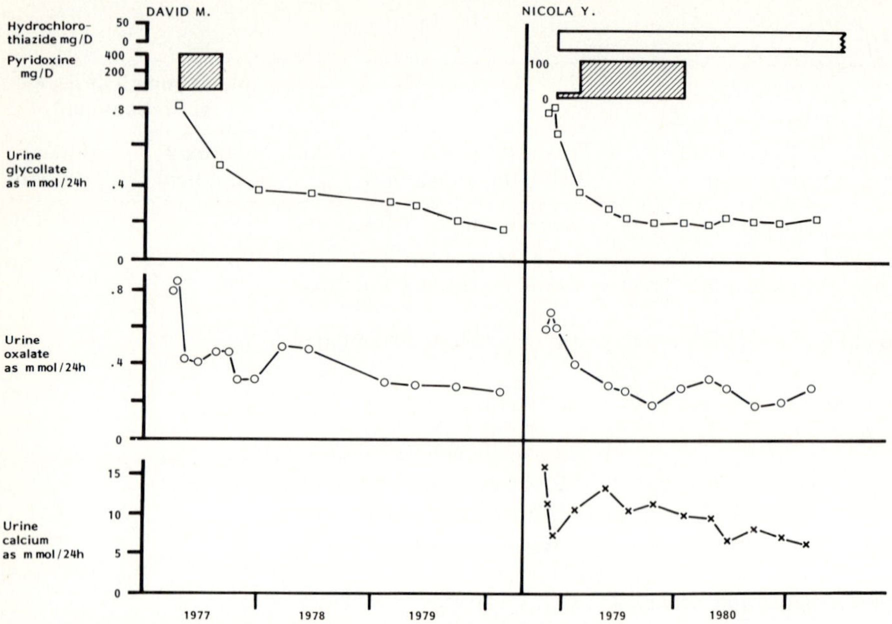

Figure 12. Serial urinary glycollate, oxalate (and calcium) levels in two patients with mild metabolic hyperoxaluria who responded to high dose pyridoxine and did not relapse when this was stopped. *(Reproduced from Harrison AR et al, 1981, with permission.[34])*

parathyroidism would have made this seem unnecessary. Yet he had quite a bad stone history despite mild hyperparathyroidism and probably the hyperoxaluria was the greater cause of the urolithiasis.

Medullary Sponge Kidney, Hypercalciuria, and Hyperoxaluria With Temporary Response to High Dose Pyridoxine

This patient is to be described in detail elsewhere and therefore only an outline of the case is given here. Simon M was born May 7, 1965. He passed a stone in January 1983 and intravenous urography (IVU) showed bilateral renal stones. He was found to have severe hypercalciuria and was given a diet severely restricted in milk and cheese, low in oxalate, and high in water. He changed from hard to softened drinking water. Nevertheless, the stones increased in size and he was refered to St. Peter's Hospitals in July 1984. Plain x-ray films showed diffuse bilateral nephrocalcinosis suggestive of medullary sponge kidney and this was confirmed by IVU; 24-hour urinary oxalate was 0.63 and glycollate 0.75 mmol. Treatment was started with 10 mg/-day of pyridoxine in July 1984 and, as there was no fall in urinary oxalate, the dose was progressively raised and reached 800 mg/day by November 1984. In March 1985, urinary oxalate fell to 0.32 mmol/24 hr but thereafter despite continuing the same high dose of pyridoxine gradually rose again

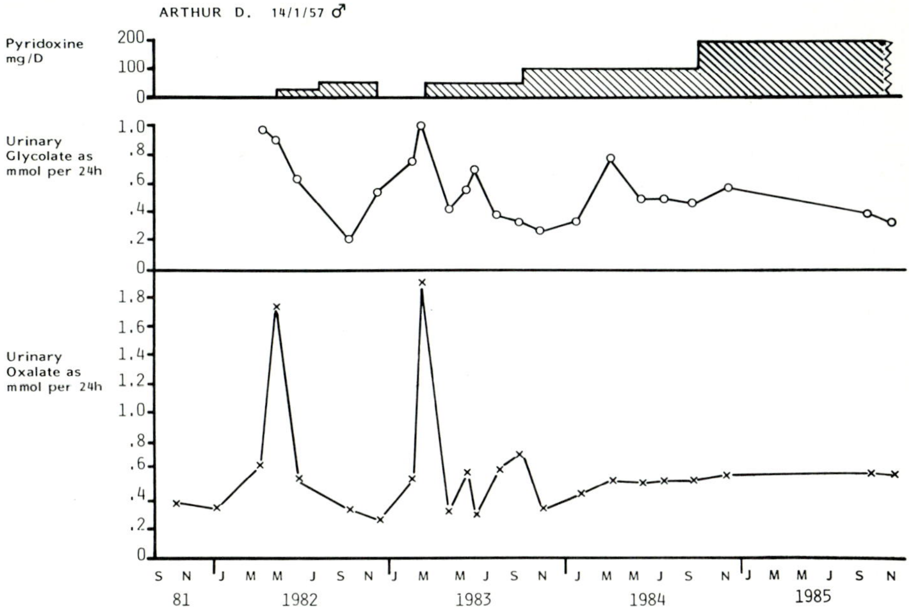

Figure 13. Serial urinary glycollate and oxalate levels in patient showing mild metabolic hyperoxaluria. He developed the hyperoxaluria under observation, responded to low dose pyridoxine, and relapsed when this was stopped. He responded a second time, but the dose of pyridoxine needed has been rising.

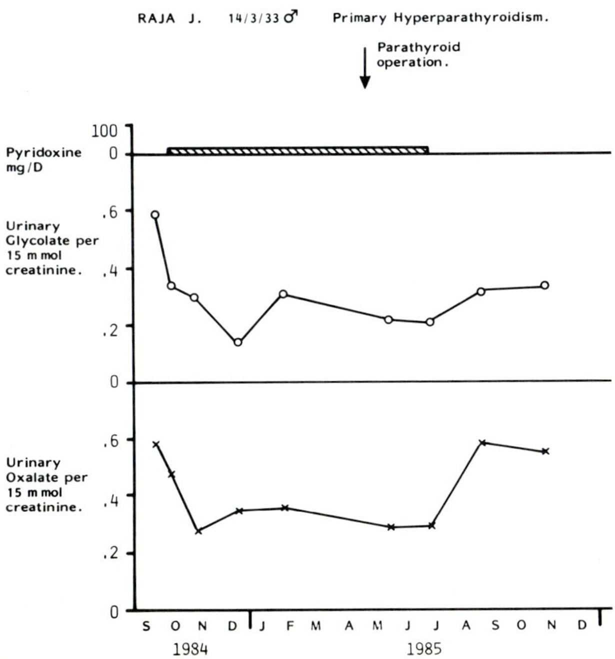

Figure 14. Serial urinary glycollate and oxalate levels in a patient with mild metabolic hyperoxaluria and primary hyperparathyroidism. With only 20 mg/day of pyridoxine, the urinary oxalate and glycollate fell to normal but rose again soon after stopping it.

and reached 0.84 mmol/24 hr by December 1985. Urinary pyridoxic acid measurements confirmed that he was taking almost the full dose of pyridoxine. Because of the inadequate response to pyridoxine, he was started on bendrofluazide 5 mg/day in October 1984 and also on milk of magnesia in January 1985.

This case is remarkable for several reasons. First, before automated urinary oxalate assays were available, this measurement would not have been performed because the diagnosis of medullary sponge kidney and hypercalciuria would have been considered sufficient explanations for the stone formation. Hence the hyperoxaluria, probably the most important factor, would have been missed. Second, the combination of medullary sponge kidney with hypercalciuria and hyperoxaluria associated with raised urinary glycollate seems of great theoretical interest. Third, the hyperoxaluria appeared to be completely resistant to pyridoxine therapy but a delayed reduction to normal urinary oxalate excretion did occur, but only lasted for some 4 months.

Conclusions

1. There is a clear lesson that there is a need to measure urinary oxalate in all cases of calcium oxalate urolithiasis even if a cause other than hyperoxaluria has already been identified.
2. One is bound to consider whether mild hyperoxaluria as described above is a variant of inherited primary hyperoxaluria. Thus both show the predominance of males over females and similar spectra of response to pyridoxine. On the other hand, no case of the former has been familial and most cases are apparently not present from birth. This last point would seem to separate mild metabolic hyperoxaluria clearly from the inherited hyperoxalurias, but a word of caution is needed in view of the finding that Scott C (discussed earlier) did not show his primary hyperoxaluria at 1 week of age but did so 5 weeks later.

PYRIDOXINE FOR ALL OXALATE STONE FORMERS?

The cases described above are bound to revive the question of whether all calcium oxalate stone formers might benefit from pyridoxine therapy as previously suggested by others.[48] The author believes that the findings that such treatment is effective in reducing urinary oxalate and stone recurrence rate is suspect[1] and should be disregarded and that there is a need to reassess this question. Figure 15 shows that when a group of normal volunteers was given pyridoxine (600 mg/day), there was no fall in urinary oxalate or glycollate.[49] The situation could be different in the calcium oxalate stone formers, however, and this needs assessing using modern and precise meth-

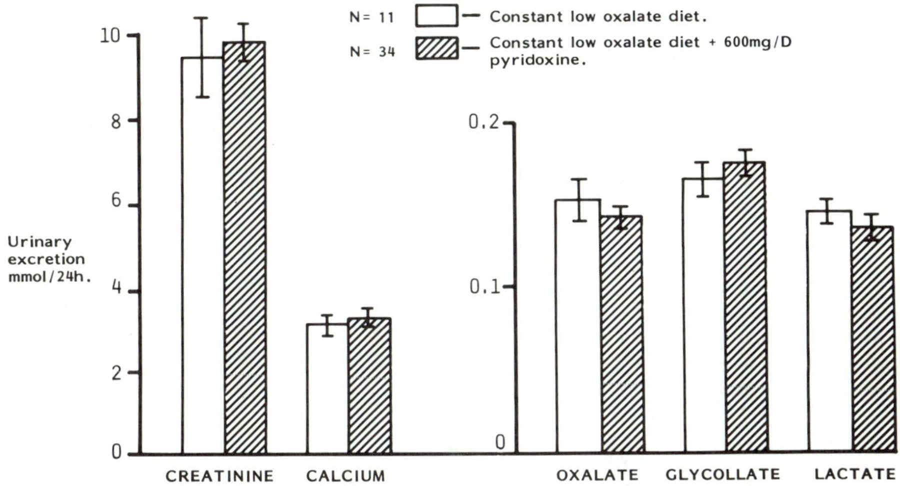

Figure 15. Mean (and SEM) 24-hr urinary excretions of four normal adults before and on 600 mg/day of pyridoxine. Note the lack of effect of the pyridoxine. N = number of 24-hr urine collections studied. *(Reproduced from Rose GA, 1985, with permission.[57])*

ods of urinary oxalate assay. It should be stressed, however, that if one wishes to lower urinary oxalate it might be much more important in these patients to insist upon low oxalate diets than to give pyridoxine.

HYPEROXALURIA CAUSED BY STEATORRHEA

Steatorrhea has been known to be associated with hyperoxaluria for some 15 years.[50,51] The cause is thought to be overabsorption of dietary oxalate and there seems little doubt that this occurs.[52,53] The theory is that the excessive free fatty acids in the small bowel bind with calcium to form calcium soaps and hence the oxalate is not precipitated and is available for absorption in the large bowel. If this was the sole cause of the hyperoxaluria, it should easily be cured by exclusion of dietary oxalate, a relatively simple task because the number of foods involved is fairly small. In my admittedly rather limited experience, however, the hyperoxaluria may be very difficult to control even in patients who appear to be keeping meticulously to low fat and low oxalate diets. The reason for this is not at all clear. Figure 16 shows that in a series of 51 patients with steatorrhea, all of them had raised urinary oxalate but the urinary glycollate values were virtually normal. This would seem to exclude pyridoxine deficiency as a cause of the hyperoxaluria (see above). Notwithstanding, six of these patients who persisted in having hyperoxaluria despite a low oxalate diet were given high dose pyridoxine without any fall in the urinary oxalate. Urinary pyridoxic acid mea-

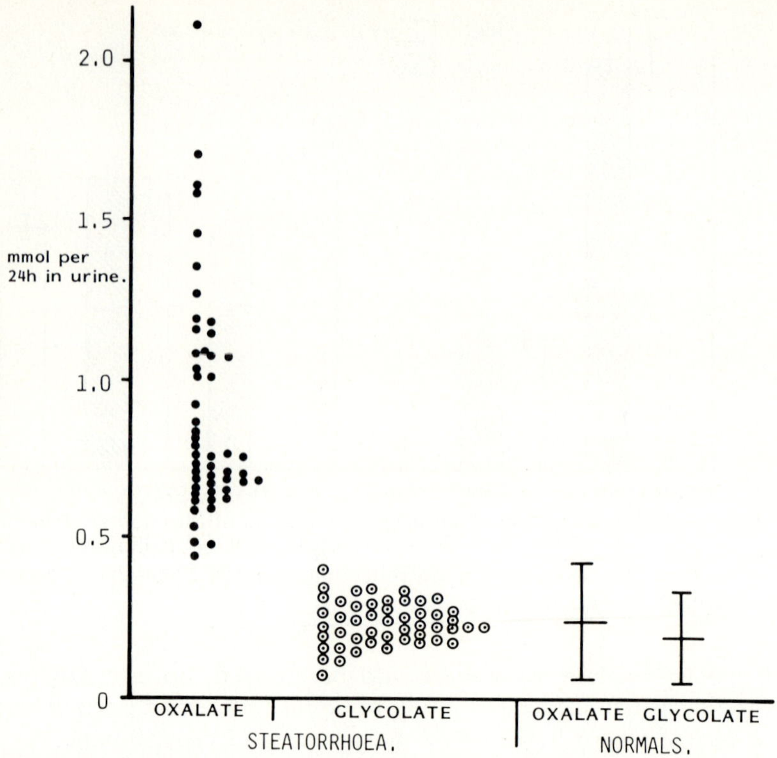

Figure 16. Urinary glycollate and oxalate on 51 patients with steatorrhea due to various causes and comparison with the normal range. Note that hyperoxaluria was found in every case but urinary glycollate excretions were virtually normal suggesting overabsorption of oxalate from the gut as the probable cause and not lack of pyridoxine.

surements in two of these cases confirmed that they both took and absorbed the pyridoxine. One wonders whether oxalate may be generated by microorganisms in the intestinal tract caused by either abnormal substrate or abnormal strains of bacteria, but no evidence of this has been offered as yet. Whatever the cause of the hyperoxaluria, it can pose a very difficult therapeutic problem. The diet should obviously be low in oxalate but it should also be low in fat.[54] Some have suggested the use of oral aluminum hydroxide[55] or cholestyramine[56] and even high calcium intake in order to reduce the absorption of oxalate.

REFERENCES

1. Rose GA: The medical treatment of renal lithiasis. In Wickham JEAW (ed): Urinary Calculous Disease, chap 6. New York, Churchill Livingstone, 1979

2. Robertson WG, Peacock MC: The cause of idiopathic calcium stone disease: Hypercalciuria or hyperoxaluria? Nephron 26:105, 1980
3. Kasidas GP, Rose GA: Metabolic hyperoxaluria and its response to pyridoxine. In Ryall R, Brockis JG, Marshall V, Finlayson B (eds): Urinary Stone, chap 26. New York, Churchill Livingstone, 1984
4. Herbert RW, Hirst EG, Percival EGV, et al: The constitution of ascorbic acid. J Chem Soc. 1933[2]:1270, 1933
5. Buttery JE, Ludwigsen N, Braiotta E, Pernall RR: Determination of urinary oxalate with commercially available oxalate oxidase. Clin Chem 29:700, 1983
6. Kasidas GP, Rose GA: Spontaneous in vitro generation of oxalate from L-ascorbate in some assays for urinary oxalate and its prevention. In Schwille PO, Smith LH, Robertson WG, Vahlensieck W (eds): Urolithiasis and Related Research. New York, Plenum, 1985, pp 653–656
7. Kasidas GP, Rose GA: Continuous flow assay for urinary oxalate using immobilized oxalate oxidase. Ann Clin Biochem 22:412, 1985
8. Kasidas GP, Rose GA: Measurement of plasma oxalate in healthy subjects and in patients with chronic renal failure using immobilized oxalate oxidase. Clin Chim Acta 154:49, 1986
9. Glazer HS: A study of urinary excretion of xanthurenic acid and other tryptophane metabolites in human beings with pyridoxine deficiency induced by deoxypyridoxine. Arch Biochem 33:243, 1951
10. MacGibbon BM, Mollin DL: Sideroblastic anaemia in man: Observations on seventy cases. Br J Haematol 11:59, 1965
11. Molony CJ, Parmalee AH: Convulsions in young infants as a result of pyridoxine (vitamin B_6) deficiency. JAMA 154:405, 1954
12. Gershoff SN, Faragalla FK, Nelson DA, Andres SB: Vitamin B_6 deficiency and oxalate nephrocalcinosis in the cat. Am J Med 27:72, 1959
13. Gershoff SN, Faragalla FK: Endogenous oxalate synthesis and glycerine serine deoxypyridoxine inter-relationships in vitamin B_6 deficient rats. J Biol Chem 234:2391, 1959
14. Gershoff SN, Mayer AL, Kulczcki LL: Effect of pyridoxine administration on the urinary secretion of oxalic acid, pyridoxine and related compounds in mongoloids and non-mongoloids. Am J Clin Nutr 7:76, 1959
15. Hunt AD, Stokes SJ, McCrory WW, Stroud HH: Pyridoxine dependency: A report of a case of intractable convulsions in an infant controlled by pyridoxine. Paediatrics 13:140, 1954
16. Horrigan DL, Harris JW: Pyridoxine responsive anemia. Adv Intern Med 12:103, 1964
17. Barber GW, Spaeth GL: Pyridoxine therapy in homocystinuria. Lancet 1:337, 1967
18. Frimpter GW, Haymovitz A, Horwith M: Cystothioninuria. N Engl J Med 268:333, 1963
19. Mason DY, Emerson PM: Primary acquired sideroblastic anaemia: Response to treatment with pyridoxal-5-phosphate. Br Med J 1:389, 1973
20. Schaumburg J, Kaplan J, Windebank A, et al: Sensory neuropathy from pyridoxine abuse. N Engl J Med 309:445, 1983
21. Berger A, Schaumburg HC: More on neuropathy from pyridoxine abuse. N Engl J Med 311:986, 1984
22. Zegher F de, Przyrembel H, Chalmers AA, et al: Successful treatment of infan-

tile type I primary hyperoxaluria complicated by pyridoxine toxicity. Lancet 2:392, 1985
23. Biehl JB, Vimitz HJ: Studies on the use of a high dose of isoniazid. Am Rev Tuberc 70:430, 1954
24. Hollister LE, Moore FF, Forrest F, Bennett JL: Antipyridoxine effect of D-penicillamine in schizophrenic men. Am J Clin Nutr 19:307, 1966
25. Fitzpatrick JM, Kasidas GP, Rose GA: Hyperoxaluria following glycine irrigation for transurethral prostatectomy. Br J Urol 53:250, 1981
26. Silverberg DS, McIntyre JWR, Ulan RA, Gavin EA: Oxalic acid excretion after methoxyfluorane and halothane anaesthesia. Canad Anaesth Soc J 18:496, 1971
27. Nime FA, Hutchins GM: Oxalosis caused by aspergillus infection. Johns Hopkins Hosp Bull 133:183, 1971
28. Kasidas GP, Rose GA: A new enzymatic method for the determination of glycollate in urine and plasma. Clin Chim Acta 96:25, 1979
29. Fitzhugh OG, Nelson AA: Comparison of the chronic toxicity of triethylene glycol with that of diethylene glycol. J Indust Hyg Toxicol 28:40, 1946
30. Wallace MR, Mason K, Gray J: Urine oxalate and calcium in idiopathic renal stone formers. NZ Med J 2:87, 1981
31. Marangella M, Fruttero B, Bruno M, Linari F: Hyperoxaluria in idiopathic calcium stone disease: Further evidence of intestinal hyperabsorption of oxalate. Clin Sci 63:381, 1982
32. Baggio B, Gambaro G, Favaro S, Borsatti A: Prevalence of hyperoxaluria in idiopathic calcium oxalate kidney stone disease. Nephron 35:11, 1983
33. Marickar YMF, Rose GA: Relationship of stone growth and urinary biochemistry in long-term follow-up of stone patients with idiopathic hypercalciuria. Br J Urol 57:613, 1985
34. Harrison AR, Kasidas GP, Rose GA: Hyperoxaluria and recurrent stone formation apparently cured by short courses of pyridoxine. Br Med J 1:2097, 1981
35. Yendt ER, Cohanim M: Response to a physiological dose of pyridoxine in type I primary hyperoxaluria. N Engl J Med 312:953, 1985
36. Koch J, Stokstad ELR, Williams HF, Smith LHC: Deficiency of 2-oxyglutarate carboligase activity in primary hyperoxaluria. Proc Natl Acad Sci USA 57:1123, 1967
37. Helin I: Primary hyperoxaluria: An analysis of 17 Scandinavian patients. Scand J Urol Nephrol 14:61, 1980
38. Nath R, Thind SK, Murthy MSR, et al: Molecular aspects of idiopathic urolithiasis. Molec Aspects Med 7:1, 1984
39. Gibbs DA, Watts RWE: The action of pyridoxine in primary hyperoxaluria. Clin Sci 38:277, 1970
40. Dent CE, Stamp TCP: Treatment of primary hyperoxaluria. Arch Dis Child 45:735, 1970
41. Rose GA, Arthur LJH, Chambers TL, et al: Successful treatment of primary hyperoxaluria in a neonate. Lancet 1:1298, 1982
42. Morris MC, Chambers TL, Evans PWG, et al: Oxalosis in infancy. Arch Dis Child 57:224, 1982
43. Wilson RE: A report from ACS/NIH renal transplant registry. Renal transplantation in congenital and metabolic disease. JAMA 232:148, 1975
44. O'Regan P, Joekes AM, Constable AR, et al: Successful renal transplantation in primary hyperoxaluria. Postgrad Med J 56:288, 1982

45. Scheinman JI, Najarian JS, Mauer SM: Successful strategies for renal transplantation in primary oxalosis. Kidney Internat 25:804, 1984
46. Silver L, Brebdler H: Use of magnesium oxide in management of familial hyperoxaluria. J Urol 106:274, 1971
47. Hallson PC, Rose GA, Sulaiman S: Magnesium reduces calcium oxalate crystal formation in human whole urine. Clin Sci 62:17, 1982
48. Hallson PC, Rose GA: A simplified and rapid enzymatic method for determination of urinary oxalate. Clin Chim Acta 55:29, 1974
49. Mayer GG, Chase T, Faruar B, et al: Metabolic studies on the formation of calcium oxalate stones, with emphasis on vitamin B_6 and uric acid metabolism. Bull N Y Acad Sci 44:28, 1968
50. Dowling RH, Rose GA, Sutor DJ: Hyperoxaluria and renal calculi in ideal disease. Lancet 1:1103, 1971
51. Admirand WH, Earnest DL, Williams HE: Hyperoxaluria and bowel disease. Trans Assoc Am Phys 84:307, 1971
52. Stauffer JQ, Humphreys MH, Weir GJ: Acquired hyperoxaluria with regional enteritis after ileal resection. Ann Intern Med 79:383, 1973
53. Tiselius HG, Ahlstrand C, Lundstrom B, Nilsson MA: 14C-oxalate absorption by normal persons, calcium oxalate stone formers and patients with surgically disturbed intestinal function. Clin Chem 27:1682, 1981
54. Andersson H, Jagenburg J: Fat-reduced diet in the treatment of hyperoxaluria with ileopathy. Gut 15:360, 1974
55. Earnest DL: Perspectives on incidence, etiology, and treatment of enteric hyperoxaluria. Am J Clin Nutr 30:72, 1977
56. Smith LH, Fromm H, Hoffman AF: Acquired hyperoxaluria, nephrolithiasis and intestinal disease. N Engl J Med 286:1371, 1972
57. Rose GA: Other causes of stone disease. In Whitfield HN, Hendry WF (eds): Text-Book of Genito-Urinary Surgery, chap 59. New York, Churchill Livingstone, 1985
58. Rose, GA: Urinary Stones: Clinical and Laboratory Aspects. Lancaster, England, MTP Press, 1982

Problems of Sexual Differentiation
Diagnosis and Management

G. William Bates and Winfred L. Wiser

"Is it a boy or a girl?" asks a new mother immediately after giving birth. Those attending the birth, as well as the new father, grandparents, and friends, ask the same question. Gender assignment is the first step in establishing identity.

With increased availability and use of amniocentesis, the question of gender identification is answered often before birth. The suspense and surprise of the sex of the newborn at birth is removed by prenatal sexual determination.

Problems of gender ambiguity occur rarely, but when there is a problem with sexual assignment, the physician responsible for making a sexual assignment must be prepared with a knowledge of the mechanisms of sexual differentiation and the endocrine events of puberty to make a rational sexual assignment. Moreover, the physician responsible for making the sexual assignment must understand the possibilities of genital reconstructive surgery and the actions of exogenous steroid hormones.

MECHANISMS OF SEXUAL DIFFERENTIATION

Human genotypic sex is established at the moment of conception by random chance. Fertilization of the ovum by an X chromosome-bearing sperm

---

Supported in part by a grant from the Vicksburg Hospital Foundation.

or Y chromosome-bearing sperm occurs with equal probability; the formation of a 46XX or 46XY embryo is an independent event and may or may not occur again in the same couple. After fertilization, human embryos of both sexes develop in an identical fashion for the first 2 months and only thereafter do anatomic and physiologic development diverge to give rise to male and female phenotypes. Little was known of this process of sexual differentiation until Jost reported his findings from studies of sexual differentiation of the castrated fetal rabbit.[1,2] The Jost studies became central dogma of sexual differentiation.

According to Jost, sexual development is a sequential, ordered, and relatively simple process and depends exclusively on the presence and function of the fetal testis (Fig. 1). In short, when testes are present (and fully functional), sexual development will occur along male lines. When ovaries are present, sexual development is female. If the testes fail to secrete protein and steroid hormones, development will occur along female lines.

The human embryo develops a pair of indifferent gonads and two sets of internal genital anlage, the Wolffian ducts and Müllerian ducts, which become subsequently the male and female internal genital tract. This occurs during the first 35 days of embryonic life. At approximately 40 days of gestation, germ cells migrate from the yolk sac into the genital ridges of the embryo. At this stage of development, male and female gonads appear identical. In male embryos, the cell-surface antigens, the HY antigens, direct subsequent events in the development of the testes.[3]

In addition to undifferentiated gonads, human embryos at 35 days of gestation have identical external genitalia. The external genitalia consist of (1) the genital tubercle, (2) the genital folds, and (3) the genital swellings. Eventually, these embryogenic structures will become the male or female genitalia.

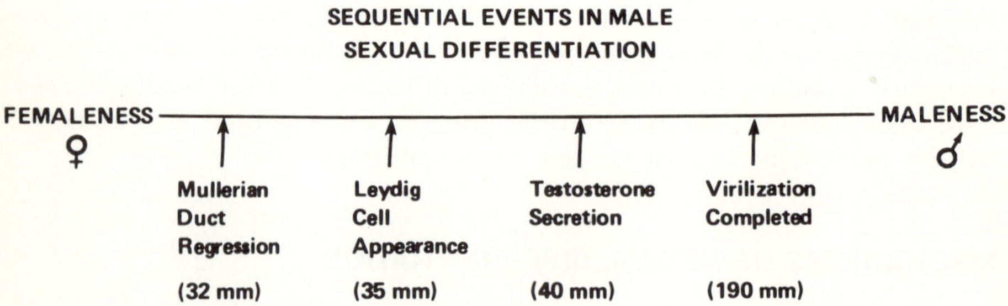

Figure 1. The sequential events in human male sexual differentiation as gestational age increases. The failure of any of the events will result in abnormal male sexual development. The failure of all of the events will result in female sexual differentiation even if the fetus has a male genotype.

Male Development

Once germ cells migrate to the male gonads, the germ cells line up to form the spermatogenic cords. Sertoli cells appear along the spermatogenic cords, and Leydig cells appear in the connective tissue of the testes.

The first event in male sexual development is secretion of Müllerian inhibiting factor. This substance acts locally on the Müllerian ducts to cause their involution and ultimate disappearance.[4] The inhibiting factor is a glycoprotein with a molecular weight of approximately 70,000 daltons; it appears to be species specific.[5]

Müllerian duct suppression is an active process. Men with persistent Müllerian duct syndrome are described in the literature.[6] Characteristically, these men have normal male external and internal genitalia as well as fallopian tubes and a uterus. Another feature of this disorder is failure of the initial phase of testicular descent from the abdominal cavity into the scrotum. This suggests that Müllerian inhibiting factor plays an early role in sexual differentiation and a later role in male sexual development.

Male pseudohermaphrodites with normal testicular function or those with an abnormality of testosterone production have no female internal genitalia structures (fallopian tubes, uterus, and upper vagina) as the result of normal testicular Müllerian inhibiting factor secretion.

Soon after the testes secrete Müllerian inhibiting factor, the Leydig cells begin secreting testosterone. Testosterone has local action on the Wolffian ducts and systemic action on the external genital anlages which give rise to male and female external genitalia.

Testosterone, secreted by each testis, has local action on its ipsilateral Wolffian duct. Under the influence of testosterone, the Wolffian ducts differentiate into epididymis, vas deferens, and seminal vesicles. In the absence of local testosterone secretion, when either ovaries are present or there is failure of testosterone secretion by the testes, the Wolffian ducts fail to develop and will undergo involution. Moreover, in cases of unilateral testicular agenesis, there is unilateral absence of the epididymis, vas deferens, and seminal vesicle on the side of the testicular agenesis.

Testosterone has systemic actions on the central nervous system (CNS) and the anlage of the external genitalia. (More will be said later about the CNS effects.) Testosterone enters the cells of the external genital anlage and is converted by the enzyme, 5α-reductase, to dihydrotestosterone. Dihydrotestosterone is a more potent androgen than testosterone. This hormone binds to the androgen receptors of the external genital anlage to stimulate their subsequent differentiation and development into the male external genitalia.[7]

The genital tubercle develops into the glans penis. The genital folds develop into the penile shaft and envelop the urethra carrying it to the distal tip of the glans penis. The genital swellings develop into the scrotum that becomes the subsequent receptacle for the testes later in fetal life.

Testosterone is essential for differentiation of the male external genitalia. In the absence of testosterone, either as the result of normal ovarian development in the female or as the result of failure of testosterone secretion by the testes, the external genitalia develop along female lines. Development of the male penis and scrotum commences shortly after the onset of virilization of the Wolffian duct. Anatomic development of the male internal and external genitalia is completed largely by the end of the first trimester of pregnancy.[8] Descent of the testes begins in the first trimester of pregnancy and continues over a 7-month period of time. Final descent into the scrotum occurs near 36 weeks of gestation.[9]

Testosterone enters target tissues by a passive diffusion process through the cell membrane. Once testosterone enters the cell, some is converted by 5α-reductase to dihydrotestosterone and some is bound as testosterone. Testosterone and dihydrotestosterone are bound to high affinity cystosolic androgen receptors and moved into the nucleus of the target cell.[10]

Testosterone and dihydrotestosterone have differential action on different target cells. This fact is known by identification of a group of individuals who are deficient in the enzyme 5α-reductase.[7] Affected individuals with this condition are males with abnormal sexual development. At birth, they are given a female sexual assignment because of the female-appearing external genitalia. Despite the appearance of the external genitalia, the internal genitalia are male, i.e., there are normal Wolffian structures (epididymis, vas deferens, seminal vesicles, and ejaculatory ducts). The Müllerian ducts undergo involution as the result of testicular secretion of Müllerian inhibiting factor.[11] At the expected time of puberty, affected individuals have deepening of the voice, development of a muscular male body habitus, and take a male gender identity, despite the fact that they were raised as females. However, they fail to have facial hair growth and male temporal hair recession. This natural experiment suggests that testosterone is necessary for Wolffian duct development, CNS action, and musculoskeletal development, and that dihydrotestosterone is necessary for male sexual hair growth and development of male external genitalia.

Not only is the secretion of testosterone and its subsequent conversion to dihydrotestosterone necessary for male sexual development, but the androgen receptor must be present in androgen-dependent cells. Several disorders of the androgen receptor have been identified that lead to abnormal sexual development.[12] A spectrum of disorders, ranging from complete feminization of the male[13] to development of an otherwise normal male with azoospermia.[14] Various degrees of genital ambiguity occur between these extremes.[12]

Thus, five critical events must occur early in fetal life for male sexual differentiation. These events are:

1. Testicular formation
2. Secretion of Müllerian duct inhibiting factor

3. Development of androgen receptors
4. Secretion of testosterone by the Leydig cells
5. Conversion of testosterone to dihydrotestosterone

If one of these critical events does not occur, sexual development will be female or ambiguous. The clinician can apply the critical events to develop a rational method for the diagnosis and management of patients with problems of sexual differentiation.

Female Development

In the female embryo, the Müllerian ducts develop into the fallopian tubes and uterus and contribute to the development of the vagina. The external genitalia in the female undergo little differentiation. The genital tubercle becomes the clitoris, the genital swellings became the labia majora, and the genital folds become the labia minora.

Milewich et al[15] demonstrated in the fetal rabbit that the fetal ovary begins to secrete estrogens at the same time in gestation as the fetal testes begin to secrete testosterone. If this occurs in human embryogenesis as well, the female fetus is exposed to estrogens and very little testosterone during the weeks of sexual differentiation. When the female fetus is exposed to androgens during the critical weeks of sexual differentiation, she will have genital ambiguity at birth. The external genitalia of the female fetus responds to androgens the same as the male. If the female fetus receives maximal androgen stimulation, she will have male external genitalia at birth (Fig. 2). Lesser androgen secretion results in partial virilization of the female external genitalia (Fig. 3).

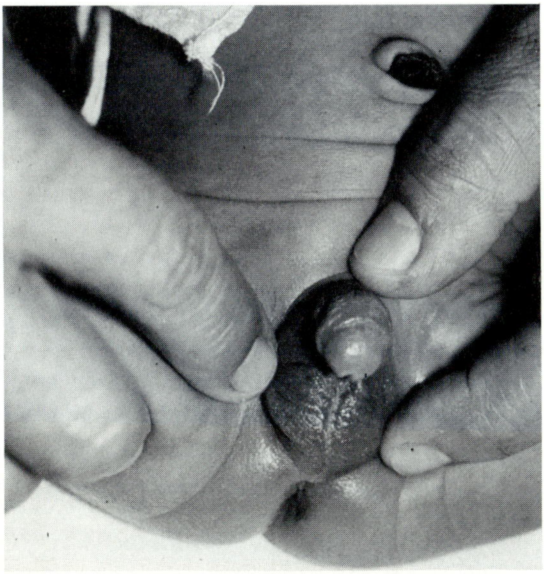

Figure 2. Complete virilization of a female fetus due to severe 21-hydroxylase deficiency. The urethral meatus is on the ventral shaft of the phallus at the distal tip. The "scrotum" is empty. *(Courtesy M. Montalvo, M.D.)*

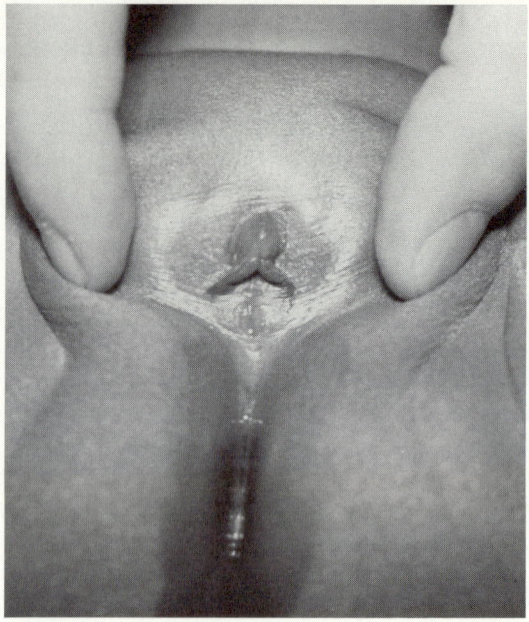

Figure 3. Six-month-old female with fusion of the posterior perineum, enlargement of the clitoris, and partial fusion of the labioscrotal folds. This is the result of moderately severe 21-hydroxylase deficiency.

EFFECTS OF PRENATAL SEX HORMONES ON GENDER-RELATED BEHAVIOR

Androgens play a critical role in the differentiation of the CNS in mammals. Deprivation by the male animal of testosterone during his critical time of brain differentiation will result in a female pattern of sexually dimorphic behavior. In contrast, a female mammal exposed to testosterone during prenatal development will, as an adult, perform similarly to a normal male in sexual behavior. Male animals, deprived of testosterone, exhibit lordosis and allow themselves to be mounted by a sexually excited male. A female animal, exposed to androgens during the species-specific critical time of brain differentiation, exhibits male mounting behavior in the presence of sexually aroused females.

The role of social learning is much greater in human behavior than in subhuman mammals but there is evidence to suggest that biologic factors influence psychosexual differentiation in humans as well. The primary models for evaluation of endocrine influences on the CNS of humans is congenital adrenal hyperplasia (CAH) in females and complete androgen insensitivity (testicular feminization) in males. In the former, the female is exposed to excess androgens during fetal life; in the latter, the male lacks androgen receptors and is unable to respond to androgens.

Erhardt and Meyer-Bahlburg[16] have identified four areas of human behavior that are influenced by the prenatal hormone environment. They are

(1) gender identity, (2) gender-role or sexual dimorphic behavior, (3) sexual orientation or erotic behavior, and (4) cognitive sexual differences.

Gender identity is formed soon after birth and gender identification typically depends on a person's sex of rearing even when this differs from the genetic sex.[16-18] By the end of the second year of life, a child's gender identity is firmly embedded and remains, even if secondary sexual characteristics of the opposite sex appear at the time of puberty. For example, if a person is raised as a girl but at the time of puberty she develops a low voice, grows a beard, and has clitoral enlargement of a phallic size (Fig. 4), she retains her female gender identity. Similarly, persons raised as males who develop gynecomastia and fail to develop a muscular, male body habitus retain their male gender identity.

The only group of individuals with pseudohermaphroditism that make a gender identity change are males with 5α-reductase deficiency. Despite their female-appearing external genitalia, during fetal life the CNS is exposed to a normal quantity of testosterone.

Because gender identity largely depends on the sex of rearing, it is important to make a sexual assignment at birth or soon thereafter that will be consistent with the most rational adult sexual function. This decision must be based on the appearance of the external genitalia, the prognosis for effective cosmetic and reconstructive surgery, and the expected effects

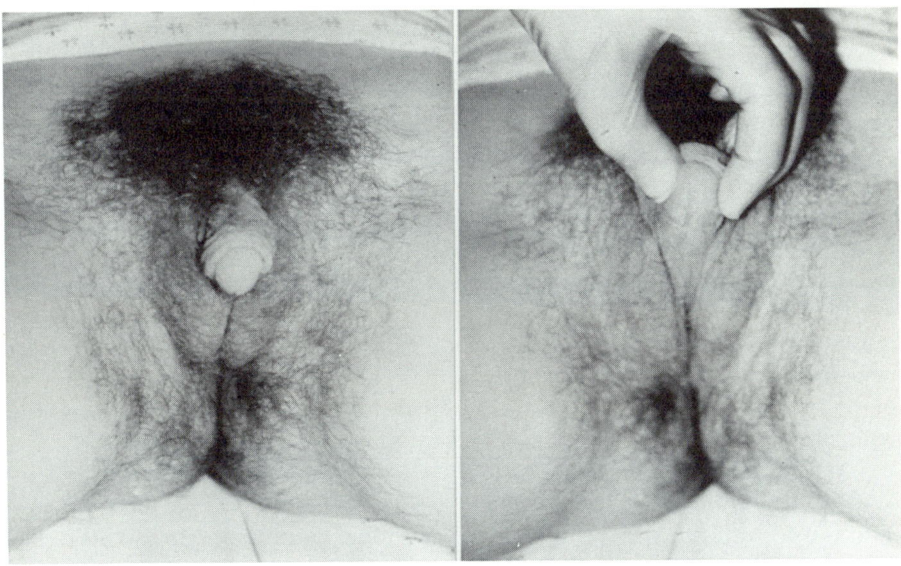

Figure 4. Sixteen-year-old male pseudohermaphrodite, raised as a female. At birth and during childhood, she had ambiguous genitalia. At the expected time of puberty, the external genitalia became more masculinized and she had male voice changes. The biochemical defect is partial 17-ketosteroid reductase deficiency.

of endogenous sex-steroid hormone secretion and exogenous sex-steroid hormone administration.

For example, girls with severe CAH may have significant virilization of the external genitalia but with surgical reconstruction of the perineum and treatment with corticosteroids are capable of female sexual function and reproduction. On the other hand, genotypic males with abnormalities of testosterone synthesis or testosterone action have a poor prognosis for male sexual function, despite efforts at surgical reconstruction and hormone replacement.

Parents of children with genital ambiguity need specific guidance and reassurance concerning their child's gender identity. Parents have difficulty accepting a child with uncertain gender identity. Parents must have a clear sexual assignment as soon as possible after birth.

The sexual orientation of persons with genital ambiguity usually proceeds along the lines of sexual rearing. Males with complete androgen insensitivity, raised as females, develop female sexual orientation at the time of puberty. These females marry and enjoy a normal heterosexual relationship. Money et al[19] have observed a greater frequency of bisexuality and homosexuality in children and adolescents with severe CAH. They attribute this sexual orientation to the prenatal exposure of the female brain to high androgen concentrations.

RECOGNIZING DISORDERS OF SEXUAL DIFFERENTIATION

Female Pseudohermaphroditism

Female pseudohermaphroditism results when the female fetus is exposed to excessive androgens during the critical weeks of sexual differentiation. The androgen source can be endogenous (from mother or fetus) or exogenous from maternal ingestion of androgenic compounds. Since the genotype in female pseudohermaphrodites is 46XX, functional ovaries are present. Thus, the Müllerian ducts are not suppressed and the internal genitalia are female. The fallopian tubes, uterus, and upper vagina develop in a normal manner. The Wolffian ducts, which require high concentration of local testosterone, fail to develop. Thus, female pseudohermaphrodites have female internal genitalia and because of the androgen excess have ambiguous external genitalia.

Congenital Adrenal Hyperplasia

The most common cause of female pseudohermaphroditism is CAH. The most common form of CAH is 21-hydroxylase deficiency. Less common, but more serious, are 11β-hydroxylase deficiency which results in virilization and hypertension and 3β-01-dehydrogenase deficiency. The latter is a rare enzymatic disorder that usually results in death soon after birth.

21-Hydroxylase deficiency occurs in approximately 1 in 5000 to 7000 births. The presenting feature in the female is ambiguous external genitalia or, in severe cases, complete virilization of the external genitalia with an empty scrotum (Fig. 2). The severity of the virilization depends upon the timing of the androgen excess during fetal life and the severity of the androgen excess. If excessive androgens were secreted by the fetal adrenal gland early in the process of sexual differentiation, there will be fusion of the labioscrotal folds, clitoral enlargement, and anatomic changes of the urethra and vagina.

Clitoral enlargement depends upon the quantity of androgen excess rather than the timing. Androgen excess during the late stages of gestation will stimulate clitoral growth and have no effect on the fusion of the labioscrotal folds, whereas androgen excess in early gestation may have little effect on the clitoris but may alter the external genitalia. This particular point is useful in distinguishing fetal androgen excess disorders from those that occur later in life.

In addition to external genital changes, patients with CAH may present with metabolic disorders such as salt wasting and hypertension. Those infants with salt wasting usually become apparent within a few days of birth. They become lethargic, stop feeding, and develop vomiting. If they do not receive corticosteroids and electrolyte replacement therapy promptly, death will occur rapidly. As soon as a child with ambiguous genitalia is identified, the physician must consider a salt-wasting form of adrenal hyperplasia as the etiology of the genital ambiguity. This is the only condition associated with ambiguous genitalia which requires immediate treatment.

CAH is the result of an autosomal dominant disorder of steroid hormone biosynthesis that prevents the infant from adequate synthesis of glucocorticoids. Because of an enzyme deficiency, usually 21-hydroxylase, the conversion of progesterone and 17α-hydroxyprogesterone to deoxycorticosterone and 11-deoxycortisone is impaired. Cortisol synthesis is inadequate. As a result, adrenocorticotropic hormone (ACTH) secretion is increased by negative feedback in response to low cortisol levels to further stimulate cortisol production. As a byproduct of cortisol production, there is further increase in androgen production, particularly of dehydroepiandrosterone (DHEA). DHEA serves as the substrate for testosterone production which causes virilization of the external genitalia.

Excess adrenal androgen production can be managed by the administration of cortisone or cortisol substitutes. These exogenous hormones effectively meet the physiologic cortisol requirements and suppress anterior pituitary ACTH secretion. Endogenous cortisol production is suppressed, the excess DHEA production is suppressed, and no further virilization occurs.

If a female with mild virilization at birth is not recognized and treated immediately, she will have continuing enlargement of the clitoris, precocious sexual hair growth, and excessive height compared with her peers (Fig. 5). Ultimately, however, she will have short stature because of premature closure of the epiphyseal plates.

A male with adrenal hyperplasia may not be identified at birth because there is no "excess" virilization of the external genitalia. During childhood, however, he may have precocious sexual development and accelerated somatic growth. If he is not treated promptly, his adult height will be severely compromised.

Female Pseudohermaphroditism Resulting from Exogenous Hormones

The administration of androgens, especially impeded androgens, to pregnant women during the critical weeks of sexual differentiation can lead to virilization of the female fetus. This is manifested mostly by fusion of the labioscrotal folds. Several case reports in the early 1960s established the link between the administration of progestins (impeded androgens) for prevention of abortion and genital anomalies.[20] These drugs are no longer used for this purpose.

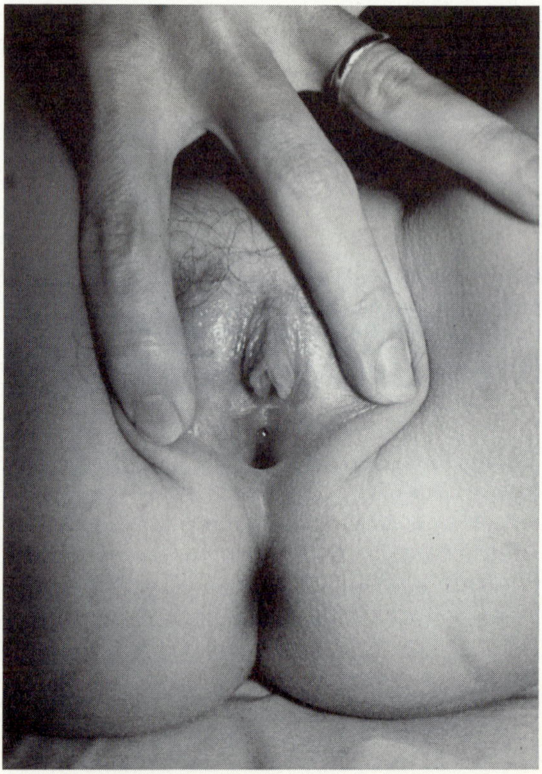

Figure 5. Precocious pubarche in a 5-year-old girl as a result of CAH. Note the clitoral enlargement, elongation of the posterior perineum, and partial fusion of the anterior vaginal introitus. These anatomic changes occurred during fetal life.

However, the inadvertent administration of progestin-containing oral contraceptives to pregnant women still poses a risk. Recently female pseudohermaphroditism associated with danazol exposure was reported.[21] Since danazol is a commonly used drug for the treatment of endometriosis, pregnancy should be excluded before this impeded androgen is prescribed.

Male Pseudohermaphroditism

Male pseudohermaphroditism results when a 46XY individual has absence of male external genitalia or inadequate virilization of the external genitalia. The genetic causes of male pseudohermaphroditism are:

1. Failure of androgen synthesis
2. Failure of androgen action
3. 5α-Reductase deficiency
4. Embryonic testicular regression

Failure of Androgen Synthesis. Five enzymatic reactions are necessary for the synthesis of testosterone from cholesterol. The enzymes required to complete this process are 20,22-desmolase, 3β-01-dehydrogenase, 17α-hydroxylase, 17,20-desmolase, and 17-ketosteroid reductase. The first three enzymes are present in both the adrenal glands and the gonads; the latter two are primarily gonadal enzymes. Thus, infants with 20,22-desmolase deficiency, 17α-hydroxylase deficiency, and 3β-01-dehydrogenase deficiency will have defects in cortisol production as well as testosterone production.

In infants with 20,22-desmolase deficiency and 17α-hydroxylase deficiency, the external genitalia will be female because of inability to synthesize *any* androgens. Death occurs rapidly in infants with 20,22-desmolase deficiency.

17α-Hydroxylase is associated with failure to form 17α-hydroxylated corticosteroids, androgens, and estrogens. Because of accumulation of deoxycorticosterone, hypertension occurs. At the expected time of puberty, there is no androgen or estrogen secretion so the external genitalia remain infantile. Gonadotropins are elevated. In 46XY individuals with 17α-hydroxylase deficiency, the testicles secret Müllerian duct inhibiting factor at the appropriate time. Absence of the uterus and upper vagina associated with hypertension in a child raised as a girl should suggest male pseudohermaphroditism because of 17α-hydroxylase deficiency. Appropriate treatment would include cortisol replacement, estrogen administration to induce breast development and development of the rudimentary vagina, and the administration of a limited course of testosterone to induce axillary and pubic hair growth. Vaginal construction may be required. This will be discussed later.

17,20-Desmolase deficiency is a rare enzymatic disorder in which persons cannot convert C_{21} steroids (progesterone and cortisols) to C_{19} steroids (androgens). If the enzymatic block is complete, 46XY individuals will have a phenotypic appearance identical to those with 17α-hydroxylase deficiency. Hypertension will not be a feature, however. Most commonly, the block is incomplete and 46XY individuals will have varying degrees of genital ambiguity depending upon the severity of the enzymatic block. Moreover, structures that develop from the Wolffian ducts are absent or rudimentary. The phallus is hypoplastic. Kaufman et al[22] reported a significant increase in phallic length in a 5-year-old 46XY male with 17,20-desmolase deficiency during the administration of testosterone. What effect testosterone will have on sexual function at puberty remains uncertain.

17-Ketosteroid reductase deficiency occurs with greatest frequency of the testosterone synthesis disorders. 17-Ketosteroid reductase catalyzes the conversion of androstenedione to testosterone and the conversion of estrone to estradiol 17-β. When 17-ketosteroid reductase is deficient or absent, there is incomplete masculinization of the male. Since the testicles secrete Müllerian inhibiting factor, the Müllerian-derived structures, i.e., fallopian tubes, uterus, and upper vagina are absent. Virilization of the male internal genitalia depends upon the degree of enzyme deficiency.

Females with this disorder will have incomplete secondary sexual development at the time of puberty. Because both testosterone and estradiol 17β production are affected, sexual hair growth and breast development are incomplete.

46XY individuals with 17-ketosteroid reductase deficiency may receive a sexual assignment at birth of either male or female depending upon the severity of genital ambiguity. If a female sexual assignment is made, gonadectomy before the onset of puberty is imperative as there will be further virilization because of the androgenic actions of androstenedione, albeit a weak androgen, and testosterone (Fig. 4). Exogenous estrogens administered at the expected time of puberty will stimulate breast development.

Because of the clinical similarities of individuals with 17-ketosteroid reductase deficiency and partial androgen insensitivity syndrome (Reifenstein's syndrome), it is possible that individuals who have been given a diagnosis of partial androgen insensitivity syndrome actually have 17-ketosteroid reductase deficiency. This differential can be made by measuring plasma concentrations of androstenedione and testosterone. The plasma testosterone concentration is in the normal range or elevated in those individuals with partial androgen insensitivity syndrome, whereas testosterone concentration is decreased in those individuals with 17-ketosteroid reductase deficiency. If further diagnostic steps are required, administration of exogenous gonadotropins or gonadotropin-releasing hormone will stimulate increased production and secretion of androgens. Androstenedione will accumulate in individuals with 17-ketosteroid reductase deficiency.

Failure of Androgen Action. Testosterone circulates in plasma bound to albumin or sex-steroid binding globulin. Only 1 to 3 percent of testosterone is free to enter cells.[12] Testosterone diffuses easily across cell membranes to enter the cytosol. In cells containing testosterone receptors, the hormone is bound and transported to the nucleus where androgen action is initiated. In the disorders that result from failure of androgen action, there is partial or complete absence of the androgen receptors. Thus a spectrum of disorders result in 46XY individuals ranging from complete androgen resistance syndrome (testicular feminization syndrome) in which the affected individual has a female phenotype with feminization at the expected time of puberty to an otherwise normal male with oligospermia. Between these extremes, lie a group of individuals with incomplete virilization of the external genitalia. The mode of inheritance is either as an X-linked recessive or an X-linked dominant disorder. The disorder has not been described in 46XX individuals.

A group of eponyms appear in the literature to describe varying degrees of genital ambiguity in affected individuals. Modern thinking, however, lumps these into a single disorder called Reifenstein's syndrome. Aiman et al[14] described the disorder of incomplete androgen resistance that is manifested only by defects in spermatogenesis. Subsequently, Aiman and Griffin reported that as many as 40 percent of males with idiopathic infertility due to azoospermia or oligospermia may have partial androgen resistance.[23]

Complete Androgen Resistance. Complete androgen resistance is the most fascinating of these disorders and validates the experimental observations made by Jost. Due to the complete lack of androgen receptors, 46XY individuals with this disorder fail to virilize during the critical weeks of sexual differentiation. Since androgen receptors are absent throughout the body, the Wolffian ducts fail to differentiate into male internal genitalia and the brain fails to develop a "male program." However, testicular secretion of Müllerian inhibiting factor occurs in a normal fashion. Thus, at birth, the newborn has normal appearing female external genitalia and a female sexual assignment is made.

At the expected time of puberty, breast development occurs as the result of testicular secretion of testosterone. Some testosterone undergoes peripheral aromatization to estradiol-17β which stimulates breast development (Fig. 6). A striking feature of this disorder at puberty is the absence or sparsity of sexual hair (Fig. 7). The person with this disorder presents with a complaint of failure to establish menses. On examination, absence of a vagina and uterus is discovered.

Measurement of plasma gonadatropins, androgens, and estrogens reveals elevated gonadatropins, a normal androstenedione concentration, a testosterone concentration in the normal or above normal male range, and estradiol-17β concentration in the normal female range. Since the testicles function in a normal fashion at the expected time of puberty and induce feminization, they should be left in situ until secondary sexual development is complete. The testicles in individuals with complete androgen insensitiv-

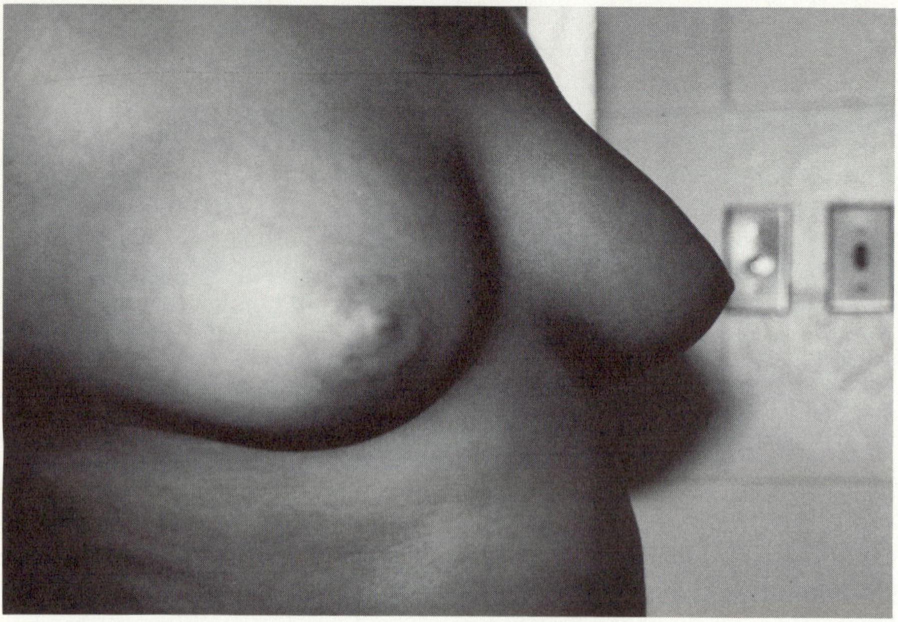

Figure 6. Sixteen-year-old male pseudohermaphrodite resulting from complete androgen insensitivity. Breast development occurred spontaneously at age 13 years.

ity have a 25 percent probability of becoming malignant gonadoblastomas and should be removed after puberty is complete. Malignant transformation has not been reported in children or adolescents. Gonads should not be removed before puberty even if the diagnosis has been made beforehand.

Most affected individuals require vaginal lengthening, either by use of a mechanical dilator or by surgical construction, in order to achieve normal female sexual function. Moreover, once the gonads are removed, exogenous estrogen replacement therapy is required to maintain estrogen-dependent tissues and to prevent symptoms of estrogen withdrawal.

Bakan[24] speculates that Queen Elizabeth I of England, the virgin queen, was affected with complete androgen resistance. Relying on physical descriptions of Elizabeth I and on reports of her behavior, Bakan makes strong arguments to support this hypothesis. Elizabeth I, in her will, forbade that her body be examined or embalmed.

Partial Androgen Resistance (Reifenstein's Syndrome). Varying degrees of genital ambiguity result from varying degrees of partial androgen resistance. The greater the degree of androgen resistance, the greater the tendency to feminize the external genitalia and develop gynecomastia at the time of puberty. Affected individuals do not respond to exogenous testos-

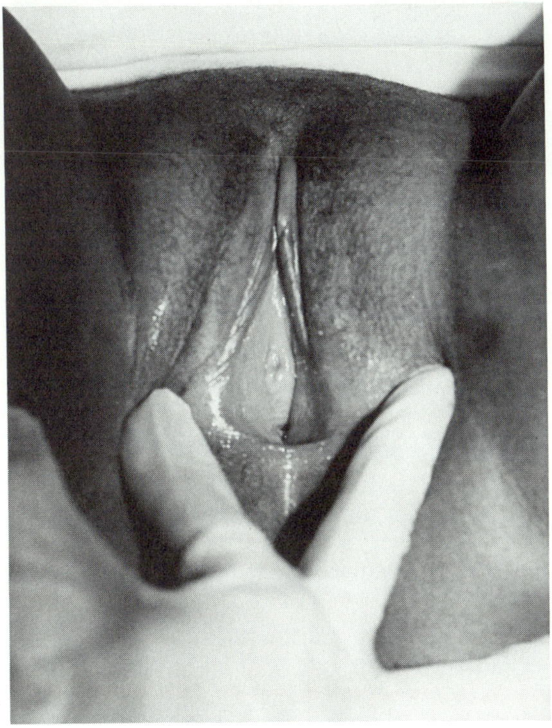

Figure 7. External genitalia of the male pseudohermaphrodite in Figure 6. Note the scant sexual hair. The vagina terminates blindly 4 cm inside the introitus.

terone administration. Therefore, it is imperative that an appropriate sexual assignment be made at birth or shortly thereafter. If a female sexual assignment is made (and that is usually the most appropriate assignment unless the phallus is well developed), the gonads should be removed before puberty. This step prevents subsequent partial virilization at the time of puberty. The person presented in Figure 8 was raised as a male. He had difficulty adjusting to his sexual assignment.

5α-Reductase Deficiency. Dihydrotestosterone, the 5α-reduced metabolite of testosterone, is a more potent androgen than its precursor hormone, testosterone. 5α-Reductase is the enzyme that catalyzes this reaction. 5α-Reductase is concentrated largely in the genital skin and to a lesser extent in the scalp and facial skin. The metabolism of testosterone to dihydrotestosterone occurs locally in the skin once testosterone enters skin cells.

Walsh et al[25] and Imperato-McGinley et al[7] described individuals deficient in 5α-reductase. Affected individuals are 46XY males with normally virilized Wolffian ducts. The external genital structures are female and the ejaculatory ducts terminate in the vagina. The sexual assignment at birth is usually female.

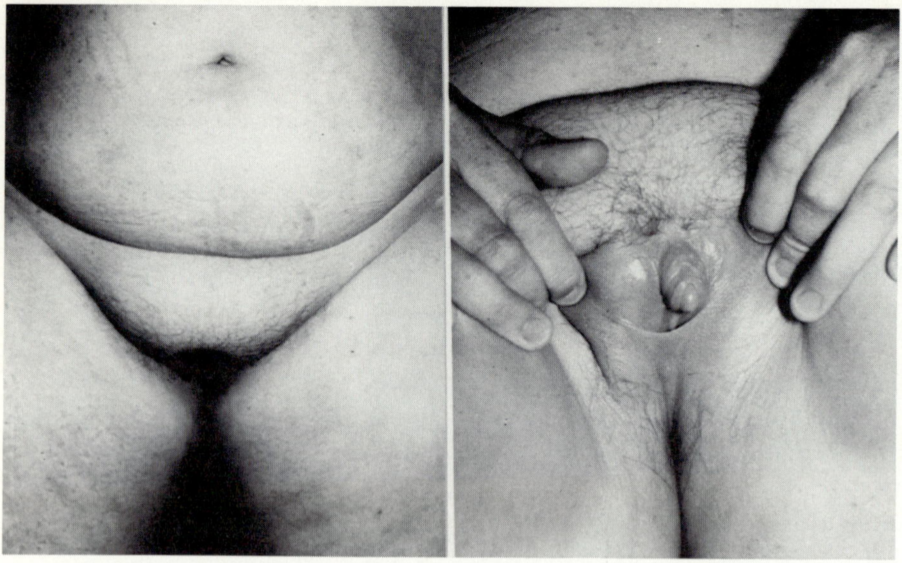

Figure 8. A male pseudohermaphrodite with partial androgen resistance. He was given a male sexual assignment at birth and has poor gender identity as an adult.

At puberty, virilization of the musculoskeletal system occurs and body hair growth begins. These individuals have less beard growth, temporal hair recession, and acne than unaffected males. Ejaculatory volumes are small and the individuals are usually infertile. Unlike individuals with androgen resistance or defects in testosterone synthesis, individuals with 5α-reductase deficiency exhibit male sexual behavior at puberty and reorder their sexual assignment.

If the diagnosis of 5α-reductase deficiency is made in a child given a female sexual assignment, then removal of the testicles should be performed before puberty to preserve the female identity. Exogenous estrogen is required at puberty to initiate female secondary sexual development.

On the other hand, individuals with 5α-reductase deficiency seem to make the transition from female to male smoothly at puberty. Price et al[26] report improved virilization in four males with 5α-reductace deficiency when given high dose testosterone therapy. In their subjects, there was increased penile growth, increased ejaculatory volume, and increased growth of facial and body hair.

Embryonic Testicular Regression. A condition of true agonadism characterized by a female phenotype, 46XY karyotype, and gonadal absence was described by Overzier and Linden.[27] Subsequently, Edman et al[28] reviewed the literature and described the condition as embryogenic testicular regression. The etiology of the testicular regression is unknown. It is assumed that the testicles either never develop and function, leading to a phenotypic female with female internal genital structures, or that the testicles develop, partially function, and undergo regression. If regression occurs immediately after secretion of Müllerian inhibiting factor, the external genitalia are female and the internal genitalia are absent. If regression occurs after the Leydig cells secrete testosterone but before virilization is complete, there are varying degrees of genital ambiguity. If virilization is completed before testicular regression occurs, the scrotum will be empty at birth.

Coulam[29] made an extensive study of one adult woman with embryogenic testicular regression and discovered a 46XY chromosome complement in surgically removed Müllerian derived tissues, i.e., uterine horns and fallopian tubes.

SEXUAL ASSIGNMENT

The first question one should ask in making a sexual assignment in a newborn with genital ambiguity is: "Is the phallus adequate for male sexual function?" If the phallus is rudimentary and does not exhibit an erectile response to stimulation, the sexual assignment should be female. The most common error committed in making a sexual assignment is to force the phenotypic sex to agree with the genotypic sex.

The obstetrician and pediatrician can begin in the delivery room by searching for a vaginal opening. If the vagina is identified and a cervix is seen, the sexual assignment should always be female. In completely virilized female pseudohermaphrodites, the sexual assignment should always be female because these persons have ovaries that contain ova and a female internal reproductive tract. They are capable of female sexual function and reproduction with proper medical and surgical management.

Most male pseudohermaphrodites should receive a female sexual assignment. The degree of incomplete virilization manifested at birth is going to be perpetuated at the time of puberty. This cannot be fully rectified with exogenous testosterone administration and reconstructive surgery.

On the other hand, when a female sexual assignment is made in a male pseudohermaphrodite, early gonadal removal, early surgical management of the rudimentary phallus, and appropriate hormonal and surgical management at puberty give an excellent final result, both physical and psychologic.

A definitive sexual assignment should be made before the end of the first year of life and if possible the definitive sexual assignment should be made before the newborn leaves the nursery. This is best for the child and its parents.

MEDICAL AND SURGICAL MANAGEMENT

Usually medical and surgical therapy are required to successfully manage children with genital ambiguity. The goals of therapy are (1) to establish a firm gender identification for the child and its parents, (2) to allow the transition from childhood to adulthood to be congruent with the established gender identification, and (3) to insure sexual function that is congruent with the established gender identification. A plan of management to accomplish these goals should be developed soon after birth.

The following questions should be asked in formulating a management plan.

1. What is the diagnosis?
2. What are the immediate exogenous hormonal requirements to offset the underlying defect and prevent further virilization? (female pseudohermaphrodites)
3. What surgical procedure(s) must be performed in the first year of life to establish a firm gender identification?
4. What effects will the gonads have on the transition from childhood to adulthood? If the effects are opposite of the established gender identification, when should the gonads be removed?
5. What are the exogenous hormonal requirements to affect secondary sexual development?
6. What surgical procedure(s) must be performed in midadolescence to complete secondary sexual development and to insure sexual function?

Female Pseudohermaphrodites

When the diagnosis is female pseudohermaphroditism as a result of CAH, the physician will initiate replacement glucocorticoid therapy. Next, the clitoris should be reduced in size by clitoral recession. Williamson[30] reported genital surgery as early as the 15th day of life in a group of female pseudohermaphrodites. The perineum may require surgical revision. Incision of the urogenital sinus can be performed successfully in infancy but exteriorization of the vagina should be delayed until after puberty. Azziz et al[31] reported no differences in long-term sexual function in 42 women with CAH, some of whom were treated in infancy and some of whom were treated at adolescence, by a procedure designed to exteriorize the vagina. If repeat operations were performed, the higher success rate was achieved after age 16 years.

At the expected time of puberty in young women with CAH, the requirement for glucocorticoid therapy may increase to facilitate secondary sexual maturation and ovulation. Revision of the perineum to open the vaginal introitus must be performed by midpuberty to enable the affected young woman to establish heterosexual relationships that can lead to coitus (Fig. 9).

Finally, the question of fertility and reproductive capacity must be addressed. More severe forms of CAH, both 21-hydroxylase deficiency and 11β-hydroxylase deficiency, are associated with reduced fertility.[32] Adequate perineal revision for coitus and adequate hormonal replacement to establish ovulation are required.

Male Pseudohermaphrodites

The greatest challenge for the physician confronted with a male pseudohermaphrodite and his family is to make a sexual assignment that is opposite the genotypic sex. The extent of the genital abnormality present at birth will be continued at puberty. Thus, it is wishful thinking to expect the genital abnormality to improve at the time of puberty. Regardless of the cause, disorders of testosterone synthesis or disorders of androgen action, the administration of testosterone will not improve the external genital development. The administration of testosterone may worsen the extent of geni-

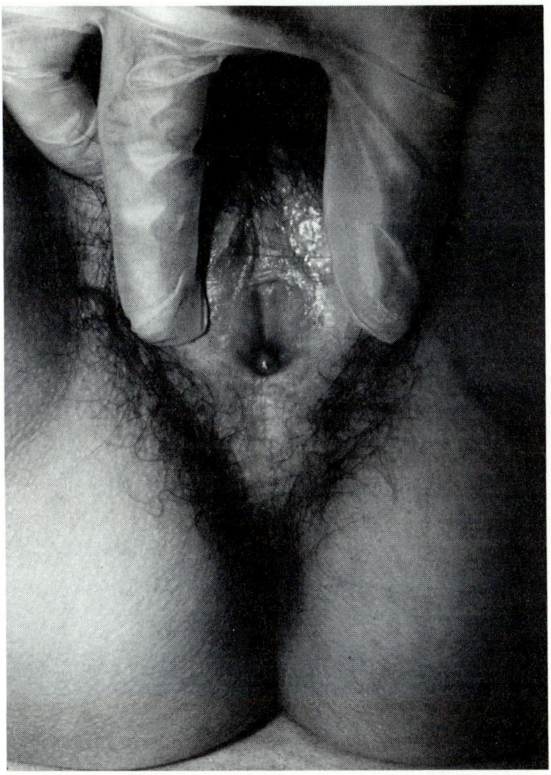

Figure 9. Fifteen-year-old female with 21-hydroxylase deficiency. Clitoral excision was performed in early childhood. Note the elongation of the posterior perineum which obscures the vagina.

tal ambiguity in those with defects in testosterone synthesis because exogenous testosterone will elongate the phallus (clitoris) but will not further virilize the labioscrotal folds or reposition the urethra along the phallus.

When the decision is made to make a female assignment for a male pseudohermaphrodite, the decision should be made to remove the gonads before the onset of puberty. Further testosterone secretion should be prevented. (The only exception to this directive is the male pseudohermaphrodite with complete androgen insensitivity. In this clinical situation, the testes will bring about complete feminization. The testicles should be removed after feminization is complete, however.)

At the time of gonadal removal, it is appropriate to shorten the clitoris. Further reconstructive surgery should be delayed until after breast development has been completed.

At the expected time of onset of female puberty, age 10 to 12 years, exogenous estrogen administration should be initiated. Estradiol-17β, 1 mg/day, is begun orally. After 2 to 4 months, the dose of estradiol-17β should be increased to 2 mg/day. Continue this dosage until the breasts have reached a Tanner IV developmental stage. Once this developmental milestone is achieved, add a progestin (17α-medroxyprogesterone acetate, 10 mg/day) for 10 days each month. This addition of progestin will complete breast development.

When feminization is complete, the physician turns attention to reconstruction of the external genitalia. Usually, the surgeon must revise the labioscrotal folds, shorten the clitoris (if this was not done during childhood), and construct a vagina. We advocate a modification of the classic McIndoe procedure for vaginal construction.[33] An example of a preoperative and postoperative perineal revision with a vaginoplasty is presented in Figure 10.

SUMMARY

Before the sixth week of gestation the fetal genitalia are indifferent. Development of the external and internal genitalia along male lines requires functional testes that secrete Müllerian inhibiting factor and testosterone, receptors for testosterone, and the enzyme 5α-reductase to convert testosterone to dihydrotestosterone in the genital skin. The absence of any one of these requirements results in female genital development or ambiguous genitalia.

Conversely, the inappropriate secretion or exposure of testosterone in a female fetus results in virilization of the external genitalia. This can produce a female pseudohermaphrodite with complete virilization or one with ambiguous genitalia.

A management plan that includes an appropriate sexual assignment should be made soon after birth. This plan must include medical and sur-

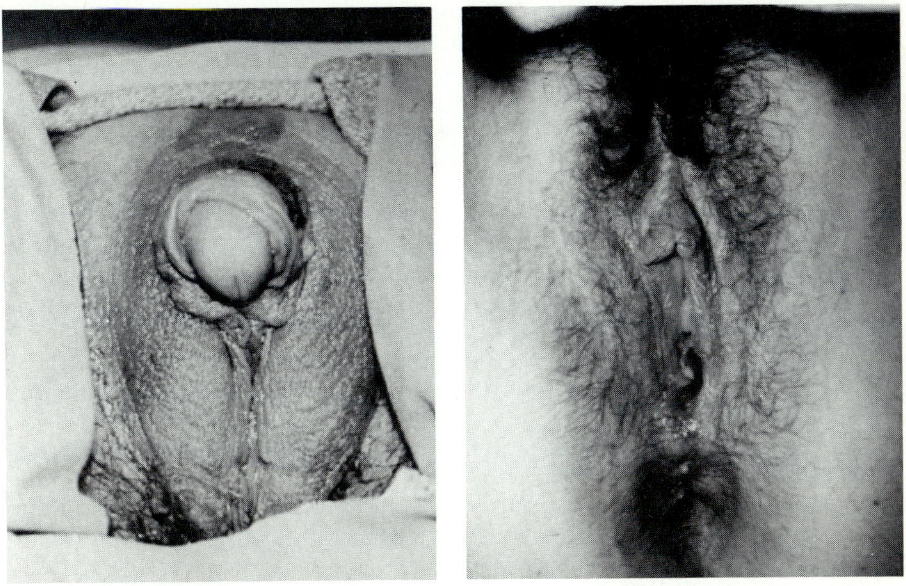

Figure 10. A. Seventeen-year-old male pseudohermaphrodite, raised as a female, with phallic enlargement and labioscrotal fusion. **B.** Cosmetic and functional outcome following perineal revision, clitoral resection, and vaginal construction.

gical management that leads to sexual function congruent with the sexual assignment.

REFERENCES

1. Jost A: The role of fetal hormones in prenatal development. Harvery Lecture 55:201, 1961
2. Jost A: A new look at the mechanisms controlling sex differentiation in mammals. Johns Hopkins Med J 130:38, 1972
3. Haseltine FP, Ohno S: Mechanisms of gonadal differentiation. Science 211:1272, 1981
4. Jost A: Problems of fetal endocrinology: The gonadal and hypophyseal hormones. Rec Prog Horm Res 8:379, 1953
5. Josso N: Anti-Müllerian hormone: New perspectives for a sexist molecule. Endocr Rev 7:421, 1986
6. Sheehan SJ, Tobbia IN, Ismail MA, et al: Persistent Müllerian duct syndrome. Review and report of three cases. Br J Urol 57:548, 1985
7. Imperato-McGinley J, Guerrero L, Gautier T, Peterson RE: Steroid 5α-reductase deficiency in man: An inherited form of male pseudohermaphroditism. Science 186:1213, 1974
8. Wilson JD, George FW, Griffin JE: The hormonal control of sexual development. Science 211:1278, 1981

9. Wilson JD, Griffin JE, George FW, Leshin M: The role of gonadal steroids in sexual differentiation. Rec Prog Horm Res 37:1, 1981
10. Wilson JD: Recent studies on the mechanisms of action of testosterone. N Engl J Med 287:1284, 1972
11. Imperato-McGinley J, Gautier T, Richards M, Shackleton C: The diagnosis of 5α-reductase in infancy. J Clin Endocrinol Metab 63:1313, 1986
12. Griffin JE, Wilson JD: The syndromes of androgen resistance. N Engl J Med 302:198, 1980
13. Wilkins L: Abnormal sex differentiation: Hermaphroditism and gonadal dyogenesis. In The Diagnosis and Treatment of Endocrine Disorders in Childhood and Adolescence, 2nd ed. Springfield, IL, Charles C. Thomas, 1957, pp 258–291
14. Aiman J, Griffin JE, Gazak JM, et al: Androgen insensitivity as a cause of infertility in otherwise normal men. N Engl J Med 300:223, 1979
15. Milewich L, George FW, Wilson JD: Estrogen formation by the ovary in the rabbit embryo. Endocrinology 100:187, 1977
16. Ehrhardt AA, Meyer-Bahlburg NFL: Effects of prenatal sex hormones on gender-related behavior. Science 211:1312, 1981
17. Roslyn JJ, Fonkalsrud EW, Lippe B: Intersex disorders in adolescents and adults. Am J Surg 146:138, 1983
18. Speroff L, Glass RH, Kuse NG: Normal and abnormal sexual development. In Clinical Gynecologic Endocrinology and Infertility, 3rd ed. Baltimore, Williams & Wilkins, 1983, pp 335–361
19. Money J, Schwartz M, Levis VG: Adult heterosexual and fetal hormonal masculinization and demasculinization: 46XX congenital virilizing adrenal hyperplasia and 46XY androgen-insensitivity syndrome compared. Psychoneuroendocrinology 9:405, 1987
20. Wilkins L, Jones HW Jr, Holman GH, Stempfel RS: Masculinization of the female fetus associated with administration of oral and intramuscular progestins during gestation: Nonadrenal female pseudohermaphroditism. J Clin Endocrinol Metab 18:559, 1958
21. Shaw RW, Farquhar JW: Female pseudohermaphroditism associated with danazol exposure in utero. Case report. Br J Obstet Gynaecol 91:382, 1984
22. Kaufman FR, Costin G, Goebelsmann U, et al: Male pseudohermaphroditism due to 17,20-desmolase deficiency. J Clin Endocrinol Metab 57:32, 1983
23. Aiman J, Griffin JE: The frequency of androgen receptor deficiency in infertile men. J Clin Endocrinol Metab 54:725, 1982
24. Bakan R: Queen Elizabeth I: A case of testicular feminization? Med Hypoth 17:277, 1985
25. Walsh PC, Madden JD, Harrod MJ, et al: Familial incomplete male pseudohermaphroditism Type 2: Decreased dihydrotestosterone formation in pseudovaginal perineoscrotal hypospadias. N Engl J Med 291:244, 1974
26. Price P, Wass JAH, Griffin JE, et al: High dose androgen therapy in male pseudohermaphroditism due to 5α-reductase deficiency and disorders of the androgen receptor. J Clin Invest 74:1496, 1984
27. Overzier C, Linden H: Echter Agonadismus (Anorchismus) bei Geschwistern. Gynaecologia (Basal) 142:215, 1956
28. Edman CD, Winters AJ, Porter JC, et al: Embryonic testicular regression: A clinical spectrum of XY agonadal individuals. Obstet Gynecol 49:208, 1977
29. Coulam CB: Testicular regression syndrome. Obstet Gynecol 53:44, 1979

30. Williamson HO: Ambiguous genitals due to congenital adrenal hyperplasia: Surgical repair in infancy. Am J Obstet Gynecol 108:1085, 1970
31. Azziz R, Mulaikal RM, Migeon CJ, et al: Congenital adrenal hyperplasia: Long-term results following vaginal construction. Fertil Steril 46:1011, 1986
32. Mulaikal RM, Migeon CJ, Rock JA: Fertility rates in female patients with congenital adrenal hyperplasia to 21-hydroxylase deficiency. N Engl J Med 316:178, 1987
33. Wiser WL, Bates GW: Management of vaginal agenesis: A report of 92 cases. Surg Gynecol Obstet 159:108, 1984

Nuclear Imaging in Urology

Anton J. Bueschen

Development of nuclear medicine procedures for urology has occurred during the past 30 years beginning with the first renogram in 1956. Subsequently, many technical improvements have occurred including the development of gamma cameras with increasing resolution, scanning cameras in addition to the stationary cameras, a change from purely qualitative images to quantitative analysis with analog-to-digital converters and computers, and new radiopharmaceuticals. These advances have led to greatly improved radionuclide renal function tests, bone scintigraphy, radionuclide cystography, and scrotal scintigraphy which have become very helpful in the evaluation of patients with urologic disease. Less frequently used applications are liver scans, gallium scans, leukocyte scans, and adrenal scans. This chapter will review renal radionuclide examinations, bone scintigraphy, radionuclide cystography, and scrotal scintigraphy with special emphasis on important technical aspects, interpretation, and indications.

RENAL RADIONUCLIDE EXAMINATION

Selection and Dose of Radiopharmaceuticals

Numerous radiopharmaceuticals have been used for the evaluation of kidneys. Three types of radiopharmaceuticals are available: agents excreted by glomerular filtration, agents excreted by tubular secretion, and agents bound to renal parenchyma (Table 1). There is not one preferred radiopharmaceutical universally used for all purposes. The agents used most

TABLE 1. RADIOPHARMACEUTICALS USED TO ASSESS KIDNEY FUNCTION AND STRUCTURE

Agents excreted by glomerular filtration
Technetium-99m-diethylenetriaminepentaacetic acid (Tc-99m DTPA)
Iodine-125-iothalamate
Chromium-51-edetate (Cr-51-EDTA)
Ytterbium-169-DTPA (Yb-169-DTPA)
Indium-113m-DTPA
Agents excreted by tubular secretion
Iodine-131-orthoiodohippurate (I-131-OIH)
Iodine-123-orthoiodohippurate (I-123-OIH)
Agents bound to renal parenchyma
Technetium-99m-dimercaptosuccinate (Tc-99m-DMSA)
Mercury-203-chlormerodrin (Hg-203)
Mercury-197-chlormerodrin (Hg-197)
Technetium-99m-glucoheptonate (Tc-99m-GH)
Others including technetium complexes of citrate, gluconate, mannonate, ascorbate, and malate
Agents used principally for other organs and only incidentally for the kidney
Gallium-67-citrate
Technetium-99m-sulfur colloid
Bone-imaging agents

often are Tc-99m-diethylentricamine pentaacetic acid (DTPA) and I-131-orthoiodohippuric acid (OIH). The advantages and disadvantages of the radiopharmaceuticals have been reviewed and will not be presented here.[1] I have used most agents, but have found I-131-OIH very practical and therefore it will be the agent presented in this chapter.

The dose of I-131-OIH can be determined by either the weight or the age of the patient. The recommended dosage schedule as determined by age is 50 μCi for patients less than 1 year old, 100 μCi for patients 1 to 6 years old, 100 μCi per kidney for children 6 to 15 years old, and 150 μCi per kidney for older children and adults.

TECHNIQUE

Preparation of the Patient

The patient requires no special preparation for radionuclide evaluation since bowel gas and fat do not interfere with the results. The patients are studied in a normally hydrated state. To assure adequate hydration, outpatients are routinely given 300 to 500 ml of fluid to drink 30 minutes before testing.

PROCEDURE

The patients are usually in a supine position during this study, with the detector placed under the imaging table. However, the sitting position is used in the patient with a urinary conduit to promote drainage of urine and the detector is placed over the abdomen of the transplant patient.

The predetermined dose of I-131-OIH is injected intravenously, and radioactivity of the upper abdomen is then detected by the scintillation camera and recorded on computer-compatible magnetic tape for the first 27 minutes after injection of the radiopharmaceutical. During the first minute of recording, the technician observes the oscilloscope to be certain that the kidneys are in the field being recorded on magnetic tape. If not, the patient is moved to the proper position. After the 27-minute recording period, the patient is placed in the prone position so that the scintillation camera is anterior to the bladder. A 1-minute recording is made over the bladder just before voiding, 30 to 35 minutes after injection of the radiopharmaceutical, and again immediately after voiding. The residual urine in the bladder is calculated using prevoid counts, postvoid counts, and volume voided. An aliquot of diluted urine is measured in the dosimeter to establish the quantity of radiopharmaceutical in the voided urine. The quantitative analysis of I-131-OIH returned at 30 to 35 minutes is used as a measure of total renal function and includes the sum of the amount of urine voided and the amount of residual urine calculated to be present in the bladder. An additional method for evaluating total renal function utilizes a blood sample obtained 44 minutes after injection of the OIH in adults and 53 minutes after injection of the OIH in children to calculate the effective renal plasma flow.[2–4]

After the test is completed, the taped data are displayed on the oscilloscope and the regions of interest in each kidney and a background area adjacent to the kidneys are selected. An analog-to-digital converter provides quantitative information on the activity over each kidney for each 1-minute interval after the background activity is subtracted. The relative percentage of activity over each kidney is then determined for the first 5-, 10-, 15-, and 25-minute intervals after injection of the orthoiodohippurate. This is accomplished by adding the counts over the kidneys at each 1-minute interval and then determining the percentage of total counts from each kidney. The total count of the two kidneys equals 100 percent for each 1-minute interval. The total activity over each kidney during the 1- to 2-minute interval represents the relative renal plasma flow to each kidney. The percentage of activity over each kidney at later intervals represents additional factors including tubular secretion and excretory function. Scintigraphs are used to correlate anatomic abnormalities with physiologic abnormalities determined by the quantitative data. The use of intravenous injection of a diuretic during the study will be discussed in the section on urinary obstruction.

NORMAL RENAL RADIONUCLIDE EXAMINATION

Results of the study are considered to be normal if the counts over each kidney in 1 to 2 minutes are between 45 and 55 percent of the total over both kidneys, if the time of maximum activity over the kidneys occurs less than 5 minutes after injection and within 1 minute of each other, and if the 1 minute count at 25 minutes is one-third or less of the maximum counts of the same kidney. Normal values for effective renal plasma flow (ERPF) vary with age and sex in adults. The difference with sex is related to the size of the patient. The ERPF declines with increasing age of adults (Fig. 1). The normal ERPF in children is determined by the following formula:

$$\text{Normal ERPF} = 61.5 + 52.2 \text{ age} \pm 27\%$$

The percentage of the injected dose excreted in the urine at 30 to 35 minutes is greater than 66 percent.

Variation of Normal

Variations from the normal study can result from either technical problems or pathologic processes. The technical problems most often leading to abnormalities of the examination are patient dehydration and subcutaneous

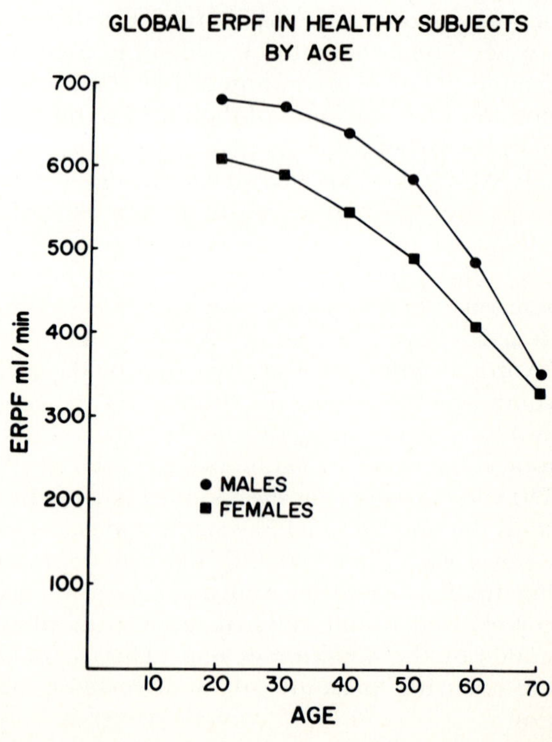

Figure 1. ERPF declines as age of patient increases and is lower in females than in males. These data were obtained from the study of a group of 420 healthy prospective kidney donors. *(From Russell CD, 1985, p 164, with permission.[1])*

infiltration of the radiopharmaceutical when it is injected. Patient dehydration often can be detected by routinely recording the volume and specific gravity of the urine voided by the patient at the end of the study. Subcutaneous infiltration of the radiopharmaceutical is detected by routinely obtaining a scintiphotograph of the injection site and having that available for the person interpreting the examination.

A delayed uptake of the radiopharmaceutical by the kidneys, delayed time of maximum activity, and delayed excretion of the radiopharmaceutical can occur with prerenal, renal, or postrenal abnormalities. Therefore, decreased renal function will be observed on the renal radionuclide examination in patients with congestive heart failure, renal artery stenosis, renal parenchymal disease, and abnormalities which cause poor evacuation from the renal pelvis and ureter. A flat renogram curve indicates an absent kidney or a nonfunctioning kidney of unknown etiology and unknown recoverability. Therefore, it must be appreciated that the radionuclide examination provides an accurate assessment of the current function of the kidneys, but other conventional radiographic and diagnostic procedures generally must be used to determine the etiology of the functional alterations.

APPLICATIONS OF RENAL RADIONUCLIDE EVALUATION

Screening

Ultrasonography and intravenous urography are the procedures most commonly used to evaluate the upper urinary tract in urologic patients. A renal radionuclide examination also can be used to screen for pathology of the upper urinary tract. None of the studies can detect all urinary tract disease. The intravenous urogram (IVU) and ultrasound are excellent screening tests for detection of renal anatomic changes such as renal masses, ureteral duplication without functional alteration, nonobstructive calculi, and transitional cell tumors. The radionuclide examination can, however, detect and quantitate functional renal changes which often cannot be appreciated from an IVU and certainly no functional changes are appreciated from ultrasound. All adult patients with hematuria should be evaluated with urography since renal masses and nonobstructive transitional cell tumors can be missed with a radionuclide evaluation.

Urinary Obstruction

The renal radionuclide examination has the following applications in the evaluation of patients with urinary obstruction:

1. Evaluates degree of renal functional alteration (total and differential function)
2. The diuretic renogram evaluates equivocal urinary obstruction to determine if obstruction has caused the dilation

3. Effectiveness of surgical relief of ureteral obstruction can be determined by comparison studies before and after relief of urinary obstruction

Urinary obstruction produces delayed time of maximum activity, delayed excretion following the maximum activity, decreased blood flow determined from the percentage of activity in the ipsilateral kidney at 1 to 2 minutes, and decreased percentage of dose excreted in the urine at 30 to 35 minutes caused by holdup of the radionuclide in the obstructed urinary tract. The patients with mild obstruction have only delayed time of maximum activity and delayed excretion and perhaps decreased return of the dose at 30 to 35 minutes, but no decreased ipsilateral blood flow. Those patients should have an excellent result from surgical relief of the obstruction. Sometimes though, it is difficult to know if the changes observed on the radionuclide and radiographic studies are caused by obstruction or other etiologies which include congenital dilation without obstruction, persistent dilation despite previous successful relief of obstruction, and infection producing depressed peristalsis. The two most used tests to evaluate equivocal urinary obstruction are pressure perfusion studies and diuresis renography.

The diuretic renogram is performed in the same manner as our other renal radionuclide examinations except that Lasix (furosemide) is injected intravenously 10 minutes after the OIH at a dose of 0.5 mg/kg up to a maximum dose of 40 mg. The diuresis created by the diuretic causes the radiopharmaceutical to be washed out of the kidney in the absence of obstruction. We obtain a ratio in each kidney of 1-minute counts at the time of maximum activity divided by 1-minute counts 27 minutes after injection of the radiopharmaceutical (peak counts/27 minutes counts). Experience has shown that a ratio of less than 1.5 suggests obstruction and a ratio of more than 2.5 represents absence of obstruction. Ratios between 1.5 and 2.5 require individual interpretation with most of those being associated with poor ipsilateral renal plasma flow. My experience with 109 renal units had ratios of more than 2.5 in 78, 1.5 to 2.5 in 15, and less than 1.5 in 16 in studying patients with only equivocal obstruction on the IVU (Figures 2 through 5).

Numerous papers have compared the diuretic renogram and the pressure perfusion study using one or the other as the standard when the test was actually done because neither one had been established as the standard.[5–15] The clinical course of the patient and preservation of renal function should provide the final answer about the reliability of the test. I have concluded the following and the recent literature is tending to support my conclusions:

1. Diuretic renography can establish the presence or absence of obstruction in most cases.

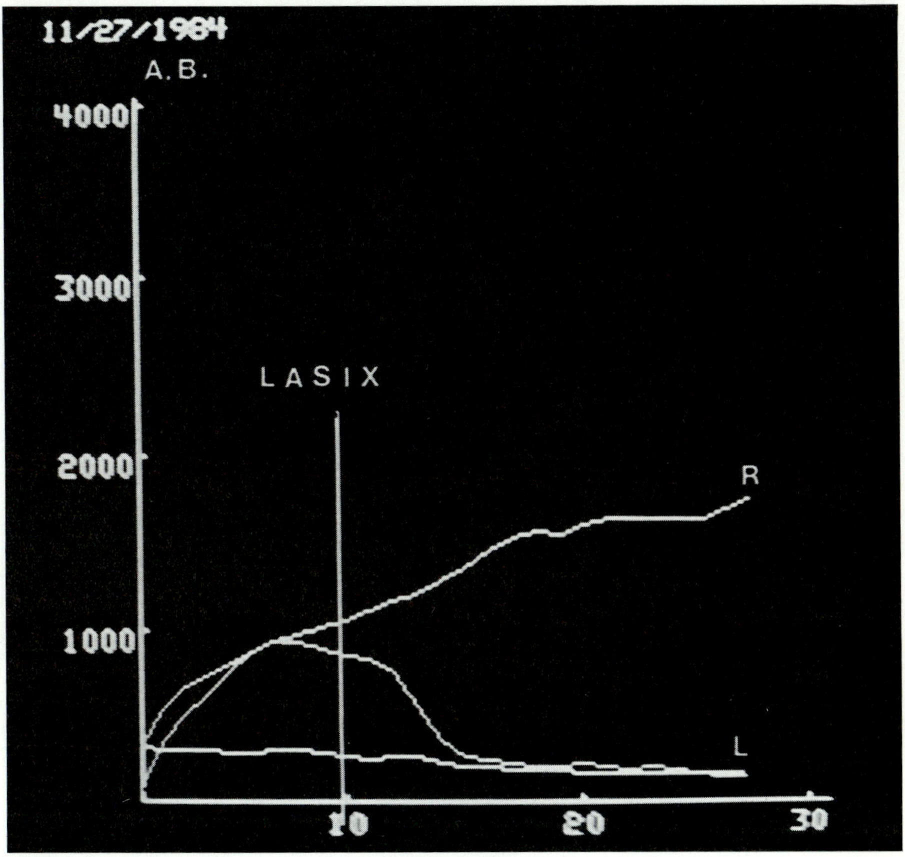

A

Figure 2. A. Lasix renogram in a 2-month-old male shows a poor response of the right kidney and a good response of the left kidney suggesting obstruction of the right kidney.

2. Good response to the diuretic cannot occur with poor ipsilateral renal function.
3. Diuretic renography is not necessary to establish the diagnosis in obvious cases of obstruction, but does provide a base line of total and differential renal function for comparison after surgical relief of the obstruction.
4. Delayed washout following injection of a diuretic can occur from vesicoureteral reflux or a distended bladder. A urethral catheter can be used during diuretic renography for those cases but is not recommended for other patients.
5. Infection of the kidney and ureter can produce diminished ureteral peristalsis and consequently a false-positive diuretic renogram.

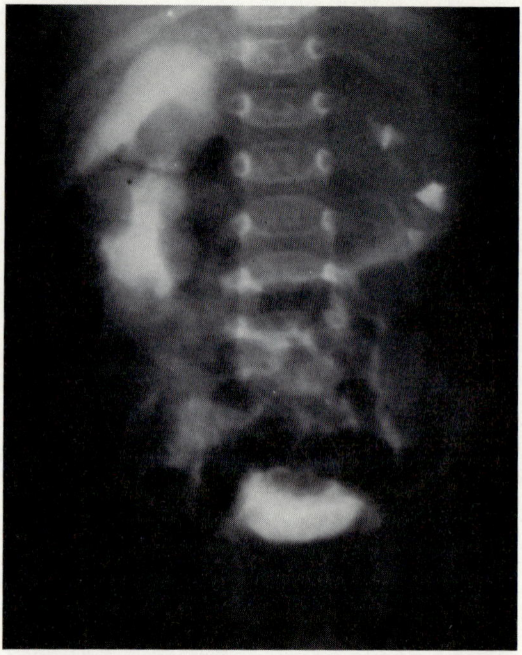

B

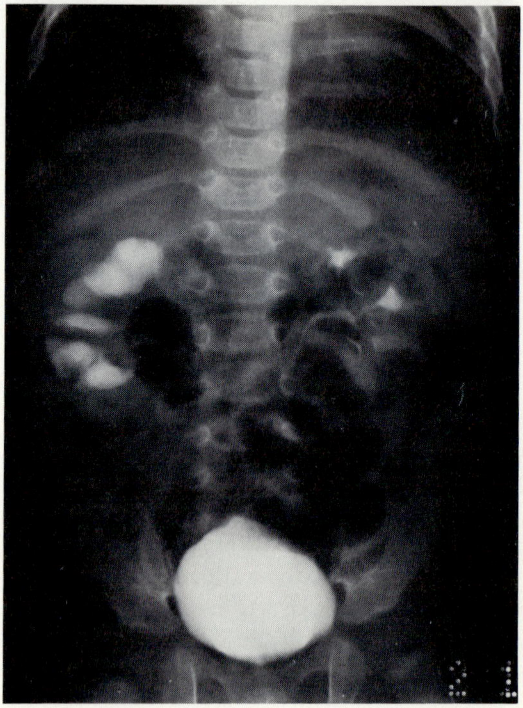

C

Figure 2. (cont.) B. IVU (40 minutes) in the same patient shows severe caliectasis on the right and a later film showed pyelectasis. **C.** IVU (40 minutes) in the same patient 2 months after a right dismembered pyeloplasty shows improved caliectasis.

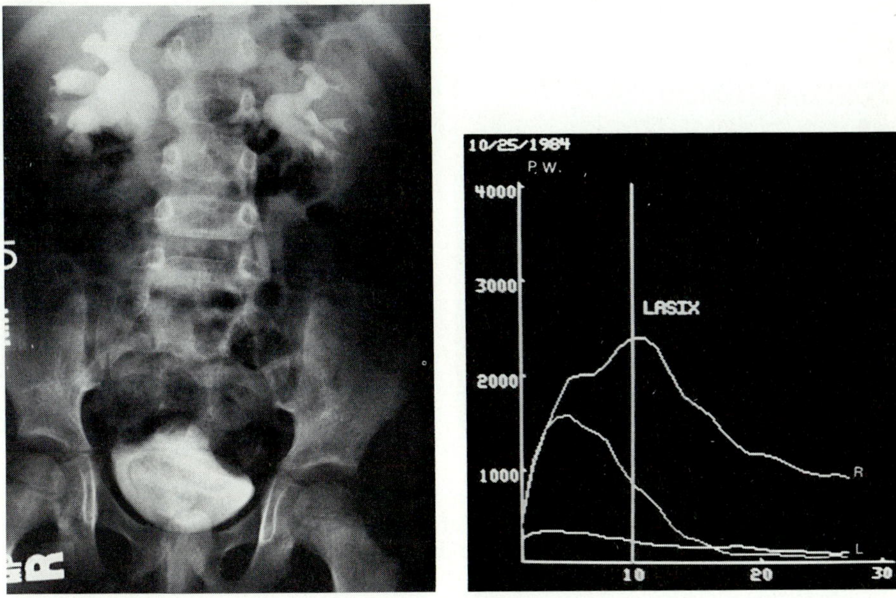

A B

Figure 3. A. IVU in a 4-year-old boy who was referred for a right pyeloplasty, shows right calycectasis and pyelectasis. **B.** Lasix I-131-OIH renogram shows symmetric and good renal plasma flow and good washout of the radiopharmaceutical after injection of the diuretic. Ratio of peak/27 min counts in the right kidney was 2.63 and total ERPF was 381 ml/min. The patient has been followed without an operation.

6. A Whitaker pressure perfusion study can provide additional help in selected cases when obstruction remains questionable after diuretic renography. It assesses outflow resistance but has the disadvantages of being invasive, providing no information about renal function, occasionally requiring general anesthesia in children, and producing more radiation exposure to the patient than a diuretic renogram.
7. The diuretic renogram and the pressure perfusion study are very helpful in the management of patients with equivocal obstruction but clinical judgment by the physician remains important.

The renal radionuclide changes which can occur following relief of obstruction are earlier maximum activity, more rapid excretion following maximum activity, increased percentage of the dose excreted in the urine at 30 minutes, and sometimes improved renal blood flow. Occasionally, a diuresis renogram is necessary to show the absence of obstruction after successful surgical correction because the patient has persistent dilation of the collecting structures.

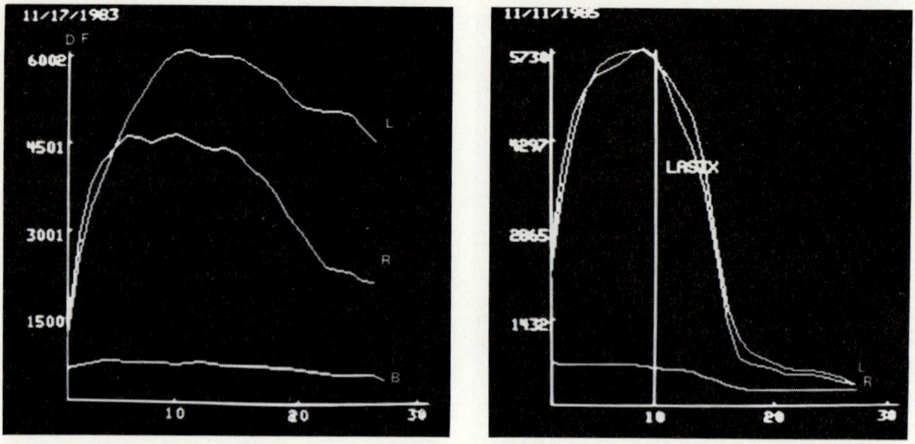

A

B

Figure 4. A. I-131-OIH renogram in a 17-year-old male who had a left pyeloplasty 6 years earlier. Renogram shows bilateral rapid uptake of radiopharmaceutical by both kidneys indicating good and equal renal plasma flow. Total ERPF, determined from 44-minute blood sample, was 620 ml/min. Peak times and drainage from the kidneys were delayed. Those delays could be due to obstruction, dilated collecting systems without obstruction, vesicoureteral reflux, or infection. Possible technical factors causing the delays are patient dehydration or subcutaneous infiltration of the radiopharmaceutical. Slightly dilated collecting systems were thought to be the cause of the delays. **B.** Diuretic renogram in the same patient shows no evidence of obstruction.

Urolithiasis

Renal and ureteral calculi may cause unilateral renal damage with unilateral stones or asymmetric renal damage with bilateral renal stones. These functional renal changes are measured easily by the radionuclide procedure. A review of 114 radionuclide studies in 77 patients with urolithiasis

Figure 5. Lasix I-131-OIH renogram in a 4-year-old girl shows poor total ERPF and a poor response to the diuretic with the ratio of counts at time of maximum activity compared to 27 minutes of less than 1.5. This patient had vesicoureteral reflux and chronic renal insufficiency. Another diuretic renogram done with bilateral ureteral catheter drainage was identical showing that the poor response to the diuretic was caused by poor renal function rather than obstruction.

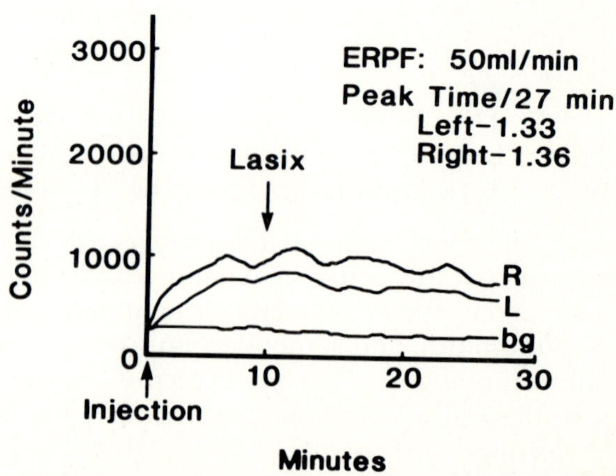

showed that ERPF, determined by the radionuclide procedure, was more accurate than was serum creatinine as an indicator of total renal function.[16] The ERPF was as low as 200 ml/min in some patients with normal serum creatinine values. In three patients who had decreased muscle mass caused by long-standing paraplegia, the serum creatinine was only 0.7 mg/dl and the ERPF was 200 to 230 ml/min.

The IVU should be part of the initial evaluation in all patients with urolithiasis so that the location of calculi and the location of obstruction can be documented. The radionuclide study provides information about the relative function of the two kidneys as well as the function of segments of the kidneys involved with stone, which is particularly helpful in patients with large renal stones and patients with bilateral stones. Differential renal function can be measured with large ureteral catheters, but this technique is time consuming and sometimes hazardous. One can quantitatively select the region of interest in one pole of the kidney and compare its function with that of another segment of equal area in the ipsilateral or contralateral kidney. Knowledge of poor function in a segment of the kidney involved with a large stone may assist the surgeon in choosing the form of therapy to be used.

A recent report studied renal function with a radionuclide examination in 33 patients who had been treated with extracorporeal shock-wave lithotripsy (ESWL).[17] There was a reduction in ipsilateral ERPF of more than 5 percent in 10 of 33 patients. The renogram showed an abnormality in 19 of 44 (46 percent) of the treated kidneys when performed 24 to 48 hours after ESWL. The authors felt that the changes were due to renal contusion and that the clinical significance was not yet known.

Vesicoureteral Reflux

The management of moderately advanced vesicoureteral reflux remains controversial. The controversy of medical versus surgical treatment is being studied by an international reflux study committee. The endpoints on which judgment of success or failure of a good treatment will rest are the development of new scars, the progression of existing scars, renal growth, the development of hypertension, recurrent rate of urinary tract infections, and changes in kidney function. The assessment of renal scars on IVU is a subjective evaluation and evaluates anatomic changes of the kidney without measuring functional changes. Alterations in blood urea nitrogen, serum creatinine, creatinine clearance, and renal concentrating ability measure alterations in total renal function. Those tests, however, do not demonstrate unilateral or asymmetric renal function alterations which frequently occur in patients with vesicoureteral reflux. Radionuclide scanning can quantitate differential functional changes which precede impaired renal growth and the development of hypertension. My experience, however, has shown only very mild if any functional change on the radionuclide study when the IVU is normal in patients with vesicoureteral reflux. Therefore, the indications for a renal radionuclide evaluation are an abnormality of the IVU or an evaluation of the upper urinary tract without using contrast medium or with less radiation exposure than received from an IVU.

Neurogenic Bladder

Periodic surveillance of the urinary tract is required to detect abnormalities resulting from neurogenic bladder dysfunction in spinal cord injury patients. The routine urologic evaluation often includes IVU, cystography, urine culture, serum creatinine, blood urea nitrogen, and residual urine volume determinations. Since the patient preparation often used for the IVU can be cumbersome for the patient and may disrupt the patient's bowel routine for several days, we compared the IVU to the renal radionuclide examination in a group of 200 spinal cord injury patients.[18] The results of the study suggested that a renal radionuclide examination and a plain film of the abdomen be used for screening upper urinary tract abnormalities in lieu of an IVU. No severe urographic abnormalities were undetected by the radionuclide study. The radionuclide study was abnormal in the presence of a normal IVU in 54 patients and the IVU was abnormal in the presence of a normal radionuclide study in 21 patients. The radionuclide study was equal or better than the IVU in detecting abnormalities of the upper urinary tract, in addition to the advantage of not requiring bowel preparation. Additional experience has confirmed our initial conclusions and the interpretation of renal scintigraphy in spinal cord injury patients has been defined more clearly.[19]

Renovascular Hypertension

The identification of renovascular hypertension was one of the first uses of radionuclides in the evaluation of renal function. Unfortunately, the early reports involved utilization of the twin probe renogram technique because the scintillation camera with multichannel collimation and computer-assisted analysis of the radionuclide study were not available. The use of the twin probe renogram technique resulted in a high incidence of false-negative and false-positive results. The introduction of the renal scintillation camera study greatly decreased the incidence of false-negative results, but still yielded a 26 percent incidence of false-positive I-131-OIH studies.[20] The criteria for a positive OIH renal scintillation camera study include decreased 1- to 2-minute counts over one kidney; delayed peaking of counts over a kidney or over a portion of a kidney; delayed emptying of a kidney or a portion of a kidney; and a marked difference in renal size. With the use of this study, it is possible to select equal areas of interest in segments of a kidney to assist in the detection of segmental renal artery stenosis. A renal radionuclide evaluation can show improvement or changes in differential renal function following percutaneous angioplasty.

Renal Transplantation

All of the potential living related renal donors have a renal radionuclide examination to determine total and differential renal function. Differential renal function cannot be ascertained as accurately from the other tests used including creatinine clearance, IVU, and renal arteriography. This initial evaluation also gives a good indication of the initial level of function anticipated in the recipient.

The renal radionuclide study aids in the evaluation of the functional status of the transplanted kidney. It has been very helpful in the evaluation and management of complications such as acute tubular necrosis, acute rejection, chronic rejection, ureteral obstruction, renal artery occlusion, and urinary extravasation (Fig. 6).[21,22] An excretion index (EI) is plotted with the ERPF to help in the differential diagnosis of some of the clinical problems following a renal transplant. The EI is a ratio of the percent of the dose excreted by a patient to the expected excretion for the patient's ERPF level. Chronic rejection is usually associated with a slow decline in ERPF with the EI remaining normal until the ERPF falls to about 120 ml/min. Renal artery stenosis has a similar pattern. It develops over a period of months and a rising blood pressure is associated with a gradual decline in ERPF and a

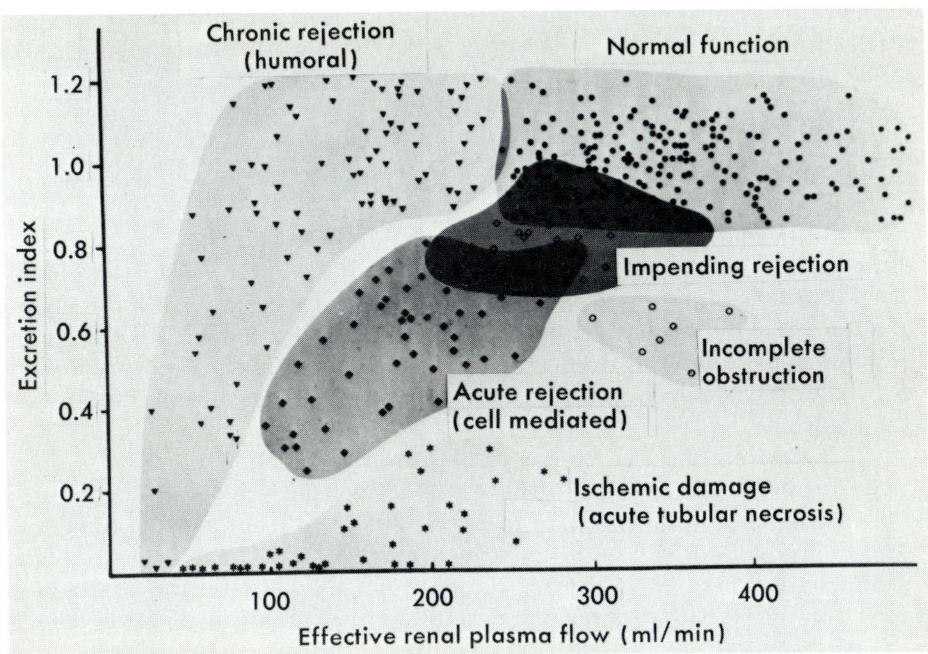

Figure 6. Plot of ERPF versus EI data from transplanted kidney patients with various clinical problems. *(From Russell CD, 1985, p 240, with permission.[1])*

normal EI. Acute rejection begins with a prolongation of cortical transit time and impaired excretory function resulting in a decreasing EI. This is followed quickly by a decline in ERPF. Acute tubular necrosis demonstrates a decreased ERPF and a disproportionately low EI. Incomplete ureteral obstruction is recognized by radiopharmaceutical visualized on the delayed scintigraphs and urinary extravasation is recognized by a collection of radiopharmaceutical outside the urinary collecting system.

Renal Masses

Renal masses previously were usually detected by excretory urography, but now are often incidental findings during ultrasonography or computed tomography (CT) of the abdomen. Rarely a radionuclide study using TC-99m-glucoheptonate or Tc-99m-dimercaptosuccinic acid can help to confirm the presence or absence of an equivocal renal mass. The greatest usefulness of a radionuclide examination for renal masses is to evaluate differential and segmental renal function before removing a renal tumor in patients with questionable renal functional reserve.

Trauma

Radionuclide studies are not part of the routine diagnostic armamentarium in the evaluation of acute urologic injuries. They are helpful in the evaluation of chronic problems related to ureteral injuries. Measurement of differential renal function aids in choosing the optimal reconstructive procedure or nephrectomy.

BONE SCINTIGRAPHY

Technique and Interpretation

Bone scintigraphy was first reported in 1959, but it did not become widely used for detection of metastatic disease until the early 1970s with the introduction of bone-seeking complexes of technetium-99m.[23,24] The radionuclide most commonly used is technetium-99m-methylene diphosphonate. It is readily available and less expensive than the previously used radiopharmaceuticals.

Bone scintigraphy is begun 1 to 3 hours after injection of the radiopharmaceutical. Normal patients will have only about 3 percent of the technetium-99m-methylene diphosphonate in the circulation 3 hours after injection and the remainder will be in the skeleton or will have been excreted. The kidneys are visualized in normal patients, but the visualization of the kidneys diminishes with decreasing renal function or greatly increased skeletal uptake. Younger patients with excellent renal function, however, can clear their kidneys of the radiopharmaceutical within 3 hours after injection. Therefore, if one is interested in evaluating the urinary tract with bone scintigraphy, one or two earlier images should be obtained. The detection of renal abnormalities as incidental findings during bone scintigraphy has been reported.[25,26] The routine radionuclide bone scan, however, is an unreliable test for detecting ureteral obstruction, especially bilateral obstruction.[27] False-positive reports of ureteral obstruction occur not infrequently in patients with compound calyces or with a capacious extrarenal pelvis.

Bone scintigraphy is a very sensitive test compared to bone roentgenography, but nonspecificity of bone scanning is a problem. Even minor alterations of bone physiology and bone pathology such as arthritis, fracture, osteomyelitis, previous surgery, and regional osteoporosis can produce false-positive bone scans. The standard roentgenogram is relatively insensitive. A minimum of 30 to 50 percent of bone mineral must be lost before such lesions become visible on radiographs. Metastases to the spinal column are even more difficult to demonstrate with estimates of 50 to 75 percent of bone destruction being necessary before visualization is possible.[24] The appearance of a lesion on a scintiscan may precede radiographic visualization by 3 to 6 months. In patients with positive roentgenograms, the scan will not infrequently show that the amount of metastatic disease present is more than appreciated from the roentgenogram. Bone scans have a small percentage (3 to 8 percent) of false negatives. The false-negative studies usually occur in patients with highly anaplastic tumors or in patients with slow growing lesions where reactive bone does not form or is not detectable.

The incidence of false-negative bone scans in patients with highly anaplastic tumors can be decreased by appreciating the condition known as a superscan. A superscan occurs occasionally in patients with widespread, symmetric skeletal metastases from prostrate cancer in whom nearly all of the isotope is taken up by skeletal metastases and little remains to be excreted by the kidneys. This condition should be suspected when there are no kidney images, the quality of the scan seems better than usual, and for a given patient dose/kg and a fixed scanning time the scintigram is darker and for a fixed scanning count it takes less time. A quantitative index, the T-12 index, has been used to recognize the superscan.[28] The T-12 index is obtained by quantitating the activity in a region of interest over the lower dorsal spine and comparing it with the activity in a region in the soft tissue over the pelvic crest. The T-12 index is about 5 for both normal patients and patients with almost any degree of isolated metastases. The index is 10 (twice normal) as renal function diminishes to 0 and is 15 to 25 (three to five times normal) for the superscan category.

Practical Applications of Bone Scintigraphy

Prostate Cancer. Bone scintigraphy has been widely used in patients with prostate cancer since distant metastases are present in about 40 percent of patients with clinical prostatic cancer when the disease is first diagnosed and almost 80 percent of patients who die of prostatic cancer have skeletal involvement. Bone scans are indicated in the initial evaluation for staging prostatic cancer and to evaluate the source of pain (Fig. 7). Serial studies are helpful but often misleading in evaluating response to endocrine or chemotherapy, and consequently probably should not be done unless it is required by a protocol or the patient has new pain. A bone scan is not helpful after definitive treatment for localized disease unless the patient has developed pain or an elevated acid phosphatase.[29]

The initial evaluation of patients with prostate cancer should be as thorough as possible because treatment varies depending upon the stage of the disease and some of the complications (impotence and incontinence) of definitive treatment of early stages are not acceptable if the patient actually has metastatic disease. The bone scan is recommended because it is the most sensitive test for the detection of bone metastases.[30]

A bone scan can be very helpful in identifying the source of pain. A patient with a metastatic lesion in the spine and referred pain can have the source of pain demonstrated on a bone scan leading to palliative radiotherapy to the proper site.

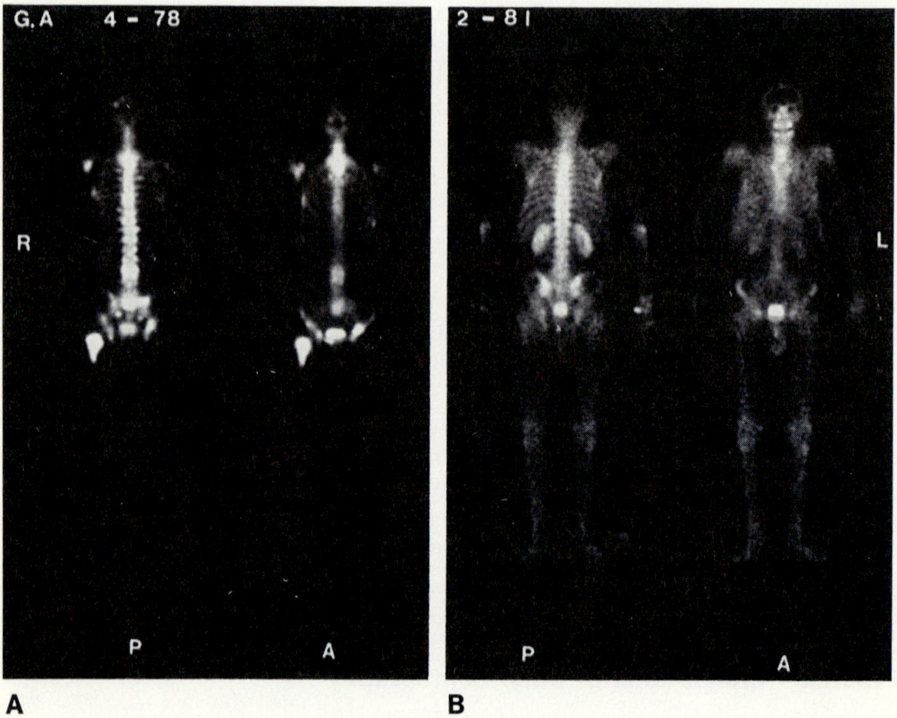

Figure 7. A. Bone scan in a patient with prostate cancer shows multiple areas of increased uptake of technetium-99m-methylene diphosphonate due to metastases and very poor renal visualization. Patient was treated with diethylstilbesterol. **B.** Bone scan in the same patient 3 years later shows no evidence of metastasis and good renal visualization. Incidentally, he is continuing to do very well 5 years after this bone scan.

Serial scanning to evaluate accurately the degree of progression or regression of disease is not always reliable.[31,32] The factors that may produce changes are (1) change in staff, (2) change in equipment, (3) change in the radiopharmaceutical agent, (4) change in the details of the protocol, and (5) change in the methods used to present the images. All those changes can occur within a hospital, but are more likely to be present when comparing serial studies done in different hospitals.

Levenson and associates found serial scanning to be very unreliable in 46 patients with stage D2 disease.[32] Most responding patients did not demonstrate improvement in bone scan or radiographs, but virtually all improving bone scans occurred in patients with tumor response. Disease progression usually was associated with worsening bone scans or radiographic findings. Because of a "flare" phenomenon, a worsening scan or radiograph could not be regarded as definite proof of tumor progression. In patients with a partial response, bone radiographs rarely improved and bone scans were better in only one third of the patients whereas worsening scans occurred in one fourth of patients with objective partial response. Pollen reported a better correlation with the bone scan with 79 percent (11 of 14) of responding patients showing improved scans.[33]

Serial follow-up bone scans after definitive therapy of localized prostatic cancer seems to be unnecessary.[29] Serial bone scans became positive in 19 percent of 100 patients followed after treatment for localized prostatic cancer. None of the patients, however, had a positive scan in the absence of either an elevated serum acid phosphatase or bone pain.

Kidney Carcinoma. Bone scintigraphy is used too often in the initial evaluation of patients with renal cell carcinoma. A review of only 12 cases of renal cell carcinoma concluded that the bone scan should be included in the initial evaluation of patients with renal tumors.[34] More recent reports of renal cell carcinoma, however, suggest that bone scintigraphy should not be expected to be very helpful in the evaluation of patients in the absence of skeletal symptoms, other metastatic lesions, and abnormal alkaline phosphatase.[35–38]

Three clinical reports concluded that bone scintigraphy is not helpful in the absence of other observations suggesting osseous metastases. Rosen and Murphy reviewed the records of 40 patients who had bone scintigraphy during the initial evaluation of renal cell carcinoma.[35] Only 3 of 40 (7.6 percent) had metastases detected by bone scan. Of those three patients, one had bone pain as the initial symptom, one had a lung metastasis, and only one was asymptomatic and had only a bone metastasis. Lindner and associates reviewed 53 patients and Blacher and associates reviewed 85 patients who had renal cell carcinoma and bone scans.[36,37] Neither study had any patients where osseous metastases were diagnosed solely on the basis of the bone scan.

Two other large series of renal tumor patients suggest that the bone scan should not be helpful. A review of 1668 renal cell carcinoma patients at the Mayo Clinic showed that 87 (5.2 percent) of the patients had bone metastases at the time of diagnosis and only 24 of those did not have symptoms referrable to bone metastases.[38] An autopsy series of 1451 cases of renal cell carcinoma showed bone metastases in 542 cases (37 percent).[39] However, metastases were confined to the bone in only 33 cases and 11 of those had metastasis to only one bone. Therefore, it seems very unlikely that a bone scan will detect bone metastases in a patient without other evidence of metastases and absence of bone pain.

Bladder Carcinoma. Bladder tumors metastasize to bone very rarely, especially compared to prostate and kidney tumors. Bone scans are recommended only for the unusual patient with skeletal symptoms.

Testis Tumors. Germ cell tumors rarely metastasize to bone before other obvious metastases. Seminoma is more likely to metastasize to bone if the patient has other known metastases.[40] A bone scan is recommended for the evaluation of seminoma if the patient has other metastases because the treatment would more likely include chemotherapy rather than radiotherapy if bone metastases were recognized.

Wilms' Tumor. Skeletal metastases are rare at diagnosis. Bone scans are indicated only when the tumor is found to be the clear cell sarcoma type which is associated with bony spread.[41]

Neuroblastoma. Bone is a common site of metastasis in patients with neuroblastoma. Therefore, bone scintigraphy is a helpful and important part of the evaluation of neuroblastoma.[42]

SCROTAL SCINTIGRAPHY

The cause of acute scrotal pain or swelling in a child or young adult is often either testicular torsion or epididymitis. Recognition and prompt treatment of testicular torsion is very important. Often a clinical examination permits the clinician to be confident of the presence or absence of testicular torsion, but frequently the diagnosis is equivocal. The diagnosis of testicular torsion by scrotal scintigraphy was first reported in 1973.[43] The test basically identifies poor blood flow. Scrotal scintigraphy technique has been improved during the past decade and recent reports have indicated accuracy of almost 100 percent.[44–51] It is a simple, rapid, noninvasive, reliable, and inexpensive test.

Technique and Interpretation

It is important for the nuclear physician to examine the scrotum and accurately localize the testicles. Technetium-99m-pertechnetate is rapidly injected intravenously. Multiple 3- to 5-second dynamic images are obtained for the angiographic phase, followed by static images to show the "blood pool" or "tissue phase." A pinhole collimator is used to obtain high resolution magnified static images.

The scintigraphic pattern of testicular torsion depends on the duration of torsion (Table 2 and Figs. 8 through 12). The dynamic images demonstrate activity from the pudendal arteries which do not pass through the spermatic cord. The static images show central areas of activity from the testicular artery and peripheral activity from the pudendal artery branches. The halo or rim of missed torsion is complete and symmetric compared to the incomplete and asymmetric rim seen with epididymitis. An abscess and hydrocele will show decreased activity in the static images but the clinical findings should help to clarify the diagnosis.

In summary, two basic patterns are seen, one with "cold" lesions with or without a surrounding rim of increased activity and the other with diffuse or focal increased blood flow and blood pool activity without any cold component. The cold lesions are seen with testicular torsion, abscess, hematoma, and hydrocele. The lesions with increased activity without any cold component are seen with epididymitis, torsion of appendages, and minor trauma. The diagnosis of spontaneous detorsion must be made from the clinical history.

Practical Applications

Scrotal scintigraphy is a very easy and helpful test for the evaluation of any acute scrotal pain or swelling of equivocal etiology. A clear clinical diagnosis of testicular torsion should be treated surgically without delay for a scrotal scan. Scrotal scintigraphy is also indicated for nonacute cases with ques-

TABLE 2. SCROTAL SCINTIGRAPHIC PATTERNS

Diagnosis	Dynamic Images	Static Images
Testicular torsion		
Early phase (1st 6 hr)	Decreased activity or normal	Decreased activity: no halo
Midphase (6–24 hr)	Increased activity	Decreased activity: halo
Late or missed (>24 hr)	Increased activity	Decreased activity: complete halo
Spontaneous detorsion	Normal or slightly increased activity	Normal or slightly increased activity
Acute epididymitis	Increased activity	Incomplete halo
Torsion of testicular appendage	Increased activity	Increased activity

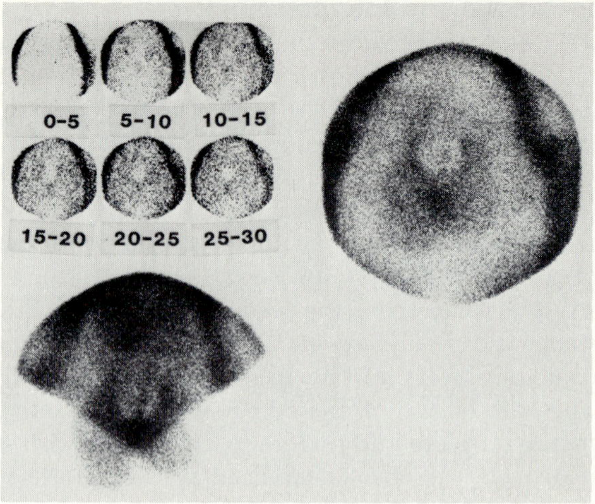

Figure 8. Normal scrotal scintigram. *(From Holder, LE, Melloul M, and Chen D: Semin Nucl Med 11:232, 1981, with permission.)*

tionable testicular viability after corrective detorsion and orchiopexy and with questionable abscess with epididymo-orchitis.

RADIONUCLIDE CYSTOGRAPHY

Radionuclide cystography for the detection of vesicoureteral reflux was first reported in 1959, shortly after the appreciation of the significance of reflux in children. The application of radionuclide cystography became popular during the early 1970s, mainly as a result of reports by Conway and associates.[52–54]

A prospective study comparing radionuclide to roentgenographic cystograms for detecting vesicoureteral reflux in 100 children using Tc-99m-pertechnetate with the gamma camera showed that radionuclide cystography was better than roentgenographic cystography.[52] Reflux was found in 44 of 200 possible renal units. In seven children (nine renal units), definite reflux was visualized only during the radionuclide examination. Reflux was seen only during roentgenograms in nine units, in four of which reflux was into the distal ureter only and appeared on only a single film of the roentgenographic series. Reflux into the distal ureter usually is not appreciated from radionuclide cystography. It was therefore concluded that more of the significant reflux was detected with the radionuclide study than with roentgenographic cystography.

The radiation exposure of children with vesicoureteral reflux is an important consideration when serial evaluations are being done over a period of several years. The radionuclide cystogram produces much less radiation exposure than the conventional radiographic cystogram. The dose to the bladder is estimated to be about 1 mrad/min for the usual μCi dose of Tc-

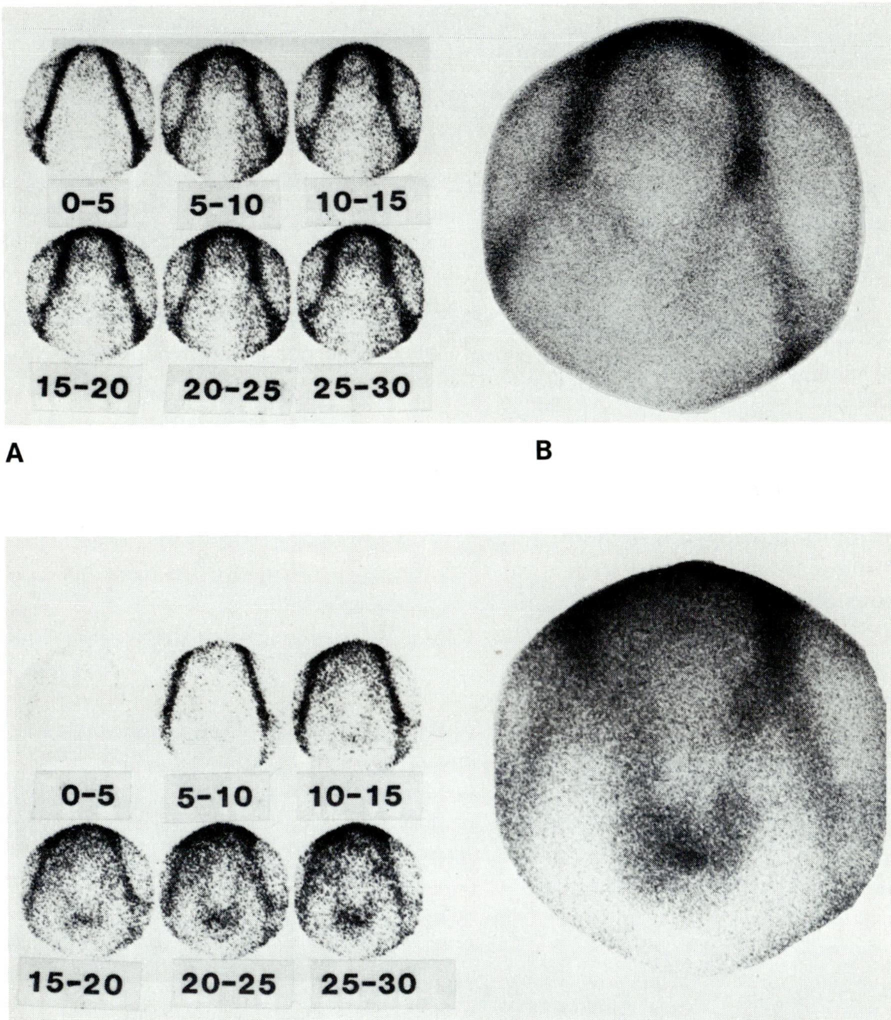

C D

Figure 9. A, B. Dynamic and static scrotal scintigram of a patient with acute testicular torsion. Dynamic scintigrams show no flow through right testicular or deferential vessels. Static scintigram shows an avascular right testicle and no halo. **C, D.** Scrotal scintigram of the same patient following surgical correction of right testicular torsion shows increased blood flow to the right testicle. *(From Holder LE, Melloul M, and Chen D: Semin Nucl Med 11:232, 1981, with permission.)*

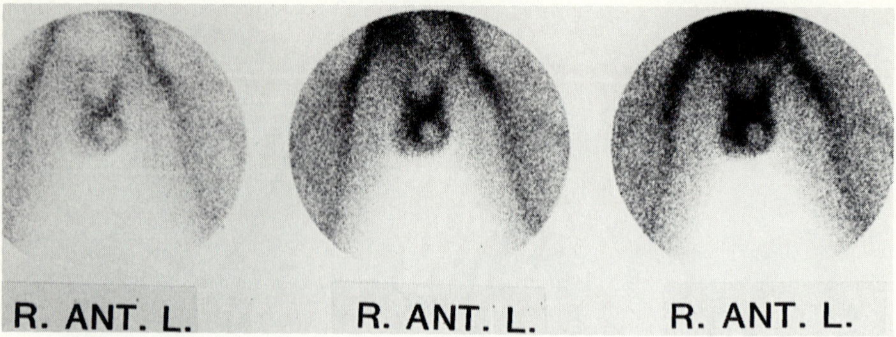

Figure 10. Scrotal scintigram shows a late or missed torsion with poor blood flow to the left testicle and a complete halo.

99m-pertechnetate in 200 cc of saline.[52] Therefore, the dose is 15 to 30 mrad for a 15- to 30-minute test. The dose to the gonads is probably less than 5 mrad. Radiographic cystourethrography produces a gonadal dose which ranges from 75 mrad to several rads depending on the fluoroscopy time and the number of films taken.[55]

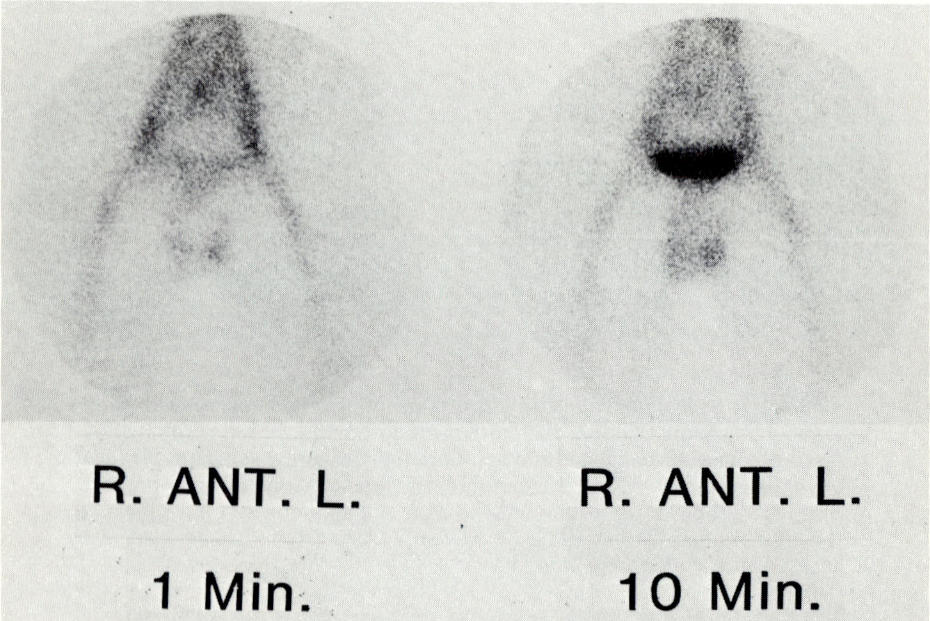

Figure 11. Static scrotal scintigram shows increased activity in left testicle shortly after manipulation and detorsion of testicle had been done in the emergency room. Scrotal scintigram confirmed satisfactory blood flow to the testicle eliminating the urgency of an operation.

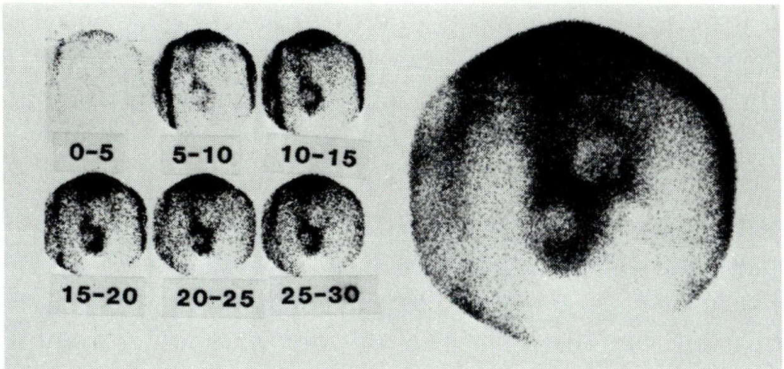

Figure 12. Scrotal scintigram of epididymitis shows increased activity in the epididymis and an incomplete halo. *(From Holder LE, Melloul M, and Chen D: Semin Nucl Med 11:232, 1981, with permission.)*

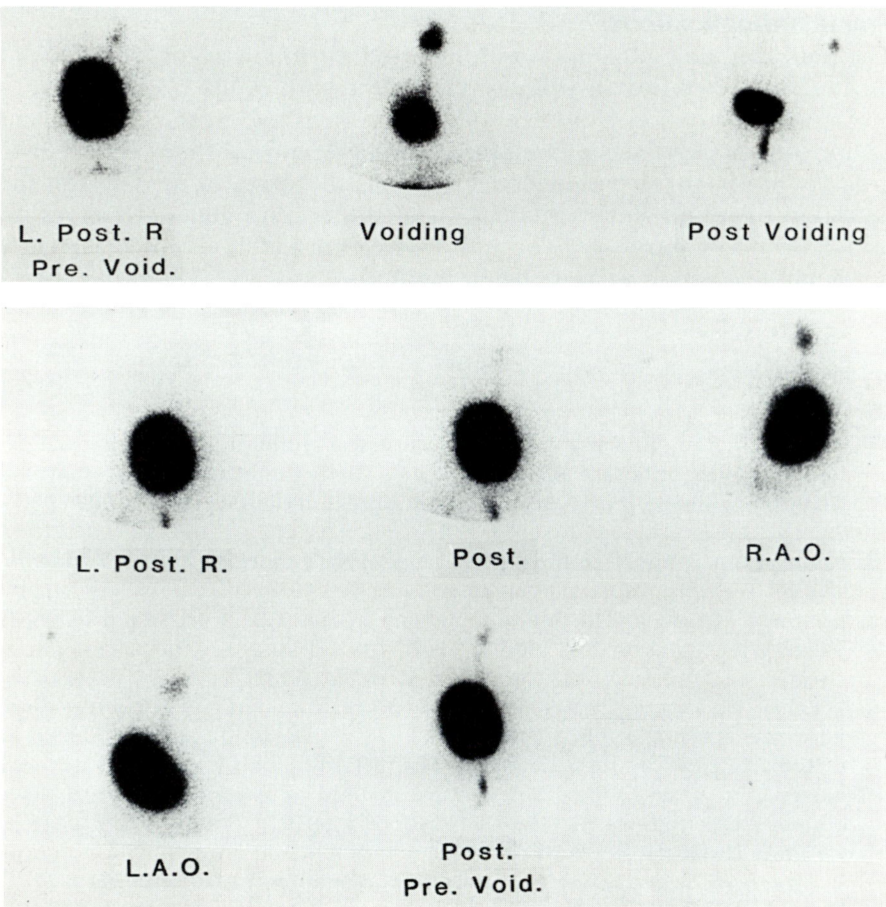

Figure 13. Radionuclide cystogram in a 2-year-old girl shows right vesicoureteral reflux which occurred at a bladder volume of 260 cc.

The radionuclide cystogram is performed with observation on a persistent scope. This enables constant monitoring without increasing radiation dosage. A high intensity is set on the gamma camera so that small amounts of radionuclide which reflux may be easily detected. Therefore, the bladder image is overexposed and appears larger than expected (Fig. 13).

The major disadvantage of radionuclide cystography is poor anatomic resolution compared to the radiographic cystogram. Therefore, it is not suitable for evaluation of the male urethra, accurate grading of reflux, and detecting minor abnormalities of the bladder wall such as small diverticula. Even though grading cannot be done by the standard method of radionuclide cystography, serial radionuclide cystograms can indicate improvement in the reflux if the reflux occurs after a larger volume of fluid has been instilled in the bladder.

Practical Applications

The radionuclide cystogram should be used for follow-up of children and for detection of reflux in siblings of children with reflux because it has a much lower radiation exposure and is very sensitive in the detection of reflux compared to the conventional radiographic voiding cystourethrogram. It has been recommended in girls as the initial screening test for detection of reflux since visualization of the urethra generally serves no useful diagnostic purpose.[56] This indication is not widely accepted currently but might become more popular in the future.

REFERENCES

1. Russell CD: Radiopharmaceuticals used to assess kidney function and structure. In Tauxe WN, Dubovsky EV (eds): Nuclear Medicine in Clinical Urology and Nephrology, chap 2. East Norwalk, Conn: Appleton-Century-Crofts, 1985, pp 7–29
2. Kontzen FM, Tobin M, Dubovsky EV, Tauxe WN: Comprehensive renal function studies: Technical aspects. J Nucl Med Tech 5:81, 1977
3. Dubovsky EV: Renal function and imaging studies. Clin Nucl Med 6:46, 1981
4. Tauxe WN, Dubovsky EV, Kidd T, et al: New formulas for the calculation of effective renal plasma flow. Eur J Nucl Med 5:51, 1982
5. O'Reilly PH, Testa HJ, Lawson RS, et al: Diuresis renography in equivocal urinary tract obstruction. Br J Urol 50:76, 1978
6. O'Reilly PH, Lawson RS, Shields RA, Testa HJ: Idiopathic hydronephrosis—the diuresis renogram: A new non-invasive method of assessing equivocal pelvioureteral junction obstruction. J Urol 121:153, 1979
7. Koff SA, Thrall JH, Keyes JW Jr: Diuretic radionuclide urography: A non-invasive method for evaluating nephroureteral dilatation. J Urol 122:451, 1979
8. Koff SA, Thrall JH, Keyes JW Jr: Assessment of hydroureteronephrosis in children using diuretic radionuclide urography. J Urol 123:531, 1980

9. Koff SA, Kogan B, Kass EJ, Thrall JH: Early postoperative assessment of the functional patency of ureterovesical junction following ureteroneocystostomy. J Urol 125:554, 1981
10. Koff SA: Ureteropelvic junction obstruction: Role of newer diagnostic methods. J Urol 127:898, 1982
11. Kass EJ, Majd M, Belman AB: Comparison of the diuretic renogram and the pressure perfusion study in children. J Urol 134:92, 1985
12. Whitaker RH: Methods of assessing obstruction in dilated ureters. Br J Urol 45:15, 1973
13. Whitaker RH: An evaluation of 170 diagnostic pressure flow studies of the upper urinary tract. J Urol 121:602, 1979
14. Whitaker RH, Buxton-Thomas MS: A comparison of pressure flow studies and renography in equivocal upper urinary tract obstruction. J Urol 131:446, 1984
15. Senac MO Jr, Miller JH, Stanley P: Evaluation of obstructive uropathy in children: Radionuclide renography vs. the Whitaker test. AJR 143:11, 1984
16. Bueschen AJ, Lloyd LK, Dubovsky EV, Tauxe WN: Radionuclide kidney function evaluation in the management of urolithiasis. J Urol 120:16, 1978
17. Kaude JV, Williams CM, Millner MR, et al: Renal morphology and function immediately after extracorporeal shock-wave lithotripsy. AJR 145:305, 1985
18. Lloyd LK, Dubovsky EV, Bueschen AJ, et al: Comprehensive renal scintillation procedures in spinal cord injury: Comparison with excretory urography. J Urol 126:10, 1981
19. Kuhlemeier KV, McEachran AB, Lloyd LK, et al: Renal function after acute and chronic spinal cord injury. J Urol 131:439, 1984
20. Keane JM, Schlegel JU: The use of a scintillation camera system for screening of hypertensive patients. J Urol 108:12, 1972
21. Dubovsky EV, Logic JR, Diethelm AG, et al: Comprehensive evaluation of renal function in the transplanted kidney. J Nucl Med 16:1115, 1975
22. Diethelm AG, Dubovsky EV, Whelchel JD, et al: Diagnosis of impaired renal function after kidney transplantation using renal scintigraphy, renal plasma flow, and urinary excretion of hippurate. Ann Surg 191:604, 1980
23. Subramanian G, McAfee JG, Blair RJ, et al: Technetium-99m-methylene diphosphonate—a superior agent for skeletal imaging: Comparison with other technetium complexes. J Nucl Med 16:744, 1975
24. O'Mara RE: Skeletal scanning in neoplastic disease. Cancer 37:480, 1976
25. Biello DR, Colemen RE, Stanley RJ: Correlation of renal images on bone scan and intravenous pyelogram. AJR 127:633, 1976
26. Pilbrow WJ: The urinary tract image obtained during ^{99m}Tc bone scanning. Clin Radiol 30:71, 1979
27. Pollen JJ, Gerber K, Heil BJ, Talner LB: Detection of ureteral obstruction on radionuclide bone scans. AJR 141:567, 1983
28. Constable AR, Cranage RW: Recognition of the superscan in prostatic bone scintigraphy. Br J Radiol 54:122, 1981
29. Huben RP, Schellhammer PF: The role of routine follow-up bone scans after definitive therapy of localized prostatic cancer. J Urol 128:510, 1982
30. Schaffer DL, Pendergrass HP: Comparison of enzyme, clinical radiographic, and radionuclide methods of detecting bone metastases from carcinoma of the prostate. Radiology 121:431, 1976

31. Constable AR: Invited review: Bone scintigraphy in nephro-urology. In Joekes AM, Constable AR, Brown NJG, Tauxe WN (eds): Radionuclides in Urology: Proceedings of the 5th International Symposium held 2–4 Sept., 1981 at the Royal Society, London. New York, Academic Press, 1982, p 313
32. Levenson RM, Sauerbrunn BJL, Bates HR, et al: Comparative value of bone scintigraphy and radiography in monitoring tumor response in systemically treated prostatic carcinoma. Radiology 146:513, 1983
33. Pollen JJ, Gerber K, Ashburn WL, Schmidt JD: Nuclear bone imaging in metastatic cancer of the prostate. Cancer 47:2585, 1981
34. Cole AT, Mandell J, Fried FA, Stabb EV: The place of bone scan in the diagnosis of renal cell carcinoma. J Urol 114:364, 1975
35. Rosen PR, Murphy KG: Bone scintigraphy in the initial staging of patients with renal cell carcinoma: Concise communication. J Nucl Med 25:289, 1984
36. Lindner A, Goldman DG, deKernion JB: Cost effective analysis of prenephrectomy radioisotope scans in renal cell carcinoma. Urology 22:127, 1983
37. Blacher E, Johnson DE, Haynie TP: Value of routine radionuclide bone scans in renal cell carcinoma. Urology 26:432, 1985
38. Forbes GS, McLeod RA, Hattery RR: Radiographic manifestations of bone metastases from renal carcinoma. AJR 129:61, 1977
39. Saitoh H: Distant metastasis of renal adenocarcinoma. Cancer 48:1487, 1981
40. Johnson DE, Appelt G, Samuels ML, Luna M: Metastases from testicular carcinoma. Urology 8:234, 1976
41. D'Angio GJ, Duckett JW Jr, Belasco JB: Tumors: Upper urinary tract. In Kelalis PP, King LR, Belman AB (eds): Clinical Pediatric Urology, 2nd ed, chap. 33. Philadelphia, Saunders, 1985
42. Howman-Giles RB, Gilday DL, Ash JM: Radionuclide skeletal survey in neuroblastoma. Radiology 131:497, 1979
43. Nadel NS, Gitter MH, Hahn LC, et al: Pre-operative diagnosis of testicular torsion. Urology 1:478, 1973
44. Chen DCP, Holder LE, Melloul M: Radionuclide scrotal imaging: Further experience with 210 patients. Part 1. Anatomy, pathophysiology, and methods. J Nucl Med 24:735, 1983
45. Chen DCP, Holder LE, Melloul M: Radionuclide scrotal imaging: Further experience with 210 new patients. Part 2. Results and discussion. J Nucl Med 24:841, 1983
46. Haynes BE, Bessen HA, Haynes VE: The diagnosis of testicular torsion. JAMA 249:2522, 1983
47. Kogan SK, Lutzker LG, Perez LA, et al: The value of the negative radionuclide scrotal scan in the management of the acutely inflamed scrotum in children. J Urol 122:223, 1979
48. Lutzker LG: The fine points of scrotal scintigraphy. Semin Nucl Med 12:387, 1982
49. Stage KH, Schoenvogel R, Lewis S: Testicular scanning: Clinical experience with 72 patients. J Urol 125:334, 1981
50. Thomas WEG, Cooke PH, Davies ER, et al: Dynamic radionuclide scanning of the testis in acute scrotal conditions. Br J Surg 68:621, 1981
51. Valvo JR, Caldamone AA, O'Mara R, Rabinowitz R: Nuclear imaging in the pediatric acute scrotum. Am J Dis Child 136:831, 1982
52. Conway JJ, King LR, Belman AB, Thorson T Jr: Detection of vesicoureteral re-

flux with radionuclide cystography. Am J Roentgenol Radium Ther Nucl Med 115:720, 1972

53. Conway JJ, Belman AB, King LR, Filmer RB: Direct and indirect radionuclide cystography. J Urol 113:689, 1975
54. Nasrallah PF, Conway JJ, King LR, et al: Quantitative nuclear cystogram. Urology 12:654, 1978
55. Leibovic SJ, Lebowitz RL: Reducing patient dose in voiding cystourethrography. Urol Radiol 2:103, 1980
56. Majd M: Nuclear medicine. In Kelalis PP, King LR, Belman AB (eds): Clinical Pediatric Urology, 2nd ed. Philadelphia, Saunders, 1985.

Shock and the Urologic Patient

Charles T. Fitts

BASIC PHILOSOPHY

The function of the circulatory system is to provide adequate perfusion of the tissues of the body. When it fails to do so, shock is present. There are several basic principles known concerning this problem that do not change from year to year and are vital to the successful clinical management of this problem. These principles have been established by years of investigative work in laboratories around the world and are as follows:

1. The conditions which may effectively interfere with adequate tissue perfusion are diverse and numerous. They may be obvious and directly related to the circulation (heart failure caused by arrhythmia) or obscure and only indirectly related to the circulation (hypoglycemic shock caused by excessive insulin).
2. There is no single treatment for shock. Treatment is specifically related to the cause, as, for instance, abolishment of the arrhythmia or raising the blood sugar in the two examples above.
3. The body can tolerate inadequate tissue perfusion for a limited period of time, which varies with the individual. Shock which is allowed to persist beyond this time in a given individual is almost invariably fatal no matter what the treatment.
4. The restoration of tissue perfusion before irreversible damage usually results in no permanent harm and is most often successfully

accomplished by identification of the specific cause or causes and correction of same.

An awareness of these principles allows one to keep some rather complex situations comfortably simplified. For instance, it becomes rather clear that much of the published research on shock states falls into one of three broad categories.

Category I involves data generated from experiments in which animals are placed in shock from a known cause, e.g., hemorrhage, endotoxin, burn, and the data are used for diagnostic purposes involving shock from that specific cause. Examples would be experiments with shock caused by hemorrhage which documented consistent lowered pH in the blood or experiments with shock caused by endotoxin administration which documented early elevated pH in the blood. Such data can be of great use to clinicians in establishing the specific shock-inducing problem existing in a given patient.

Category II involves data generated from experiments in which animals are placed in shock from a known cause, e.g., hemorrhage, endotoxin, burn, in which primary therapy directed at the specific insult is evaluated. An example would be shock induced by hemorrhage and various volume replacement regimens compared with each other for efficacy. Such data can be of great use to clinicians in establishing the most effective therapy for a specific shock-inducing problem.

Category III involves data generated from experiments in which animals are placed in shock from a known cause, e.g., hemorrhage, endotoxin, burn, in which primary therapy directed at the specific insult is deliberately withheld until it is felt that the damage is "irreversible." Secondary therapy aimed at correcting this irreversible state is then evaluated. An example is to induce hemorrhagic shock in animals, then prolong the period of hypotension before returning the shed blood long enough to insure that no animals will recover despite returning the shed blood. At this point treatment "X" is provided in addition to the return of the shed blood in one group. Increased survival in this group is interpreted as new and effective "therapy for shock." Such experiments are also not infrequently carried out with treatment administered *before* the induction of shock.

It is this category III research that must be carefully weighed by the clinician as it is extraordinarily contrived and complicated by clinical standards. There is practically no direct clinical relevance to those studies involving pretreatment. The opportunity for the clinician to deal with the other situations set up in category III research exists in only two sets of circumstances.

1. The patient was late in coming to medical attention and shock has been prolonged unduly.
2. The physician is unable to arrive at a correct diagnosis.

In these circumstances, specific therapy is either too late or not recognized as such. What is the likelihood that the clinician will be able to rescue this situation by applying the latest published category III therapy? As of the date of publication, an example would be the administration of an endorphin-blocking agent such as nalaxone.[1] In 1985 it probably would have been the administration of prostaglandin inhibitors,[2] in 1984 it probably would have been the use of cryoprecipitate to reverse fibronectin deficiencies.[3] In 1983 it was the administration of pharmacologic doses of steroids.[4] It seems safe to predict that therapy will change again next year. The fact of the matter is that there is no consensus of scientific data that shows any one treatment to be consistently effective in bringing about increased survival in animals in a category III experiment. Certainly there is no consensus concerning such nonspecific therapy in human shock. The regimen that has come closest to claiming this honor has been pharmacologic doses of steroids in septic shock. Even here, however, there is not clear agreement among published clinical data concerning the effect of such treatment on survival in humans with septic shock.[5] Certainly continued laboratory efforts to solve the problem of widespread cellular deterioration should and must continue; however, the clinician must maintain a clear and accurate understanding of the current status in this difficult area.

The reason for continued failure to find a cure-all for an animal that has suffered a prolonged period of inadequate tissue perfusion does not seem too difficult to imagine. Once perfusion has persisted to the point where metabolism cannot be maintained, cell death must occur including the denaturization of protein within the matrix. The chances of successfully reversing this process must be roughly the same as those involved in converting a hard boiled egg back into a viable chick embryo.

The job of the clinician in the management of shock then focuses heavily upon correct diagnosis of the specific cause followed by prompt treatment, the nature of which is determined by the cause of the shock.

DIAGNOSIS AND INITIAL MANAGEMENT

The diagnosis of shock is twofold. First, one establishes that inadequate tissue perfusion is present, then the specific cause is sought.

The establishment of the initial diagnosis should be instinctive and routine. It is based upon the clinician's ability to recognize the activation of the stereotyped sympathoadrenal-mediated response to inadequate tissue perfusion. This emergency mechanism causes immediate observable changes. Arteriolar constriction shunts blood away from skin, viscera, and muscle while preserving flow to heart and brain. Obvious physical findings as a result are cool, pale, clammy skin and no urine output. The heart beats faster and stronger in response to sympathoadrenal discharge. Respiratory effort is deepened and the rate increased. These measures may successfully defend the blood pressure temporarily thus technically allowing for shock to be present in the absence of a significantly lowered blood pressure. This does not usually last long, however, and as a standard clinical rule, shock presents with lowered blood pressure more often than not. Any previously normotensive patient with a systolic blood pressure below 90 mm Hg should be considered in shock until proved otherwise.

The diagnosis of the specific etiology of shock is not entirely a scientific entity but is still partially an art. Every clinician should have developed in his mind a set of priorities for this emergency that allows him to take effective rapid steps to *simultaneously* approach a diagnosis and initiate therapy. The key to this approach involves estimates of probabilities and safety factors. There are two specific causes of shock which together make up the majority of cases encountered. These two cases are volume deficit and pump failure. Accordingly it is logical that the initial management of shock immediately focuses on an assessment of these two problems. In these terms it is well to remember a simple set of principles. The heart is a pump that pumps what comes to it. It cannot pump what does not come to it. If it does not pump what does come to it, it is failing. (Armed with these self-evident truths alone a surgeon can enter a room full of physiologists, participate in an hour long discussion of circulatory dynamics and emerge with only superficial abrasions.) Venous return is therefore the logical point at which to begin the assessment. It is for this reason that the placement of a central venous line close to but not in[6] the right atrium is the most helpful initial step. Two things are immediately accomplished. One is able to give drugs and fluids intravenously and can, in addition, assess the question of whether the right heart is or is not successfully pumping what comes to it. If the right heart is in fact successfully pumping what comes to it, central venous pressure (CVP) should measure 10 cm H_2O or less. Therefore, in the absence of a significant elevation of CVP over this level or most certainly with even lower CVP values, an immediate bolus of fluid (isotonic saline or Ringer's lactate) can be given intravenously. If on the other hand, CVP is markedly elevated (greater than 15 cm H_2O) or becomes so after fluid administration, one must assume that pump failure is operative. At this time, aggressive fluid input is stopped and cardiac assessment assumes priority. This use of CVP has held up over the years as a safe and practical initial step to take in shock, especially in young, previously healthy patients with early shock. In older patients or as shock persists and complications such as adult respiratory distress syndrome or renal failure occur, the need for measurement of left heart filling pressure may arise. This currently requires the Swan-Ganz balloon flotation catheter. With this instrument in place left-sided, cardiac filling pressure can be determined as well as serial cardiac outputs with the thermodilution technique. Cardiac output and blood pressure measurements can then be used to derive values for total peripheral resistance. Basically, however, this device is used to cover the possibility that the left and right sides of the heart may not necessarily function equally and measurement of filling pressure in one side alone could fail to detect failure of the other side. It should be mentioned here that the placement of a Swan-Ganz catheter is an invasive procedure not without complications. It is not indicated in every patient in shock but generally should be reserved for those patients with known or suspected myocardial, pulmonary, or renal dysfunction. Currently, venous return and filling pressure are now called preload. Measures which increase venous return or filling pressure are said to increase preload and generally are judged favorable. It should be remembered, however, that increasing preload above 15 to 18 mm Hg for the left ventricle or 15 cm H_2O for the right ventricle will not increase cardiac output in the normal heart. Another old familiar concept that has acquired a new name is peripheral resistance or that resistance against which the heart must work to expel blood. The new name is afterload and, in general, when attempting to maximize cardiac performance, it is considered favorable to take measures which diminish afterload within limits and to increase preload within limits.

This immediate, combined diagnostic-therapeutic attack upon the questions of hypovolemia and pump failure should be the foundation of the initial management of shock. The less common causes of shock must be considered as part of the process, however, and ruled in or out as soon as possible. The successful accomplishment of this objective is assured by different routines adopted by individuals and is certainly part of the art of medicine and not susceptible to rigid considerations. It should be sufficient to note that at a minimum, sepsis, anaphylaxis, adrenal insufficiency, hypoglycemia, pericardial tamponade, tension pneumothorax, drug overdose, and acute gastric dilatation are considered in each case.

TREATMENT OF HEMORRHAGIC SHOCK

The treatment of shock caused by hemorrhage begins as already mentioned with the combined therapeutic-diagnostic cornerstone of establishing a large bore (16-gauge or bigger) centrally placed venous line and measuring filling pressure (preload) while administering crystalloid solutions. External hemorrhage may be obvious at this time and should be controlled by pressure. If shock is caused by hemorrhage, the CVP should usually be low and rises little with fluid infusion while arterial pressure responds with a rise. Once the diagnosis of hemorrhagic shock is established, proper treatment consists of immediate aggressive fluid replacement. The preponderance of evidence at this time establishes Ringer's lactate and blood to be the fluids of choice.[7] At this time there is no known safer or more effective fluid to use initially than the crystalloid Ringer's lactate. Furthermore, extensive work during the past has established that in hemorrhagic shock there occurs a deficit in extracellular fluid which is greater than the volume of shed blood.[8,9] The use of sodium-containing fluids in addition to blood replacement has been shown to increase survival.[10] Therefore, the initial use of Ringer's lactate will prove to be wise in almost any circumstance. If blood loss is held to a relatively low level and resuscitation is rapid, it is best to replace blood loss only with Ringer's lactate (at about a 3:1 or 4:1 ratio) as long as the hematocrit does not drop below 30 thereby avoiding the risks of blood transfusions. There seems to be reasonable support for the belief that a hematocrit between 30 and 35 is quite efficient since raising the level higher gives little extra oxygen-carrying capacity to blood and the rheologic properties at this level are superior to those at higher levels. On the other hand, if hemorrhage is severe or continuing, the initial use of Ringer's lactate has helped restore tissue perfusion while blood was being properly typed and crossed. Also, as already pointed out, the crystalloid would have been needed in addition to the blood anyway for most effective therapy.

The role of colloid solutions in the treatment of hemorrhagic shock appears to have steadily decreased as experimental and clinical studies continue to accumulate a preponderance of data that no colloid solutions are superior to blood and Ringer's lactate in survival results and most are associated with increased risks and expense.[11–13] That means currently there is no reason to give albumin, plasmanate, dextran, hetastarch, or any other colloid solution.

There are measures that should be routinely considered when the number of blood transfusions begins to grow since dilutional coagulopathy and bleeding can become problems. In general it is considered advisable to give one unit of fresh frozen plasma after five units of packed red blood cells. Although platelet measurements may indicate more or less need for platelet transfusions, a good rule of thumb is to consider giving 12 platelet packs per 10 units of packed red cells.

The use of vasoactive drugs in the treatment of uncomplicated hemorrhagic shock has never been shown to increase survival in either animal or human studies.

The determination of arterial pH, Pco_2, and Po_2 is of great help in estimating the status of tissue perfusion. In shock caused by hemorrhage, aerobic glycolysis is shifted to anaerobic glycolysis as less oxygen is available to the tissues. This prevents the oxidation of glucose all the way to CO_2 and H_2O (with a consequent severe drop in energy production) and an accumulation of lactic acid. The resulting metabolic acidosis is generally accompanied by a normal Po_2. It must be realized that these relatively normal blood gas values reflect the situation with a successful compensatory increase in rate and depth of respiration which is an integral part of the response to hemorrhage. Even slight pulmonary pathology may lead to rapid deterioration in these values, if it interferes with the compensatory effort and uncovers the fact that the lungs are dealing with inadequate tissue perfusion along with the rest of the body.[14] Accordingly, the clinician must be aggressive in protecting pulmonary function and the administration of oxygen is indicated. Successful restoration of adequate tissue perfusion is invariably accompanied by a rapid and satisfying return of the pH of the blood to a normal value. Direct efforts to correct this metabolic acidosis by the administration of alkalizing agents such as sodium bicarbonate are generally unrewarding. Further evidence of successful resuscitation includes a return of arterial pressure to normal, CVP within normal limits, slowing of the pulse, warming of the skin, and restoration of urinary output to 30 cc/hr or more in the adult. Failure to achieve such results in a case of hemorrhagic shock should lead one to consider serious continued hemorrhage, a significant complicating factor or a misdiagnosis.

TREATMENT OF SEPTIC SHOCK

Sepsis may be the cause of inadequate tissue perfusion and the combination is termed septic shock. Of the particular types of shock, this one has more reason to concern the urologist than most since the urinary tract is the most common source of gram-negative infection and urinary tract instrumentation or surgery frequently precedes the event. Approximately 20 percent of patients with gram-negative bacteremia develop septic shock, while only 5 percent of patients with gram-positive bacteremia do so. Since gram-negative bacteremia is four to five times more common than gram-positive bacteremia, it is easy to understand that some refer to the problem as gram-negative shock.

Septic shock is a more complex problem than almost any other type of shock and presents some highly distinctive clinical and laboratory findings, knowledge of which is vital to successful management.

The pathophysiology of septic shock has not been entirely delineated but major deficiencies in peripheral utilization of substrates including at least glucose, oxygen, and amino acids are consistently documented.[15-17] How these deficiencies are brought about is controversial. There is evidence that the complement system, B-endorphin production by the pituitary, prostaglandins, and peripheral shunting participate in the process among others. By whatever mechanism, the end result of the impaired peripheral utilization results in cellular deprivation, increased capillary permeability with attendant volume loss, and possibly direct myocardial depression later. One of the unique features of septic shock is the initial response of the body to this situation. The cardiac output is elevated, the total peripheral resistance is decreased, and metabolic *alkalosis* is present while arterial blood pressure is low and urine output is decreased to absent. Except for the lowered blood pressure and decreased urinary output, these findings are the opposite of those noted in hemorrhagic shock. The patient clinically presents with warm pink skin and obvious hyperdynamic circulation. Mild lethargy and confusion are frequent. This is the early stage of septic shock, that stage when therapy has the greatest likelihood of success. If effective intervention is not carried out during this stage, the patient progresses at a variable rate to a more severe stage in which the hemodynamic findings convert to decreased cardiac output, increased total peripheral resistance, and severe metabolic acidosis. The patient now takes on the classic picture of inadequate tissue perfusion, i.e., the skin is cold, clammy, and pale and pulse weak and thready. Therapy in this stage has much less chance of success. Accordingly, it is of great importance that the clinician make the diagnosis early and institute therapy promptly.

The clinical diagnosis of early septic shock is made in the presence of:

1. Hypotension
2. Probable or known source of infection
3. Fever and/or leukocytosis and/or chills
4. Altered mental status
5. Hyperventilation

Confirmatory laboratory findings include respiratory alkalosis, increased cardiac output, and decreased total peripheral resistance. A lowered platelet count sometimes occurs, especially in children.

The treatment of septic shock is best started with the insertion of a large bore intravenous needle preferably in a central venous position. The need for a Swan-Ganz catheter is likely, although young patients with early shock from an obvious, rapidly correctable cause may not require it. Crystalloid solutions should be administered until systemic blood pressure or CVP or pulmonary wedge pressure rise sharply while an appropriate broad-spectrum antibiotic coverage aimed at the likely spectrum of organism is started intravenously. Blood, urine, sputum, and other cultures and Gram stains as indicated are obtained and major efforts directed at uncovering any focus of infection that may be drained. The computed tomography scan has become extremely useful in such a search when the physical findings are not obvious. These three measures are the standard of treatment—fluids, drainage, antibiotics—and if applied early should reverse the shock. If shock is found late or progresses rapidly because of complicating factors, therapy becomes much more difficult and less likely to succeed. The role of pharmacologic doses of steroids in the management of this problem is controversial. Laboratory data have accumulated over many years in animal models of various forms of septic shock in which steroid administration has been beneficial more often than not. In addition there is an equally impressive accumulation of evidence documenting specific effects of steroids such as inhibition of leukocyte aggregation, stabilization of lysosomal membranes, and decrease in capillary permeability, all of which have theoretical benefits in septic shock.

A clinical trial of steroids in septic shock including a prospective study with definite increased survival in the steroid-treated patients has been published.[4] A more recently published prospective clinical study, however, does not reveal increased survival in the steroid-treated groups.[5] A large multicenter study is now in effect hopefully to answer this question. It is this author's opinion that the data in both of the above publications as well as other data support the use of methylprednisolone sodium succinate (30 mg/kg of body weight) intravenously over 10 to 15 minutes after the establishment of the diagnosis of septic shock, to be repeated 4 hours later if shock persists.

The use of vasoactive drugs has never been shown to increase survival in septic shock. Nevertheless, human nature being what it is, there is always a current acceptable drug to utilize when therapy is failing. That currently accepted drug is dopamine, having replaced isuprel in the last few years, which in turn had replaced aramine, which in its turn had replaced norepinephrine.

Although many other drugs are being utilized in studies of septic shock with some favorable results, currently the most exciting prospect is the B-endorphin antagonist naloxone which has emerged from successful animal studies[18] and is beginning to be reported clinically.[1,19]

REFERENCES

1. Rock P, Silverman H, Plump D, et al: Efficacy and safety of Naloxone in septic shock. Crit Care Med 13:28, 1985
2. Fink M, MacVittie T, Casey L: Inhibition of prostaglandin synthesis restores normal hemodynamics in canine hyperdynamic sepsis. Ann Surg 200:619, 1984
3. Saba T, Niehaus G, Scovill W, et al: Lung vascular permeability after reversal of fibronectin deficiency in septic sheep: Correlation with patient studies. Ann Surg 198:654, 1983
4. Schumer W: Steroids in the treatment of clinical septic shock. Ann Surg 184:333, 1976
5. Sprung C, Caralis P, Marcial E, et al: The effects of high-dose corticosteroids in patients with septic shock. A prospective, controlled study. N Engl J Med 311:1137, 1984
6. Fitts C, Barnett L, Webb C, et al: Perforating wounds of the heart caused by central venous catheters. J Trauma 10:764, 1970
7. Shires G: Pathophysiology and fluid replacement in hypovolemic shock. Ann Clin Res 9:144, 1977
8. Shires T, Coln D, Carrico J, Lightfoot S: Fluid therapy in hemorrhagic shock. Arch Surg 88:688, 1964
9. Crenshaw C, Carrizara P, Allsman A, Shires G: Changes in extracellular fluid during acute hemorrhagic shock in man. Surg Forum 13:6, 1962
10. Baxter C, Maynard D: Prevention and recognition of surgical renal complications. In Jenkins MT (ed): Common and Uncommon Problems in Anesthesiology. Philadelphia, F.A. Davis, 1969
11. Moyer C, Margraf H, Monafo W Jr: Burn shock and extravascular sodium deficiency: Treatment with Ringer's solution with lactate. Arch Surg 90:799, 1965

12. Sturm J, Carpenter M, Lewis F Jr, et al: Water and protein movement in the sheep lung after septic shock: Effect of colloid versus crystalloid resuscitation. J Surg Res 26:233, 1979
13. Shoemaker W, Hauser C: Critique of crystalloid versus colloid therapy in shock and shock lung. Crit Care Med 7:117, 1979
14. McLaughlin J, Suddhimondala C, Mech K Jr, et al: Pulmonary gas exchange in shock in humans. Ann Surg 169:42, 1969
15. Gump F, Long C, Killian P, et al: Studies of glucose intolerance in septic injured patients. J Trauma 14:378, 1974
16. Siegel J, Greenspan M, DelGuercio L: Abnormal vascular tone, defective oxygen transport and myocardial failure in septic human shock. Ann Surg 165:504, 1967
17. Freund H, Ryan J Jr, Fischer J: Amino acid derangements in patients with sepsis: Treatment with branched-chain amino acid rich effusions. Ann Surg 188:423, 1978
18. Evans S, Hinds C, Varley J: Effects of intravascular volume expansion on the cardiovascular response to Naloxone in a canine model of severe endotoxin shock. Br J Pharmacol 83:443, 1984
19. Groeger J, Carlon G, Howland W: Naloxone in septic shock. Crit Care Med 11:650, 1983

Current Status of Neonatal Circumcision

W.R. Turner, Jr.

Circumcision is one of the most ancient of surgical procedures and also the most common one that is done in the United States.[1] Egyptian wall paintings from around 2300 B.C. illustrate a man undergoing circumcision[2] and some authorities feel that this may have been a method of marking slaves. The ancient Hebrews of the same era practiced circumcision but for them it represented a covenant with God,[3] as is clearly outlined in the Torah. Circumcision, historically, was so widespread that Columbus is said to have encountered it in natives[4] of the New World. Obviously, it represents a time-honored and ancient ritual, but its practice today (other than as a religious rite) continues to be questioned and even condemned by the medical community. To paraphrase Winston Churchill, never has so much been written about so little.

The sheer numbers of circumcisions performed each year, estimated at 1.5 million,[1] should be of concern if, as noted by the American Academy of Pediatrics, there is no valid medical indication for neonatal circumcision. The frequency with which it is done should suggest that inevitably this procedure will result in litigation and Fink[5] notes that two law suits are in progress in California charging that circumcision was "an inhumane act, has no basis medically, is a forceable removal done with ill will for traditional, cultural, and religious reasons unrelated to medicine." All urologists are aware of numerous suits for the complications of circumcision, but these contentions represent a potentially ominous turn. If circumcision has so few genuine indications, why does it persist? Since it has sprung up in many societies, is there some tribal wisdom for it or is it simply a rite of passage? The

Alexandrian philosopher, Philo, is quoted as saying concerning circumcision, "It would serve well to investigate more wisely and seriously the causes, thanks to which this custom has prevailed and not hastily pass judgement on the recklessness of great nations."[5]

Assuredly, in older children and adults, there are valid indications for circumcision including such problems as phimosis, paraphimosis, and balanoposthitis; however, these are extremely rare occurrences in the newborn. It is quite doubtful that phimosis is a meaningful diagnosis in the neonate since the vast majority of newborns will not have a retractile foreskin[6] because of adhesions which are normally present between the glans and the foreskin until around 3 to 4 years of age.

If newborns are not routinely circumcised, it has been estimated that between 2 to 10 percent of males will ultimately require this operation.[6,7] Does this justify routine circumcision? Probably not, but recent data concerning the relationship of neonatal circumcision to urinary tract infection (UTI) shed additional light on this discussion. In a series of 5261 male neonates, Wiswell et al[8] found an infection rate of 4.1 percent in the uncircumcised compared to 0.21 percent in the circumcised. Bacteriuria was the yardstick for diagnosing a UTI and these figures represent a 20-fold increase of UTIs in the uncircumcised as compared to the circumcised. In those children with UTIs, 83 percent were less than 3 months of age. Ginsburg and McCracken[9] also noted that the vast majority of UTIs in male infants occurred in the uncircumcised male. Several authors have noted the presence of gram-negative bacteria under the foreskin of the uncircumcised male child, a finding which decreases with age and is rare by age 5 years.[10–12] The decrease in bacterial contamination of the preputial space would appear to roughly correlate with the incidence of UTI in boys, which becomes increasingly less common with the passage of years. Williams wondered if the staghorn calculi he saw in his clinic in London might possibly be caused by *Proteus* organisms harbored under the foreskin.[13] No definitive data could be collected, however, because so few neonates in England undergo circumcision. Although the risk of UTI is low whether or not neonatal circumcision is carried out,[14,15] it seems clear that the child who is uncircumcised is at greater risk for preputial bacteria and resulting UTIs. A possible explanation for this was thought to be bacterial contamination that was normally prevented by a defensive barrier under the prepuce such as preputial glands that could produce an immune barrier system in much the same manner as Stamey and Howell have described in the vagina of females.[16] However, dermatopathologic study could demonstrate no glandular structures in the inner surface of the prepuce.[17] In the absence of vesicoureteral reflux, it may fairly be asked, do these UTIs place the child's kidneys at risk? Probably not. Even though Roberts[12] has noted that pyelonephritic scarring may rarely occur without demonstrable reflux, in the great majority of cases demonstrating renal damage, UTI and vesicoureteral reflux both exist.[18] One may wonder, in view of the documented increase of UTI in uncircumcised children and in view of the certain knowledge that reflux of infected urine may lead to renal damage, if there is a population of neonates that would indeed benefit from routine circumcision? Since Noe has indicated that the incidence of males with reflux may approach that of females in frequency,[19] it is tempting to be greatly concerned about male neonates who might be prone to UTI and complications, such as children of diabetics, and to consider such groups as prime candidates for "routine" neonatal circumcision. Clearly, this cannot be answered definitively, but the recent work of Wiswell and colleagues[8] inevitably leads to the conclusion that circumcision, in certain instances, may indeed be prophylactic and need not be condemned, as frequently is the case.

Prevention of malignancy, particularly penile cancer, by circumcision has been espoused by many as yet another reason for routine neonatal circumcision. The risk of an uncircumcised male having carcinoma of the penis depends, however, upon the hygiene of the individual and, indirectly, upon the particular society being evaluated. In Denmark, the risk is about 1 in 907 and this is probably a fair representation of the risk of penile cancer in a highly civilized and hygienic Western society.[20] Moreover, King notes that proper washing will probably provide protection equal to that of circumcision, and therefore circumcision to prevent carcinoma of the penis has little merit.[21] The incidence of carcinoma of the cervix is said to be less in Israeli women who are, presumably, married to men who have been circumcised neonatally.[22,23] At present the data are still unclear about the relationship of circumcision to carcinoma of the cervix but it does not appear to support the view that circumcision protects female partners from cervical cancer.[21-24] Apt[23] has also suggested that carcinoma of the prostate is four times greater in uncircumcised Scandinavians but at present no data seem to corroborate this.[25]

Warner and Straskin have suggested that venereal disease might be prevented by circumcision but there seems to be general agreement that no such statement can be supported as a reason for routine circumcision.[7]

Cameron has presented data which suggest that uncircumcised males may be more susceptible to contracting the AIDS virus.[26]

There are many contraindications to circumcision such as hypospadias, bleeding tendency, premature birth, myelomeningocele, sickle cell disease, and blood dyscrasias, to mention a few and one must seriously question any "routine procedure" which has so many contraindications. It must also be asked if circumcision has a significant complication rate, specifically what is the risk of death. Mortality associated with circumcision varied from none in 500,000 done in New York City[15] to 0.067 percent in a series described by Speert.[27] Any statistics on complication rates of neonatal circumcision must be viewed in light of the fact that they are difficult to ascertain since the infant is usually followed by someone other than the physician doing the circumcision. It should also be noted that the complication rate is directly related to the definition of the term. For example, in one series of circumcisions, done under general anesthesia, vomiting was noted as a complication resulting in a high complication rate in that series. It is clear, however, that several types of complications do occur frequently. One of the most common is meatitis with a resulting meatal stenosis caused by the exposure of the unprotected glans to the urine-soaked diaper. Meatal stenosis has been wittily referred to by a prominent British urologist as "... the price you Americans pay for your obsession with circumcisions." Meatal stenosis that is truly obstructive is unusual. Removal of too much or too little skin also seems to be a common problem but only occasionally does it necessitate repeat circumcision or operative correction. The hidden penis syndrome is one of the more dramatic complications of circumcision and it most probably is caused by insufficient removal of the inner layer of the prepuce, thus allowing the penile shaft skin to extend over the glans penis scarring cicatricially and pushing the penis down into the fat pad. Significant bleeding postcircumcision occurs in about 1 percent of patients and one ritual circumcision patient is noted to have died secondary to the delayed transfusion.[28] In one series of 140 circumcisions, 2 children needed to be readmitted to address bleeding which clearly can occur, albeit rarely. Wound infection is uncommon,[29] although Fournier's gangrene has been reported in two children postcircumcision[30] and several lawsuits are now pending over the loss of the glans penis. Urethral fistulas can occur and sloughing of the skin and adhesions of the foreskin round out a cursory list of complications which also may occur. Even if no difficulty results from the circumcision, one must consider pain to the neonate as a complication. Many consider the neonatal nervous system so immature that pain of significant degree does not occur. Talbert and colleagues,[31] however, have shown a consistent rise in both cortisol and cortisone levels suggesting a pain response during and immediately after circumcision, so perhaps it is wishful thinking to say that the neonate does not have significant pain. Certainly, all neonates do indeed scream when the clamps are applied.[1]

If "routine circumcision" is severely questioned by the Academy of Pediatrics and by most pediatricians, why do 80 percent of American males undergo circumcision as opposed to less than 10 percent in Great Britain?[7] In 1949, Gardner noted that, in England, circumcision was most common in the upper class public school students and that the rate was vastly lower in a working class community such as Newcastle.[4] Slaby and Drizd[33] showed that the circumcised rate increases with increased economic status and whites are much more likely to be circumcised than blacks. It is obvious that social and intellectual status have much to do with the parents' desire for circumcision. Lindeke[32] and others[33] substantiated an educational bias and added that the status of the father's penis, circumcised or uncircumcised, lent great weight to the parents' decision. Often mothers did not understand what was being done and why,[34] yet most wanted circumcision despite being told that it was most likely a socially motivated operation. A further disturbing factor was that only about 7 percent of these mothers remembered being counseled about circumcision by the obstetrician.[35] The series by Metcalf et al[35] showed that parents wanted circumcision to improve hygiene in 69 percent, because of custom in 21 percent, because the father was circumcised and for physical appearance in 14 percent.[34] It is logical to ask how these parents feel about their own penile status. In Harmond's[36] series of 311 males, 6.3 percent of circumcised men wished they had not been; of 106 uncircumcised males, 47 percent wished they had been neonatally circumcised; and 50 percent of these men had been circumcised after the neonatal period. Patel[37] noted that only 20 percent of newborns were circumcised if the neonate's physician was opposed to it, while 100 percent of neonates were circumcised if the physician favored it. It is therefore obvious that most nonritual circumcision is done for social and perceived needs rather than as a scientifically based decision.

At this point in a review such as this, circumcision would probably be roundly denounced because of its unscientific basis. However, the work of Wiswell et al,[8] noting a 20-fold greater incidence of UTIs in uncircumcised males, might lend a prudent individual to the conclusion that perhaps routine neonatal circumcision is too readily being condemned. There may indeed be a role for prophylactic routine circumcision, but before one rushes to embrace this, one must look carefully at complication rates and must also make every effort to educate the parents on the pros and cons of neonatal circumcision, while making certain that the parents have understood the information that was being given and have understood that circumcision is not viewed as a medical necessity. Under these circumstances and with a consent that is clearly documented, neonatal circumcision done by a skilled individual is certainly reasonable and is much preferable to "routine circumcision" that is carried out under anesthesia at a later date because of parental wishes. It may well be that further study on circumcision may demonstrate certain neonatal populations that are particularly prone to UTIs and in these neonates, circumcision may be advocated by the physician for true medical reasons. It is probably ill advised to have a "routine" neonatal circumcision policy since by its very nature this avoids a decision-making process. There is not as yet enough evidence to justify universal circumcision for prophylaxis alone but there may well be justification for it in certain highly specified and uncommon situations. When parents are totally informed of the indications, contraindications, complications, and risks as well as the position of the Academy of Pediatrics and they still wish for neonatal circumcision to be done by a skilled practitioner, then that is a reasonable decision. Certainly, the condemnation of all neonatal circumcision seems unwise.

REFERENCES

1. Watterstein E: Circumcision. The uniquely American medical enigma. Urol Clin North Am 12:123, 1985
2. Majno G: The Healing Hand. Cambridge, Mass., The Harvard Press, 1975, p 230

3. Genesis: 17:9–14
4. Gardner D: The fate of the foreskin. Br Med J 2:1433, 1949
5. Fink AJ: Letter to editor. Pediatrics 77(2):265, 1986
6. Thompson HC, King LR, Knox E, Korones SB: Report of the ad hoc task force on circumcision. Pediatrics 56:610, 1975
7. Warner E, Straskin E: Benefits and risks of circumcision. Can Med Assoc J 125:967, 1982
8. Wiswell TE, Smith FR, Bass JW: Pediatrics 75(5):901, 1985
9. Ginsburg CM, McCracken GH: Urinary tract infections in young infants. Pediatrics 69:409, 1982
10. Bollgren I, Winberg J: The periurethral aerobic bacterial flora in healthy boys and girls. Acta Pediatr Scand 65:74, 1976
11. Winberg J, Anderson HJ, Bergstrom T, et al: Epidemiology of symptomatic urinary tract infection in childhood. Acta Paed Scand 65:74, 1976
12. Roberts JA: Does circumcision prevent urinary tract infection? J Urol 135:991, 1986
13. Williams Sir DI: Personal communication
14. Winberg J, Andersen HJ, Bergstrom T: Epidemiology of symptomatic urinary tract infection in childhood. Acta Pediatr Scand 252(suppl):1, 1974
15. Slotkowski EL, King LR: Neonatal circumcision in Illinois. Illinois Med J 162(5):421, 1982
16. Stamey TA, Howell JJ: Studies of introital colonization in women with recurrent urinary tract infections. IV. The role of local vaginal antibodies. J Urol 120:742, 1978
17. Maize JC: Personal communication
18. Smellie JM, Normand ICS: Bacteriuria, reflux, and renal scarring. Arch Dis Child 50:581, 1975
19. Noe HN: Screening for familial reflux. Semin Urol IV(2):86, 1986
20. Swafford TD: Circumcision and the risk of cancer of the penis. Am J Dis Child 139:112, 1985
21. King LR: Neonatal circumcision in the United States in 1982. J Urol 128:1135, 1982
22. Hochman A, Ratzkowski E, Schreiber H: Incidence of carcinoma of the cervix in Jewish women in Israel. Br J Cancer 9:358, 1955
23. Apt A: Circumcision and prostatic cancer. Acta Med Scand 178:493, 1965
24. Aitkin, Swan J, Biard D: Circumcision and cancer of the cervix. Br J Cancer 19:217, 1965
25. Kaplan GW, O'Connor VJ Jr: The incidence of carcinoma of the prostate in Jews and Gentiles. JAMA 196:803, 1966
26. Cameron W: Lack of circumcision linked to higher risk of catching AIDS. Baltimore Sun, Wed. Oct. 7, 1987, p. 3
27. Speert H: Circumcision of the newborn: An appraisal of the present status. Obstet Gynecol 2:164, 1953
28. Preston EN: Whither the foreskin? A consideration of routine circumcision. Can Med Assoc J 95:576, 1966
29. Griffiths DM, Atrell JD, Freeman NV: A prospective survey of the indications and morbidity of circumcision in children. Eur Urol 11:184, 1985
30. Sussman SJ, Shiller RP, Shashikumar VL: Fournier's syndrome. Am J Dis Child 132:1189, 1978

31. Talbert LM, Kraybill EN, Potter HD: Adrenal cortical response to circumcision in the neonate. Obstet Gynecol 48(2):208, 1976
32. Lindeke L, Iverson I, Fisch R: Neonatal circumcision: A social and medical dilemma. Matern Child Nurs J 15:31, 1986
33. Slaby AR, Drizd T: Circumcision in the United States. Am J Pub Health 75(8):878, 1985
34. Rand ES: The effect of an educational intervention in the role of neonatal circumcision. Obstet Gynecol 62(2):64, 1983
35. Metcalf JJ, Osborn LM, Mariana EM: Circumcision: A study of current practices. Clin Pediatr 22:575, 1983
36. Harmond GE: Circumcision: The issue behind the foreskin. J SC Med Assoc 80(11):547, 1984
37. Patel H: The problem of routine circumcision. Can Med Assoc J 95:576, 1966

Index

An italicized f or t indicates a figure or table.